Vitamin C: Important Aspects in Nutrition and Health

Vitamin C: Important Aspects in Nutrition and Health

Editor: Mavis Keller

AMERICAN
MEDICAL PUBLISHERS
www.americanmedicalpublishers.com

AMERICAN
MEDICAL PUBLISHERS
www.americanmedicalpublishers.com

Cataloging-in-Publication Data

Vitamin C : important aspects in nutrition and health / edited by Mavis Keller.
p. cm.
Includes bibliographical references and index.
ISBN 978-1-63927-824-4
1. Vitamin C. 2. Vitamin C--Health aspects. 3. Vitamin C--Physiological effect. 4. Nutrition.
5. Vitamin C--Therapeutic use. 6. Vitamin C--Metabolism. I. Keller, Mavis.
QP772.A8 V583 2023
612.399--dc23

American Medical Publishers,
41 Flatbush Avenue,
1st Floor, New York,
NY 11217, USA

ISBN 978-1-63927-824-4 (Hardback)

Contents

Preface

This book aims to highlight the current researches and provides a platform to further the scope of innovations in this area. This book is a product of the combined efforts of many researchers and scientists, after going through thorough studies and analysis from different parts of the world. The objective of this book is to provide the readers with the latest information of the field.

Vitamin C, also called ascorbic acid, is a vitamin that dissolves in water. It is commonly found in citrus fruits and some vegetables. Vitamin C plays an important role in the repair of tissues, formation of collagen and enzymatic production of some neurotransmitters. It is also essential for the functioning of the immune system and several enzymes. The deficiency of vitamin C causes scurvy. The early symptoms of scurvy include weakness, feeling tired and sore arms and legs. It could lead to bleeding under the skin, spongy gums, 'corkscrew' hair growth, and poor wound healing without proper treatment. Adequate doses of vitamin C should be supplemented in diet. However, large doses of vitamin C can cause gastrointestinal discomfort, headache, trouble in sleeping, and flushing of the skin. This book includes some of the vital pieces of works being conducted across the world, on various topics related to vitamin C. Those in search of information to further their knowledge on the role of this vitamin in nutrition and health will be greatly assisted by it.

I would like to express my sincere thanks to the authors for their dedicated efforts in the completion of this book. I acknowledge the efforts of the publisher for providing constant support. Lastly, I would like to thank my family for their support in all academic endeavors.

Editor

1

Does Vitamin C Deficiency Promote Fatty Liver Disease Development?

David Højland Ipsen, Pernille Tveden-Nyborg and Jens Lykkesfeldt *

Department of Veterinary Disease Biology, Faculty of Health and Medical Sciences, University of Copenhagen, Ridebanevej 9, Frederiksberg C, 1870 Copenhagen, Denmark; E-Mails: dhi@sund.ku.dk (D.H.I.); ptn@sund.ku.dk (P.T.-N.)

* Author to whom correspondence should be addressed; E-Mail: jopl@sund.ku.dk;

Abstract: Obesity and the subsequent reprogramming of the white adipose tissue are linked to human disease-complexes including metabolic syndrome and concurrent non-alcoholic fatty liver disease (NAFLD) and non-alcoholic steatohepatitis (NASH). The dietary imposed dyslipidemia promotes redox imbalance by the generation of excess levels of reactive oxygen species and induces adipocyte dysfunction and reprogramming, leading to a low grade systemic inflammation and ectopic lipid deposition, e.g., in the liver, hereby promoting a vicious circle in which dietary factors initiate a metabolic change that further exacerbates the negative consequences of an adverse life-style. Large epidemiological studies and findings from controlled *in vivo* animal studies have provided evidence supporting an association between poor vitamin C (VitC) status and propagation of life-style associated diseases. In addition, overweight per se has been shown to result in reduced plasma VitC, and the distribution of body fat in obesity has been shown to have an inverse relationship with VitC plasma levels. Recently, a number of epidemiological studies have indicated a VitC intake below the recommended daily allowance (RDA) in NAFLD-patients, suggesting an association between dietary habits, disease and VitC deficiency. In the general population, VitC deficiency (defined as a plasma concentration below 23 μM) affects around 10% of adults, however, this prevalence is increased by an adverse life-style, deficiency potentially playing a broader role in disease progression in specific subgroups. This review discusses the currently available data from human surveys and experimental models in search of a putative role of VitC deficiency in the development of NAFLD and NASH.

Keywords: antioxidants; obesity; oxidative stress; non-alcoholic fatty liver disease; non-alcoholic steatohepatitis; reactive oxygen species; vitamin C; vitamin C deficiency

1. Introduction

Obesity has become an epidemic with detrimental effects on health and wellbeing. In 2013, more than one-third of the world's adult population could be characterized as being overweight or obese (body mass index (BMI) ≥25 kg/m^2) [1]. Obesity has been found to result in dysfunctional adipose tissue, low-grade systemic inflammation and redox imbalance with increased oxidative stress [2–4]. As part of the so-called metabolic syndrome, known associations with obesity include a wide range of diseases, e.g., atherosclerosis, insulin resistance (IR), type 2 diabetes and non-alcoholic fatty liver disease (NAFLD) [5]. The development of NAFLD is closely linked to increased levels of circulating lipids, IR, inflammation and oxidative stress [6,7]. In agreement with a putative role of oxidative stress in the etiology of NAFLD, important antioxidant enzymes and vitamins are decreased in obese and NAFLD patients [4,8,9].

Vitamin C (VitC) is a water-soluble, chain-breaking antioxidant capable of scavenging essentially all physiologically relevant free radicals [10]. Additionally, it serves as donor of reducing equivalents in multiple enzymatic reactions, of which its role in proline and lysine hydroxylation during collagen synthesis is probably most widely known [11]. Humans and a few other species are unable to synthesize VitC, and must instead acquire it through dietary means. Inadequate dietary intake results in VitC deficiency defined as plasma levels below 23 μM [12]. Cross-sectional population studies have shown that about 10%–20% of the western population can be diagnosed with VitC deficiency and that poor VitC status is associated with increased all-cause mortality [13–17] Moreover, the prevalence of VitC deficiency in specific subgroups may be considerably higher, potentially enhancing susceptibility to oxidative stress and disease [18]. Accordingly, VitC status correlates inversely with e.g., BMI and is significantly decreased in obese compared with lean individuals [9,19–22]. Thus, the apparent link between obesity, NAFLD and oxidative stress suggests that NAFLD progression may be accelerated by poor VitC status.

The aim of this review is to discuss the current data from human and animal studies in relation to a putative role of VitC in the development of NAFLD.

2. Obesity, Systemic Inflammation and NAFLD

2.1. Obesity and Systemic Inflammation

Obesity is primarily a consequence of a sedentary lifestyle and the intake of an excess amount of calories. As a result, unused resources are accumulated as fat in adipose tissue, facilitating adipocyte hypertrophy and hyperplasia, alongside increased production of chemokines, cytokines, reactive oxygen species (ROS), hypoxia and cell death, ultimately leading to macrophage infiltration and adipocyte dysfunction [23–25]. Macrophages initiate and maintain inflammation by secreting a variety of cytokines, such as tumor necrosis factor α (TNFα) and interleukin (IL) 6 [2,23] At the same time, dysfunctional adipocytes increase their secretion of pro-inflammatory cytokines, while decreasing secretion of anti-inflammatory cytokines [24,26]. Decreased secretion of adiponectin by adipocytes and concurrent interference with the insulin signaling pathway by inflammatory cytokines promotes the development of IR [2,27,28]. Furthermore, inflammation of the adipose tissue may participate in the induction of hepatic IR as well [29]. Inflammation, IR and adipocyte hypertrophy per se can increase the rate of lipolysis and subsequent release of free fatty acids (FFA) [2,30,31]. FFAs have been shown to directly activate macrophages through Toll-like receptors 2 and 4 and enhance the production of inflammatory cytokines [32]. Thus, a vicious cycle is established: Adipocyte dysfunction induces a low-grade inflammation, which increases the release of FFA. In turn, the FFAs stimulate macrophage activation and additional production of inflammatory cytokines [5] (Figure 1). Ultimately, this may result in a state of chronic, low-grade systemic inflammation and oxidative stress [33]. Low levels of antioxidants may enhance oxidative stress, aggravating an already vulnerable state of redox imbalance.

Figure 1. Propagation of low-grade systemic inflammation from adipose tissues.

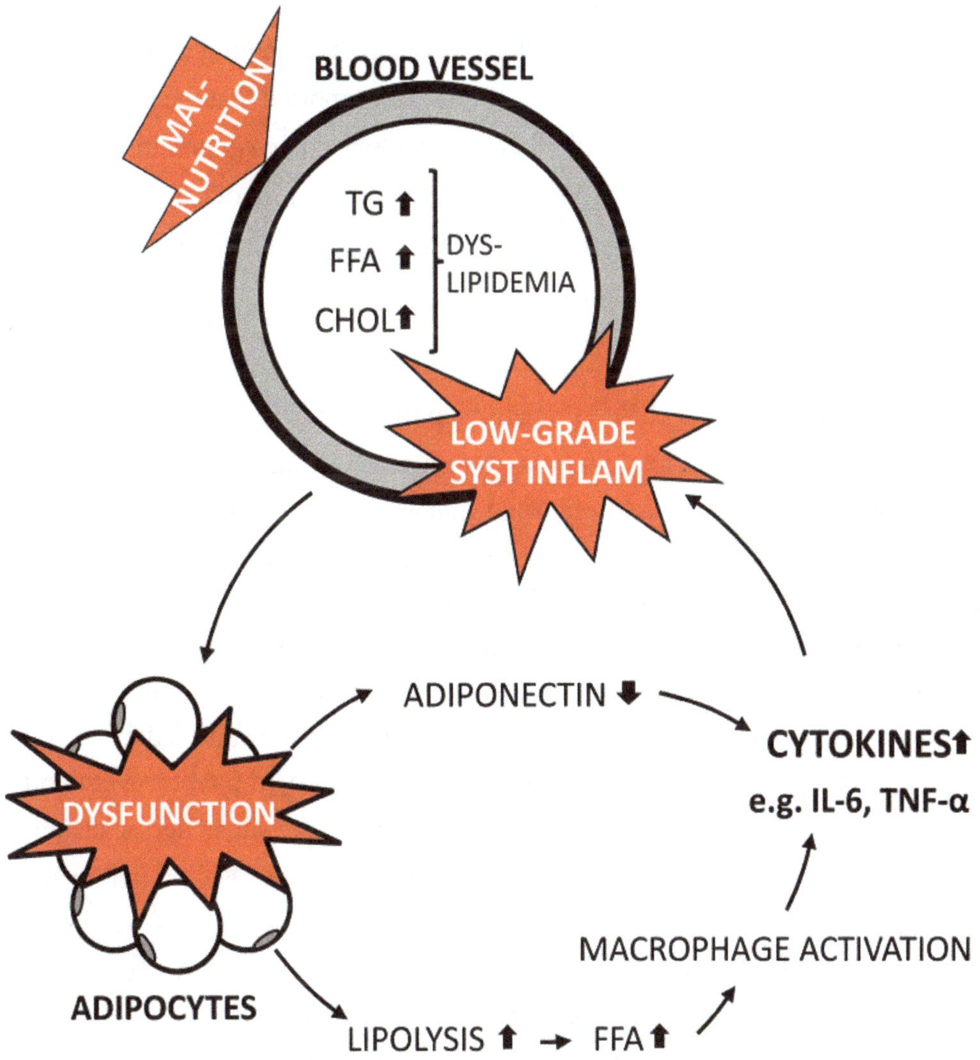

Dietary induced dyslipidemia leads to increased fat deposition and promotes hypertrophy and hyperplasia of adipocytes as well as cellular reprogramming leading to altered secretory functions of adipocytes. The tissue expansion and associated adipocyte dysfunction increases the release of inflammatory cytokines (such as IL6 and TNFα) and activates macrophages. Furthermore, release of the anti-inflammatory adipokines, e.g. adiponectin, is decreased. This induces a state of low-grade systemic inflammation, which in turn compromises insulin sensitivity and increases lipolysis in adipose tissues, increasing the release of free fatty acids (FFA) and exacerbating the dietary induced dyslipidemia. Moreover, FFAs also promote macrophage activation by binding to Toll-like receptors 2 and −4, further propagating the production of inflammatory cytokines. Thus a viscous cycle is established in which dyslipidemia and systemic inflammation is propagated through dysfunctions in adipocyte metabolism.

Multiple cross-sectional studies have found decreased levels of VitC and several other antioxidants in obese men and women, and observed an inverse correlation between VitC levels and BMI, waist circumference and body fat percentage [15,19–22]. The third Glasgow MONICA population survey investigated the plasma VitC status of men and women aged 25–74 years and found 44% of the participants (n = 1267) to be VitC deficient, with a VitC plasma concentration below 23 μM [15]. Additionally, using data from 8808 U.S. adult men and women participating in the Third National Health and Nutrition Examination Survey (NHANES III), Ford *et al.* reported that the metabolic syndrome was associated with decreased levels of VitC and other antioxidants such as vitamin E (VitE) [34]. Dietary habits may be an important factor contributing to the poor VitC status in obesity. Obese individuals have been shown to consume less dietary VitC [22]. Similarly, obese women were found to consume less fruits and vegetables compared to lean controls [35].

A putative role of VitC in inflammation has also been suggested, since VitC levels have been found to be inversely associated with inflammatory markers such as C-reactive protein (CRP) and myeloperoxidase [19,22]. Furthermore, VitC may be involved in the regulation of the key adipokine, adiponectin, supported by a recent study reporting dietary VitC intake to correlate with adiponectin levels in adolescent girls [36]. *In vitro* studies have suggested that VitC increases the secretion of high molecular weight (HMW) adiponectin in fully differentiated human adipocytes without changing total adiponectin secretion [37]. Contrary to this, however, supplementation with VitC (500 mg/day) in obese patients did not change adiponectin levels [21]. Quantification of total adiponectin, instead of the bioactive HMW isomer alone, may account for the conflicting results. Alternatively, the dose of VitC might have been too low, as 1000 mg/day was shown to improve several other metabolic parameters in patients with type 2 diabetes, *i.e.*, HbA1c, fasting blood sugar, serum insulin, triglycerides (TG) and low-density lipoprotein (LDL) [38]. Further cell studies have shown that increased oxidative stress decrease the expression of adiponectin mRNA in adipocytes and that adiponectin levels are inversely correlated with 4-hydroxynoneal, a maker of lipid peroxidation [39]. Adiponectin levels were also inversely associated with the severity of hepatic steatosis and necroinflammation [40]. Thus, a role of VitC in adiponectin regulation could have important effects on progression of inflammation, IR and NAFLD.

2.2. NAFLD

NAFLD is estimated to affect 6% to 33% (median 20%) of the world's population and constitutes the most common liver disease in the western world [41,42]. NAFLD comprises a cluster of hepatic conditions ranging from simple, initially benign and reversible steatosis to hepatocyte ballooning, Mallory bodies, fibrosis and inflammation in non-alcoholic steatohepatitis (NASH), [6,43–45]. However, in some patients, hepatic steatosis progresses to NASH, increasing the risk of hepatic cirrhosis and hepatocellular carcinoma [43,46]. NAFLD is strongly associated with obesity, dyslipidemia, IR, oxidative stress, inflammation and the metabolic syndrome [47,48]. Indeed, the prevalence of NAFLD in obese patients has been reported to be 74%, the amount of visceral adipose tissue in particular being highly correlated with increased risk of NAFLD [6,49]. The pathogenesis of NAFLD is not yet completely understood. However, it is currently believed that initial hepatic fat accumulation is followed by multiple parallel hits that promote inflammation and disease progression. The most important events believed to be involved in this process include; IR, increased FFA, dietary factors, cytokines derived from the adipose tissue and ROS formation [7].

IR is a key mechanism in hepatic dyslipidemia. Expectedly, diabetic patients have an increased prevalence of NAFLD compared to non-diabetic individuals, supporting the link between IR and NAFLD [50]. While IR increases circulating levels of FFAs, hyperinsulinemia during IR, paradoxically, apparently inhibits hepatic lipid oxidation and increases *de novo* lipogenesis [51]. Concurrently, saturation of very-low-density lipoprotein (VLDL) secretion may facilitate lipid accumulation as well [52]. In patients with NAFLD, the majority of hepatic lipids originate from circulating FFA [53]. FFA from visceral adipose tissue can drain directly into the portal vein and be transported straight to the liver. As hepatocytic FFA uptake is mediated by passive diffusion, increased FFA levels result in increased FFA uptake, which is subsequently stored as TG [6,54]. Interestingly, a meta-analysis of clinical trials investigating the effect of VitC intervention on LDL, high-density lipoprotein (HDL) and TGs in patients with hypercholesterolemia suggested that VitC supplementation can reduce the concentration of lipids in circulation (TG and LDL-C) [55]. Additionally, adipose tissue-derived cytokines may contribute to the development of NAFLD, and inflammation of the adipose tissue may indeed precede hepatic inflammation [56–58]. Adiponectin has been shown to reduce ectopic hepatic lipid accumulation, systemic IR and inflammation [59]. In addition, TNFα and IL6 have received much attention as putative key cytokines involved in hepatic lipid accumulation, inflammation and IR [60].

Dietary factors also play an important role in NAFLD. High dietary fructose, trans-fatty acids, and cholesterol have all been found to contribute to the development of dyslipidemia, hepatic fat accumulation and subsequent disease progression [7,61–65]. FFA and cholesterol not only induce hepatic lipid deposition, but may also have injurious effects in the liver, in part by inducing hepatocyte apoptosis, lipotoxicity, mitochondrial dysfunction and endoplasmic reticulum stress with subsequent ROS formation and inflammation [24,66–71]. Furthermore, activation of hepatic stellate cells and Kupffer cells, e.g., by hepatocyte apoptosis and ROS, also appear to promote disease progression through the secretion of TNFα, IL6, transforming growth factor β and collagen, which induces inflammation and fibrosis [72] (Figure 2). Indeed, increased generation of ROS and lipid peroxidation are believed to be key pathogenic components in NAFLD, perpetuating inflammation, fibrogenesis, and development of cirrhosis and hepatocellular carcinoma [73,74]. Oxidative stress alone has been found to be associated with NAFLD both in patients with, but also without type 2 diabetes [75]. VitC has been shown to decrease mitochondrial ROS formation and stimulate the activity of manganese superoxide dismutase (SOD) and glutathione peroxidase (GPx) in isolated rat liver mitochondria [76]. However, dietary intake of VitC and VitE has been reported to be lower in NAFLD patients, potentially predisposing them to oxidative stress [77,78].

Figure 2. Putative effects of vitamin C deficiency on the progression of NAFLD.

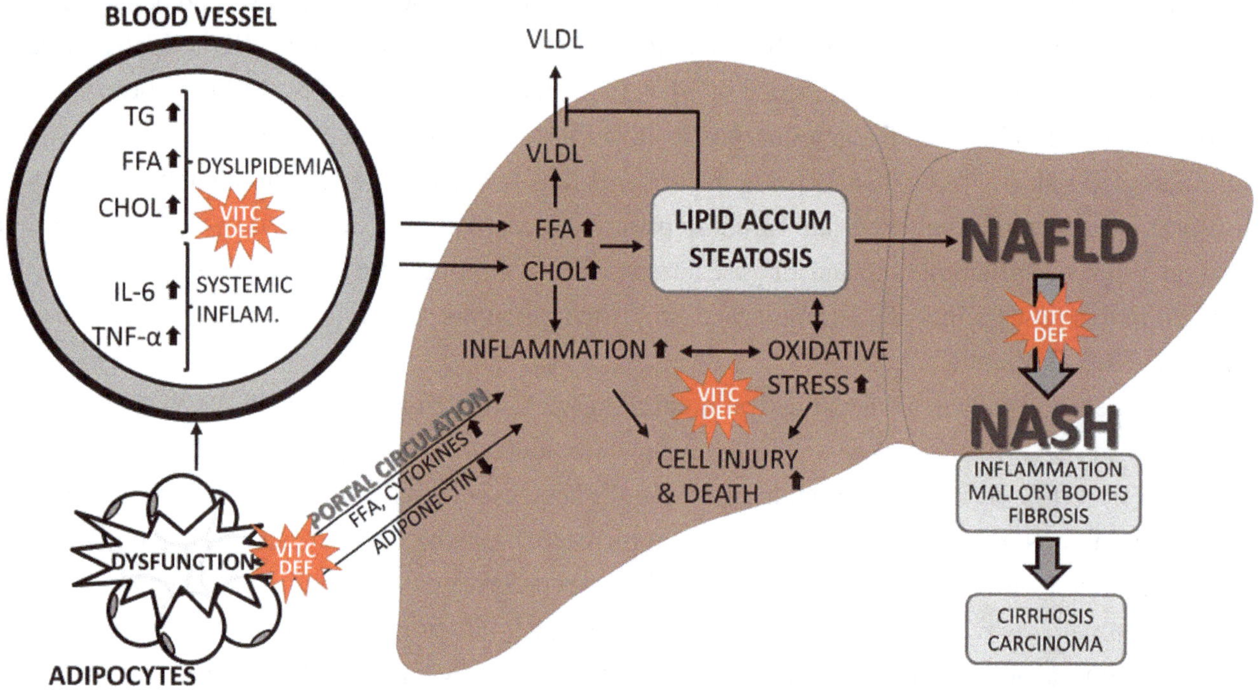

As co-factor for the 7α-hydroxylase, catalyzing the conversion of cholesterol to 7α-hydroxycholesterol, VitC deficiency may increase circulating levels of cholesterol (CHOL) by reducing its excretion through the bile. Systemic inflammation and dyslipidemia is propagated through adipocyte dysfunction, e.g., releasing fatty acids (FFA) and inflammatory cytokines to the blood stream. Moreover, by affecting adiponectin regulation, lack of VitC may further increase dyslipidemia, systemic inflammation and oxidative stress. As VitC is also a powerful antioxidant, deficiency per se promotes cellular oxidative stress, e.g., in the liver. The excess lipids induce mitochondrial dysfunction and stress of the endoplasmic reticulum (ER) further propagating hepatic oxidative stress and inflammation. FFA and CHOL is taken up by hepatocytes and processed to be exported from the liver by VLDL. When overloaded, hepatic VLDL export is saturated and lipids are accumulated in hepatocytes. Ultimately, NAFLD progression is driven by increased oxidative stress and inflammation, promoting activation of hepatic stellate and Kupffer cells, which alongside an increased hepatic production of TNFα, IL6, transforming growth factor β and collagen, amplifies the induction of cellular damage and fibrosis. Combined with key pathogenic changes taking place during the advancement from simple steatosis (NAFLD) to steatohepatitis (NASH), e.g., hepatocyte ballooning, formation of Mallory bodies and fibrosis, NASH may progress even further to hepatic cirrhosis and hepatocellular carcinoma.

Consistent with this notion, a number of investigators have found that markers of oxidative damage such as malondialdehyde (MDA) and protein carbonyls are elevated, while antioxidants like catalase and SOD are decreased in the plasma and livers of animals and humans with NAFLD [8,65,79,80].

This has led to the hypothesis that VitC therapy could prove beneficial in the treatment of NAFLD (Figure 2).

3. Does Vitamin C Deficiency Promote NAFLD?

3.1. Animal Studies of Vitamin C Deficiency

Several *in vivo* studies have investigated the role of poor VitC status in relation to dyslipidemia and NAFLD (Table 1). Like humans, guinea pigs are unable to synthesize VitC due to a non-functional gene encoding for L-gulonolactone oxidase (gulo), making them an excellent model for the study of VitC deficiency. Moreover, with regards to, e.g., cholesterol distribution, activity of enzymes involved in lipoprotein metabolism, LDL receptor binding domain characteristics and cholesterol synthesis, guinea pigs are comparable to humans in contrast to other rodents [81]. Contrary to the guinea pig, the gulo gene is functional in mice and rats and both species are able to synthesize VitC. However, the effect of VitC deficiency can be examined in genetically engineered rodent models, although the validity and human relevance of such models may be difficult to assess.

Guinea pigs kept on a diet without VitC for 4 weeks showed elevated levels of hepatic cholesterol and TG compared to control animals on a VitC supplemented diet [82]. Similarly, another study in guinea pigs showed increased hepatic triacylglycerol and cholesteryl esters after 6 weeks of VitC deficiency [83]. Scurvy can be avoided by supplementing the diet with small amounts of VitC, allowing investigators to study the long-term effects of non-scorbutic VitC deficiency. After up to 31 weeks on such a diet, guinea pigs had elevated levels of TG in the liver, thoracic aorta and serum. This was due to decreased conversion of cholesterol to bile acid, revealing a crucial role of VitC in this process [84]. Specifically, VitC is a co-factor for the 7α-hydroxylase catalyzing the conversion of cholesterol to 7α-hydroxycholesterol, constituting the rate-limiting step in bile acid formation, and thus, VitC deficiency results in reduced excretion of cholesterol in animals [85]. The addition of cholesterol to a VitC deficient diet exacerbated the effects of VitC deficiency per se by increasing the amount of hepatic TG, cholesterol, focal fibrosis and proliferation of connective tissue. Moreover, high dose (100 mg/day, p.o.) of VitC significantly diminished these changes [86]. Interestingly, dietary cholesterol also appears to have effects on the VitC status. In a long-term dietary intervention study in guinea pigs, high cholesterol fed animals consistently showed 33% (range 27%–43%) lower plasma and liver VitC concentrations compared to control animals regardless of low or high dietary VitC intake [87]. In the osteogenic disorder shionogi (ODS) rat—a mutant rat strain unable to synthesize VitC—VitC deficiency with or without cholesterol and cholic acid supplementation for 19 days increased hepatic cholesterol and total lipids [88]. Furthermore, regardless of the amount of cholesterol added to the diet, Uchida *et al.* did not find any effect of VitC relating to changes in hepatic lipids in ODS rats [89]. These discrepancies may reflect the significant differences between guinea pigs and rats in the way lipids are handled and stored [90,91]. Collectively, the above results suggest that VitC is involved in the regulation of both circulating and hepatic lipid homeostasis, supporting VitC as an important factor in the development of NAFLD.

Table 1. Animal studies of vitamin C deficiency.

Species	Age/Weight	Design	Outcome	Ref.
Guinea Pigs	200–300 g	Control (VitC 5 mg VitC/day) Deficient (0.5 mg VitC/day) High VitC (100 mg VitC/day) ± 100 mg chol/day Duration: 16 weeks	VitC deficiency, liver: TG ↑ Chol ↑ PL ↔ VitC deficiency + chol, liver: TG ↑ Chol ↑ PL ↔ Histology reveal fat infiltration, local necrosis and proliferation of connective tissue	[86]
Guinea Pigs	400–450 g	Control (1000 mg VitC/kg diet) VitC deficient (0 mg VitC/kg diet) VitC high (25,000 mg VitC/kg) Duration: 4 weeks	VitC deficiency, liver: Chol ↑ TG ↑ VitC deficiency, serum: Chol ↑ TG ↑ HDL ↓ LDL ↑ VLDL ↓	[82]
Guinea Pigs	300–450 g	Control (10 mg VitC/day) Deficient (0.5 mg VitC/day) Duration: 22, 28 or 31 weeks	VitC deficiency, liver/serum/thoracic aorta: Chol ↑	[84]
Guinea Pigs	?	Control (660 mg VitC/kg diet) Deficiency (33 mg VitC/kg diet) High (13,200 mg VitC/kg diet) Duration: 5 weeks	VitC deficiency, liver: TBARS ↑ MDA ↑ protein carbonyls ↑	[92]
Guinea Pigs	250–300 g	Control (25 mg VitC/kg/day) Deficiency (0 mg VitC/kg/day) Duration: 21 days	VitC deficiency, liver: TBARS ↑	[93]
Guinea Pigs	600–700 g	Control (500 mg VitC/kg diet) Deficiency (50 mg VitC/kg diet) Duration: 6 weeks	VitC deficiency, liver: TAG ↑ CE ↑ FC ↔	[83]
Guinea Pigs	12 weeks	High or low fat diet with different VitC: Low (100 mg VitC/kg diet) High (691 mg VitC/kg diet) Duration: 6 months	High fat diet, liver: VitC ↓	[87]

Table 1. *Cont.*

Mice, SMP30$^{-/-}$ and WT	30 days	SMP30$^{-/-}$ or WT ±1.5 mg/L VitC in water Duration: 57 days	VitC deficiency, liver: protein carbonyl ↑ SOD-activity ↑ Cu Zn-SOD protein expression ↑ TBARS ↔, CAT protein expression ↓	[94]
Mice, Gulo$^{-/-}$ or WT	20–21 weeks	16 weeks on western diet, then: Control (0.33 g VitC/L in drinking water) Deficiency (0 g VitC/L in drinking water) Duration: 3 weeks	VitC deficiency: GSH ↔ MDA ↑ F2- an F4-isoprostanes ↔	[95]
Mice, Gulo$^{-/-}$	Newborn	Control Gulo$^{+/+}$ (0 mg VitC) Deficiency Gulo$^{-/-}$ (0 mg VitC) Duration: 18 days	Gulo$^{-/-}$, liver: MDA ↑ protein carbonyl ↑ sulfhydryls ↔ GSH ↑	[96]
Rats, ODS or WT	6 weeks	ODS fed 0, 50, 300, 3000 mg VitC/kg diet ± 0.5% chol and 0.25% cholic acid WT fed 0 mg VitC/kg diet ± 0.5% chol and 0.25% cholic acid Duration: 19 days	VitC deficiency, liver: Chol ↑/↔ total lipids ↑/↔ VitC deficiency, serum: Chol ↔ HDL-C ↔ VitC deficiency + chol/cholic acid, liver: Chol ↑, total lipids ↔ VitC deficiency + chol/cholic acid, serum: Chol ↑, HDL-C ↑	[88]
Rats, ODS	6 weeks	Control 300 mg VitC/kg diet Deficient 0 mg VitC/kg diet Duration: 14 days	VitC deficiency, liver: CINC-1 ↑ Apo-A1 mRNA ↓ ApoE mRNA ↔	[97]
Rats, ODS or WT	9 weeks	Control (30 mg VitC/L in drinking water ± 0.5% chol Deficiency 0 mg/L in drinking water Duration: 3 weeks	VitC deficiency, liver: Chol ↔ TG ↔ PL ↔ VitC deficiency, serum: Chol ↑ Total lipoprotein ↓ HDL ↓IDL ↓ LDL ↑ VLDL ↓ VitC deficiency + chol did not affect serum levels further. Chol feeding, regardless of VitC status, increase hepatic lipids	[89]

CAT: Catalase. Chol: Cholesterol. CE: cholesteryl ester. CINC-1: Cytokine-induced neutrophil chemoattractant-1. FC: Free cholesterol. GSH: Glutathione. Gulo: L-gulonolactone oxidase HDL: High-density lipoprotein. IDL: Intermediate-density lipoprotein. LDL: Low-density lipoprotein. MDA: Malondialdehyde. ODS: Osteogenic Disorder Shionogi. PL: Phospholipids. SMP30: Senescence marker protein. SOD: Superoxide dismutase. TAG: Triacylglycerol. TBARS: Thiobarbituric acid reactive substances. TG: Triglyceride. VitC: Vitamin C. VLDL: Very-low-density lipoprotein. WT: Wild type; Ref.: Reference; ↓ Decrease; ↑ Increase; ↔ No change.

In accordance with a central role in the prevention of oxidative stress, VitC deficiency has been shown to cause a reduction in both expression and activity of various antioxidant enzymes with a concurrent rise in markers of oxidative stress. Thus, 3–5 weeks of VitC deficiency caused increased levels of thiobarbituric acid reactive substance (TBARS), MDA and protein carbonyls in the liver of guinea pigs [92,93]. Oxidative stress was also evident in the liver of gulo$^{-/-}$ mice without access to VitC for 57 days. Protein carbonyls, but not TBARS, were increased in the livers of these animals, alongside decreased catalase protein expression compared to WT or gulo$^{-/-}$ supplemented controls [94]. However, SOD activity was increased, likely as a compensatory mechanism [94]. Indeed, SOD appears to play an important role in NAFLD as increased hepatic fibrosis is found in NASH patients with mutations in the gene coding for SOD2 [98]. Pierce *et al.* found increased hepatic MDA in VitC deficient gulo$^{-/-}$ mice placed on a western diet, but with no change in glutathione or isoprostanes [95]. However, other authors report an increase of glutathione a long with increased MDA and protein carbonyls in livers of gulo$^{-/-}$ mice deprived of VitC for similar periods of time [96]. These differences between studies may be attributed to different diet compositions and age of the animals, *i.e.*, a western type diet and 4–5 weeks old animals *vs.* normal chow and newly born animals, respectively. The considerable number of studies reporting increased protein carbonyls, MDA and TBARS in VitC deficient animals, support that VitC has a protective effect against hepatic protein and lipid oxidation. This may be of significance as lipid oxidation has been shown to occur in NAFLD and even correlate with the severity of liver necroinflammation and fibrosis [99]. Furthermore, keeping ODS rats on a VitC free diet for 14 days resulted in increased cytokine-induced neutrophil chemoattractant-1 (CINC-1), a potent inflammatory chemokine, in serum, liver and spleen. Thus, VitC deficiency may mediate the infiltration and accumulation of neutrophils with subsequent inflammatory damage in some tissues [97].

3.2. Animal Studies of VitC Intervention and NAFLD

Methionine and choline are essential for hepatic β-oxidation and VLDL production. Expectedly, methionine and choline deficient (MCD) diets cause accumulation of intra-hepatic lipids and decreased VLDL synthesis [43]. Rezazadeh and coworkers fed rats a MCD diet for 10 weeks, and randomized animals to receive VitC or no supplementation for an additional eight weeks on the diet [100]. While VitC supplementation significantly decreased hepatocellular ballooning and inflammation, liver steatosis still persisted. At the same time, hepatic markers of oxidative stress were decreased, while SOD and catalase were increased [100]. Similar results were obtained by supplementing rats placed on a MCD diet with VitC for 10 weeks. The authors also found that VitC treatment significantly increased glutathione reductase (GR) and GPx activity [101]. Moreover, VitC treatment resulted in a significant decrease in circulating liver enzymes, TG and LDL, showing a protective effect of VitC supplementation on the MCD diet-induced dyslipidemia [100,101]. Conversely, rats fed a choline deficient diet for 4 weeks with concurrent VitC supplementation did not show any improvements in serum TG or aspartate aminotransferase, even though hepatic steatosis was ameliorated and oxidative stress reduced [102]. However, the studies differ considerably in diet composition, duration and rat strain used, confounding compatibility between findings.

Imbalance of the antioxidant status, similar to that observed in the animal studies, has also been found in patients with steatosis while antioxidant status is even further compromised in NASH [80]. Animal models utilizing MCD or choline deficient diets to induce NAFLD appear to present a similar pathology, but the pathogenesis is different from the human situation. Additionally, most animals lose weight on the MCD diet, contrary to the human situation, in which many NAFLD patients are obese. Results may therefore not be directly translatable.

Guinea pigs placed on an atherogenic diet, high in fat and cholesterol, for 4 months developed dyslipidemia with elevated serum cholesterol and phospholipids in addition to elevated hepatic levels of cholesterol, phospholipids and TG [103]. VitC deficiency exacerbated the dyslipidemia and hepatic consequences, but high VitC reduced the severity of both dyslipidemia and hepatic lipid accumulation [103]. It is noteworthy, that extremely high doses of VitC (13,200 mg/kg diet) have been shown to decrease hepatic markers of oxidation to the same degree as normal VitC doses in guinea pigs, but also cause a reduction of body weight and GR activity, similarly to what was observed in the VitC deficient animals [92]. It is possible that the very high dose of VitC caused adverse effects in the guinea pigs, e.g., gastrointestinal disturbances and osmotic diarrhea [104,105], which could affect bodyweight and general physiology, however, this was not reported by the authors. Conversely, Roomi *et al.* did not report any adverse effects of a mega-dose of VitC (25,000 mg VitC/kg diet) in guinea pigs [82]. Contrary to guinea pigs, supplementation with high levels of VitC in ODS rats did not reduce hepatic cholesterol to a greater extent that normal VitC levels did [88]. Thus, VitC treatment seemingly reduces hepatic oxidative stress, but have variable effect on hepatic steatosis, likely depending on the employed method of induction, *i.e.*, a high fat diet *versus* a MCD or MD diet (Table 2).

3.3. Epidemiological Studies of VitC Intake and NAFLD

A number of cohort studies have been carried out, investigating the dietary habits of patients with NAFLD. Results are conflicting; some studies indicate suboptimal VitC intake by NAFLD patients while others do not (Table 3). Using a 7-day food record Musso *et al.* evaluated dietary habits in patients with NASH and healthy controls. Among other differences, NASH patients consumed significantly less VitC compared to the healthy controls (84.3 ± 43.1 *vs.* 144.2 ± 63.1 mg) [77]. Males constituted the vast majority of the NASH group (24/25 patients) and though below that of healthy controls, dietary intakes were close to the recommended daily intake of 90 mg VitC/day, although this was not the case for smokers with NASH [77,106]. Contrary to this, Ferolla and colleagues found that intake of VitC in NAFLD patients diagnosed with fatty liver, did not meet recommendations when assessed in men and women using 24-h dietary recall and food frequency questionnaires (FFQ) [78]. Unfortunately, the lack of a control group impedes investigation as to whether low VitC intake was also prevalent in a comparable healthy population. Different methodology, ethnicity and patients' disease stage may account for apparent study dissimilarities. Indeed, food records may themselves lead patients to change their dietary patterns [107].

Table 2 Animal studies of VitC intervention in NAFLD.

Species	Age/Weight	Design	Outcome	Ref.
Guinea Pigs	300 g	Normal or atherogenic diet Control (10 mg/kg/day) Deficiency (1 mg/kg/day) High (25 mg/kg/day) VitC administration: Oral Duration: 4 months	Compared to control (normal diet): VitC deficiency, liver: TC ↑ TG ↑ PL ↓ serum: TC ↔ TG ↔ PL ↔ High VitC, liver: TC ↔ TG ↓ PL ↑ serum: TC ↔ TG ↔ PL ↔ Compared to control (atherogenic diet): VitC deficiency, liver: TC ↑ TG ↑ PL ↓ serum: TC ↑ TG ↑ PL ↔ High VitC, liver: TC ↓TG ↔ PL ↓ serum: TC ↓ TG ↓ PL ↓	[103]
Rats	250–300 g	Control (MCD diet for 10 weeks, then 8 additional weeks of MCD diet + vehicle) Treatment (MCD diet for 10 weeks, then 8 additional weeks of MCD diet + VitC 30 mg/kg/day) VitC administration: Oral Duration: 18 weeks	VitC, liver: ballooning ↓ inflammation ↓ steatosis ↔ SOD ↑ CAT ↑ protein carbonyls ↓ VitC, serum: AST ↓ ALT ↓ ALP ↓ γGT ↓ TC ↓ HDL ↑ LDL ↓	[100]
Rats	250–300 g	Control (MCD diet + vehicle) Treatment (MCD diet + VitC 30 mg/kg/day) VitC administration: Oral Duration: 10 weeks	VitC, liver: ballooning ↓ SOD ↑ CAT ↑ GR ↑ GPx ↑ TBARS ↓ protein carbonyls ↓ VitC, serum: AST ↓ ALT ↓ ALP ↓ γGT ↓ TC ↓ HDL ↑ LDL ↓	[101]
Rats	300–350 g	Control (CD diet + vehicle) Treatment (CD diet +30 mg VitC/kg/day) VitC administration: Oral Duration: 4 weeks	VitC, liver: prevents steatosis and reduces oxidative stress VitC, plasma: AST ↔ TG ↔	[102]

ALP: Alkaline phosphatase; ALT: Alanine aminotransferase; AST: Aspartate aminotransferase; CAT: Catalase; CD: Choline deficient; GPx: Glutathione peroxidase; GR: Glutathione reductase; γGT: Gamma-glutamyl transferase; HDL: High-density lipoprotein; LDL: Low-density lipoprotein; MCD: methionine choline deficient; PL: Phospholipids; SOD: Superoxide dismutase; TBARS: Thiobarbituric acid reactive substances; TC: Total cholesterol; TG: Triglyceride; VitC: Vitamin C; Ref.: Reference; ↓ Decrease; ↑ Increase; ↔ No change.

Han and co-workers studied the dietary intake of Korean adults [108] and reported no differences in dietary VitC intake between men and women with NAFLD and control subjects However, when adjusted for age, job, education level, exercise frequency, smoking status, energy intake and *n*–3 fatty acid intake, VitC intake was negatively associated with the risk of NAFLD in male patients (OR: 4.23; *p*-trend = 0.014) [108]. In children with steatosis or NASH, Vos *et al.* found dietary intakes of VitC to be similar [109]. However, while differences in steatosis grade were not associated with differences in VitC intake, significantly increased hepatocyte ballooning was indeed observed in children with decreased VitC consumption [109]. In another study, Mager *et al.* reported that daily recommendations of VitC were met by children with NAFLD [110]. However, impaired antioxidant status was implied as measured by low levels of red blood cell-glutathione compared to previous reports in healthy children although the conclusion is weakened by the lack of paired controls [110]. Da Silva and associates concluded that VitC intake was not different between healthy controls and adults with either steatosis or NASH [111]. In this study of 74 NASH patients and 27 healthy controls, the intake correlated with median VitC plasma concentrations, which did not differ between groups 67.6 and 72.1 μM, respectively [111]. Likewise, Madan *et al.* did not find any differences in VitC plasma levels between 29 NAFLD patients and 23 healthy controls [112]. Also, the VitC plasma concentrations were found not to correlate with hepatic inflammation or fibrosis [112]. However, in another study by Cabakan and co-workers, 105 NASH patients had reduced VitC plasma levels alongside increased plasma MDA and nitric oxide compared with steatosis patients [113]. It is possible that this reflects an ability of VitC to slow down the progression of NAFLD.

The conflicting results do not allow a definitive conclusion regarding dietary VitC intake. However, the NAFLD patients included in the studies mentioned above largely seem to have met recommended daily allowance of VitC. Unfortunately, most of the studies only examine the estimated dietary intake of VitC and have not actually measured plasma VitC concentrations. It has been suggested that assessments of dietary VitC only have a moderate relationship with plasma VitC levels, thus the two measures may not describe the VitC status in the same way [114]. Moreover, dietary questionnaires have certain limitations and underreporting is known to occur, which may also skew results [107]. As noted previously, oxidative stress is increased in NAFLD patients [75]. As such, they may have an increased demand of antioxidants, like VitC, and inadequate levels are not likely to be reflected by reports of dietary intake alone. Daily doses of VitC between 30 and 100 mg do not result in plasma saturation, leading some investigators to propose that the daily recommended dose of VitC be increased from 75 and 90 mg/day (US women and men, respectively) [105], to 200 mg/day in healthy individuals [115]. Furthermore, small differences in dietary intake of VitC between 30 and 100 mg/day can lead to vastly different plasma concentrations, as this interval represents a very steep part of the plasma concentration *vs.* dose curve [115]. Therefore, patients with a daily VitC intake in this area and even corresponding to the current recommendation may still be at risk of having plasma VitC concentrations below optimal levels. While they may not strictly be VitC deficient, plasma VitC levels between 23 and 50 μM may still leave patients vulnerable to disease, as, e.g., the relative risk of heart failure has been shown to increase significantly by every 20 μM drop in VitC plasma concentrations [116].

Table 3. Epidemiological studies of VitC status in NAFLD patients.

Design	Groups	Outcome	Ref.
Cross-Sectional	Adults Healthy controls ($n = 25$) NASH ($n = 25$)	NASH patients consumes less dietary VitC ($p = 0.0001$)	[77]
Cross-Sectional	Adults NAFLD patients ($n = 96$)	Dietary VitC intake was below recommended levels	[78]
Cross-Sectional	Adults Male healthy controls ($n = 63$) Male NAFLD ($n = 103$) Women healthy controls ($n = 116$) Women NAFLD ($n = 66$)	Dietary intake of VitC was not different in men and women with NAFLD compared with control ($p = 0.666$) Intake of VitC correlated negatively with the odds-ratio of NAFLD for male patients (OR: 4.23, p-trend = 0.014)	[108]
Cross-Sectional	Children Steatosis ($n = 39$) Borderline Z3 ($n = 27$) Borderline Z1 ($n = 36$) NASH ($n = 47$)	Dietary VitC intake was similar in all groups ($p = 0.15$) and above recommended levels High grade of steatosis was not associated with lower dietary VitC intake ($p = 0.97$) Amount of hepatocyte ballooning increases with lower dietary VitC levels ($p = 0.05$)	[109]
Cross-Sectional	Children NAFLD ($n = 38$)	Dietary VitC intake was in agreement with recommended levels	[110]
Cross-Sectional	Adults Healthy control ($n = 27$) Steatosis ($n = 33$) NASH ($n = 41$)	Plasma concentrations of VitC did not differ between groups ($p > 0.05$) Dietary intake of VitC did not differ between groups ($p > 0.05$)	[111]
Prospective	Adults Healthy controls ($n = 23$) NAFLD ($n = 29$)	Plasma VitC concentrations were not different between groups ($p = 0.65$) Plasma VitC concentrations did not correlate with inflammatory grade ($p = 0.56$) or fibrosis stage ($p = 0.53$)	[112]
Cross-Sectional	Adults Fatty liver disease ($n = 38$) NASH ($n = 67$)	Plasma VitC concentrations were lower in NASH patients ($p = 0.001$)	[113]

NAFLD: Non-alcoholic fatty liver disease; NASH: Non-alcoholic steatohepatitis; OR: Odds ratio; VitC: Vitamin C; Ref.: Reference.

3.4. Clinical Intervention Studies with VitC and NAFLD

To date, no study has directly examined the effect of VitC treatment alone in NAFLD and compared it to a placebo-treated control group. However, studies which combine VitC with other treatment form(s) have been conducted (Table 4). A 12 month, double-blinded, randomized controlled trial (RCT) examined the differences between placebo and combined treatment with VitC (500 mg/day) and E (600 IU/day) in children [117]. Both groups received lifestyle intervention, involving increased physical activity and a tailored diet aimed at inducing weight loss or maintaining weight in overweight and normal weight children, respectively. Liver brightness (as a measure of lipid accumulation), examined by ultrasound, circulating levels of liver enzymes, cholesterol and TG were reduced in both groups compared to baseline, but were not significantly different between groups [117]. Subsequently, the study was continued as an open-label study for an additional 12 months, but with fewer participants and the inclusion of a post-treatment liver biopsy [118]. Compared to baseline, both groups exhibited significant improvements in steatosis grade, lobular inflammation, hepatocyte ballooning and liver enzymes, but not in fibrosis scores. However, again there were no differences between placebo and treatment group. Thus, VitC and E supplementation are seemingly not superior to lifestyle intervention in children with NAFLD [118]. However, due to the study design, it is not possible to determine if vitamin treatment is better than no treatment at all. The authors rightfully suggested that increased fruit and vegetable consumption, augmented by the new diet, may well have minimized the effect of the vitamin treatment [118]. Indeed, VitC absorption is highly dose depended and excess amounts are effectively excreted and can therefore not facilitate additional health benefits [115]. Harrison *et al.* examined the effect of VitC (1000 mg/day) in combination with VitE (1000 IU/day) *versus* placebo after 6 months treatment of NASH patients [119]. Lifestyle interventions in both groups focused on exercise and a low-calorie diet. Hepatic inflammation, necrosis, fibrosis and liver enzymes were not significantly different between the groups. However, a significant, albeit clinically modest, intra-group improvement was observed in the vitamin treated group, with regards to hepatic fibrosis. On the basis of this result, the authors concluded that VitC and VitE treatment seemingly improves hepatic fibrosis in NASH patients [119]. However, this conclusion has been criticized; emphasizing that valid conclusion in placebo-controlled trials must be made by comparing treatment and placebo-groups rather than with historic data [120]. Interestingly, the fibrosis score was not improved in children with NAFLD, when compared to baseline [118]. Both studies implemented lifestyle changes, but doses of VitC and E, study duration and participants were different between the two studies. Additionally, the children with NAFLD had a low fibrosis score (0–1) at baseline, which may impede detection of potential improvements [118]. Importantly, liver physiology, development and the features of NASH may differ considerably between children and adults, which could affect study outcomes [121,122].

Table 4. Clinical intervention studies with VitC in NAFLD.

Design	Groups and Intervention	Outcome	Ref.
12 months, double-blinded, randomized clinical trial	Children Lifestyle intervention + placebo ($n = 43$) Lifestyle intervention + VitC (500 mg/day) and VitE (600 IU/day) ($n = 45$)	No differences between groups ($p > 0.05$)	[117]
24 months 12 month double-blinded followed by 12 month open-label, randomized clinical trial	Children Lifestyle intervention + placebo ($n = 28$) Lifestyle intervention + VitC (500 mg/day) and VitE (600 IU/day) ($n = 25$)	No differences between placebo and VitE/VitC groups ($p > 0.05$) Compared to baseline, treatment improved steatosis grade ($p < 0.001$), lobular inflammation ($p < 0.001$), hepatocyte ballooning ($p < 0.001$) and NAFLD activity score ($p > 0.001$), but not portal inflammation ($p = 0.1$) and fibrosis stage ($p = 0.6$).	[118]
6 month, double-blinded, randomized clinical trial	Adults Lifestyle intervention + placebo ($n = 22$) Lifestyle intervention + VitC (1000 mg/day) and VitE (1000 IU/day) ($n = 23$)	No differences between placebo and VitC/VitE groups ($p > 0.05$) Compared to baseline, VitC/VitE treatment improves fibrosis ($p = 0.002$)	[119]
12 months, pilot study No control group	Adults VitC (300 mg/day) and VitE (300 mg/day ($n = 23$)	Treatment decreased serum ALT ($p < 0.0001$) and hs-CRP ($p < 0.005$) and improved steatosis (6/10), necroinflammation (8/10), fibrosis (4/10).	[123]
6 month, open-label, randomized study	Adults Ursodeoxycholic acid (10 mg/kg/day) ($n = 29$) VitC (500 mg/day) and VitE (600 IU/day) ($n = 27$)	No differences between ursodeoxycholic acid and VitC/VitE treatment ($p > 0.05$)	[124]
4 years, randomized clinical trial	Adults NAFLD Placebo ($n = 36$) Treatment (1000 mg VitC/day, 1000 IU VitE/day, 20 mg atorvastatin/day) ($n = 44$) Adults Normal liver Placebo ($n = 190$) Treatment (1000 mg VitC/day, 1000 IU VitE/day, 20 mg atorvastatin/day ($n = 185$)	Treatment reduced risk of having moderate to severe hepatic steatosis (OR = 0.36, $p < 0.017$)	[125]

ALT: Alanine aminotransferase; Hs-CRP: High sensitivity C-reactive protein; NAFLD: Non-alcoholic fatty liver disease; OR: Odds ratio; VitC: Vitamin C; VitE: Vitamin E; Ref.: Reference.

In a pilot study, NASH patients were treated with VitC (300 mg/day) and VitE (300 mg/day) for 12 months and changes were compared to baseline. BMI remained unchanged, but serum alanine aminotransferase and high-sensitivity-CRP were significantly reduced by the antioxidant treatment [123]. High-sensitivity-CRP has been shown to be associated with the severity of liver pathology in NASH [126]. Ten of the 23 study participants underwent liver biopsy post-treatment and of these, steatosis improved in 6/10, necroinflammation in 8/10 and fibrosis in 4/10 [123]. However, the lack of a placebo group confounds these findings with time-induced changes and complicates the interpretation of the potential effect of the combined VitC and E treatment. The effect of ursodeoxycholic acid (UDCA) (10 mg/kg/day) compared to that of VitC (500 mg/day) and VitE (600 IU/day) was examined in a 6 month, open-label, randomized study [124]. Compared to baseline, both treatments decreased circulating levels of liver enzymes without inducing changes in liver echogenicity. Side effects were reported in the UDCA treated group, whereas no side effects were reported in the vitamin treated group [124]. This is in agreement with other studies reporting that VitC and E are well tolerated [119,123]. Foster and coworkers evaluated the combination of atorvastatin (20 mg/day), VitC (1000 mg/day) and VitE (1000 IU/day) [125]. CT-scans were used to identify NAFLD. Subsequently, the participants were divided into NAFLD patients and normal liver patients. These two groups were further allocated to either the treatment combination or placebo. The four groups were reexamined after 2 and 4 years. In patients without NALFD at baseline, the treatment had no preventive effect. However, in patients with NAFLD, active treatment significantly reduced the prevalence of fatty liver [125]. This is contrary to the result of Ersöz *et al.*, who found no improvement in hepatic echogenicity after 6 months of treatment [124]. However, considerably lower vitamin doses, duration and different radiological methods were used by Ersöz *et al.*, which may explain the conflicting results. However, improvements in hepatic steatosis may of cause, in part be contributed to atorvastatin, as hepatic steatosis is associated with dyslipidemia [127]. Indeed, active treatment with VitC, VitE and atorvastatin did reduce plasma levels of LDL and cholesterol, while HDL and TG levels remained unchanged [125]. Furthermore, treatment with atorvastatin (20 mg/day) alone, improved ultrasound echo-patterns in NAFLD patients [128]. Unfortunately, radiological techniques are not able to detect small amounts of hepatic steatosis and can therefore not distinguish between the different forms of NAFLD [129]. Consequently, the effect of the treatment on more advanced stages of NAFLD is unknown.

4. Conclusion

Controlled animal experiments support a role of VitC deficiency in the elevation of plasma and hepatic lipids, alongside increased hepatic oxidative stress, fibrosis and inflammation. In agreement, VitC treatment of liver disease-induced animals has been shown to reduce hepatic markers of oxidative stress. Clinical studies of the relationship between VitC deficiency and NAFLD have not been conducted and studies of estimated dietary intakes of VitC in NAFLD patients are conflicting. Some studies show correlations between VitC intake and NAFLD progression, while others do not. Importantly, only a few studies have addressed VitC plasma levels in NAFLD patients [111–113]. The presently available RCTs have not found an effect of VitC superior to that of placebo. However, a number of studies do demonstrate hepatic improvements compared with baseline, but the use of treatment-cocktails and concurrent life-style interventions seriously confound the analysis of VitC specific effects. Additionally, most RCTs have not recorded or reported baseline VitC concentrations and putative effects of VitC supplementation cannot be assessed in patients already saturated with VitC due to its non-linear absorption kinetics [16]. Therefore, the role of VitC in NAFLD should be investigated in future RCTs in which plasma VitC status is controlled for.

Acknowledgments

D.H.I. and J.L. are supported by the LifePharm Centre for *in Vivo* Pharmacology.

Author Contributions

The manuscript was conceived by all authors. DHI wrote the draft manuscript which was subsequently edited by all authors.

References

1. Ng, M.; Fleming, T.; Robinson, M.; Thomson, B.; Graetz, N.; Margono, C.; Mullany, E.C.; Biryukov, S.; Abbafati, C.; Abera, S.F.; *et al.* Global, regional, and national prevalence of overweight and obesity in children and adults during 1980–2013: A systematic analysis for the global burden of disease study 2013. *Lancet* **2014**, *384*, 766–781.
2. Bastard, J.P.; Maachi, M.; Lagathu, C.; Kim, M.J.; Caron, M.; Vidal, H.; Capeau, J.; Feve, B. Recent advances in the relationship between obesity, inflammation, and insulin resistance. *Eur. Cytokine Netw.* **2006**, *17*, 4–12.
3. Jankovic, A.; Korac, A.; Srdic-Galic, B.; Buzadzic, B.; Otasevic, V.; Stancic, A.; Vucetic, M.; Markelic, M.; Velickovic, K.; Golic, I.; *et al.* Differences in the redox status of human visceral and subcutaneous adipose tissues—Relationships to obesity and metabolic risk. *Metabolism* **2014**, *63*, 661–671.
4. Uzun, H.; Zengin, K.; Taskin, M.; Aydin, S.; Simsek, G.; Dariyerli, N. Changes in leptin, plasminogen activator factor and oxidative stress in morbidly obese patients following open and laparoscopic swedish adjustable gastric banding. *Obes. Surg.* **2004**, *14*, 659–665.
5. Mathieu, P.; Lemieux, I.; Despres, J.P. Obesity, inflammation, and cardiovascular risk. *Clin. Pharmacol. Ther.* **2010**, *87*, 407–416.
6. Qureshi, K.; Abrams, G.A. Metabolic liver disease of obesity and role of adipose tissue in the pathogenesis of nonalcoholic fatty liver disease. *World J. Gastroenterol.* **2007**, *13*, 3540–3553.
7. Tilg, H.; Moschen, A.R. Evolution of inflammation in nonalcoholic fatty liver disease: The multiple parallel hits hypothesis. *Hepatology* **2010**, *52*, 1836–1846.
8. Horoz, M.; Bolukbas, C.; Bolukbas, F.F.; Sabuncu, T.; Aslan, M.; Sarifakiogullari, S.; Gunaydin, N.; Erel, O. Measurement of the total antioxidant response using a novel automated method in subjects with nonalcoholic steatohepatitis. *BMC Gastroenterol.* **2005**, *5*, 35.

9. Da Silva, V.R.; Moreira, E.A.; Wilhelm-Filho, D.; de Miranda, J.X.; Beninca, J.P.; Vigil, S.V.; Moratelli, A.M.; Garlet, T.R.; de Souza Meirelles, M.S.; Vannucchi, H.; *et al.* Proinflammatory and oxidative stress markers in patients submitted to roux-en-y gastric bypass after 1 year of follow-up. *Eur. J. Clin. Nutr.* **2012**, *66*, 891–899.
10. Buettner, G.R. The pecking order of free radicals and antioxidants: Lipid peroxidation, α-tocopherol, and ascorbate. *Arch. Biochem. Biophys.* **1993**, *300*, 535–543.
11. Kivirikko, K.I.; Myllyla, R. Post-translational processing of procollagens. *Ann. N. Y. Acad. Sci.* **1985**, *460*, 187–201.
12. Smith, J.L.; Hodges, R.E. Serum levels of vitamin C in relation to dietary and supplemental intake of vitamin C in smokers and nonsmokers. *Ann. N. Y. Acad. Sci.* **1987**, *498*, 144–152.
13. Simon, J.A.; Hudes, E.S.; Tice, J.A. Relation of serum ascorbic acid to mortality among us adults. *J. Am. Coll. Nutr.* **2001**, *20*, 255–263.
14. Hampl, J.S.; Taylor, C.A.; Johnston, C.S. Vitamin C deficiency and depletion in the United States: The third national health and nutrition examination survey, 1988 to 1994. *Am. J. Public Health* **2004**, *94*, 870–875.
15. Wrieden, W.L.; Hannah, M.K.; Bolton-Smith, C.; Tavendale, R.; Morrison, C.; Tunstall-Pedoe, H. Plasma vitamin C and food choice in the third glasgow monica population survey. *J. Epidemiol. Commun. Health* **2000**, *54*, 355–360.
16. Lykkesfeldt, J.; Poulsen, H.E. Is vitamin C supplementation beneficial? Lessons learned from randomised controlled trials. *Br. J. Nutr.* **2010**, *103*, 1251–1259.
17. Frei, B.; Birlouez-Aragon, I.; Lykkesfeldt, J. Authors' perspective: What is the optimum intake of vitamin C in humans? *Crit. Rev. Food Sci. Nutr.* **2012**, *52*, 815–829.
18. Tveden-Nyborg, P.; Lykkesfeldt, J. Does vitamin C deficiency increase lifestyle-associated vascular disease progression? Evidence based on experimental and clinical studies. *Antioxid. Redox Signal.* **2013**, *19*, 2084–2104.
19. Aasheim, E.T.; Hofso, D.; Hjelmesaeth, J.; Birkeland, K.I.; Bohmer, T. Vitamin status in morbidly obese patients: A cross-sectional study. *Am. J. Clin. Nutr.* **2008**, *87*, 362–369.
20. Canoy, D.; Wareham, N.; Welch, A.; Bingham, S.; Luben, R.; Day, N.; Khaw, K.T. Plasma ascorbic acid concentrations and fat distribution in 19,068 british men and women in the european prospective investigation into cancer and nutrition norfolk cohort study. *Am. J. Clin. Nutr.* **2005**, *82*, 1203–1209.
21. Johnston, C.S.; Beezhold, B.L.; Mostow, B.; Swan, P.D. Plasma vitamin C is inversely related to body mass index and waist circumference but not to plasma adiponectin in nonsmoking adults. *J. Nutr.* **2007**, *137*, 1757–1762.
22. Mah, E.; Matos, M.D.; Kawiecki, D.; Ballard, K.; Guo, Y.; Volek, J.S.; Bruno, R.S. Vitamin C status is related to proinflammatory responses and impaired vascular endothelial function in healthy, college-aged lean and obese men. *J. Am. Diet. Assoc.* **2011**, *111*, 737–743.
23. Sun, K.; Kusminski, C.M.; Scherer, P.E. Adipose tissue remodeling and obesity. *J. Clin. Investig.* **2011**, *121*, 2094–2101.
24. Bano, G. Glucose homeostasis, obesity and diabetes. *Best Pract. Res. Clin. Obstet. Gynaecol.* **2013**, *27*, 715–726.

25. Furukawa, S.; Fujita, T.; Shimabukuro, M.; Iwaki, M.; Yamada, Y.; Nakajima, Y.; Nakayama, O.; Makishima, M.; Matsuda, M.; Shimomura, I. Increased oxidative stress in obesity and its impact on metabolic syndrome. *J. Clin. Investig.* **2004**, *114*, 1752–1761.
26. Odegaard, J.I.; Chawla, A. Pleiotropic actions of insulin resistance and inflammation in metabolic homeostasis. *Science* **2013**, *339*, 172–177.
27. Stumvoll, M.; Goldstein, B.J.; van Haeften, T.W. Type 2 diabetes: Principles of pathogenesis and therapy. *Lancet* **2005**, *365*, 1333–1346.
28. Wisse, B.E. The inflammatory syndrome: The role of adipose tissue cytokines in metabolic disorders linked to obesity. *J. Am. Soc. Nephrol.* **2004**, *15*, 2792–2800.
29. Sabio, G.; Das, M.; Mora, A.; Zhang, Z.; Jun, J.Y.; Ko, H.J.; Barrett, T.; Kim, J.K.; Davis, R.J. A stress signaling pathway in adipose tissue regulates hepatic insulin resistance. *Science* **2008**, *322*, 1539–1543.
30. Farnier, C.; Krief, S.; Blache, M.; Diot-Dupuy, F.; Mory, G.; Ferre, P.; Bazin, R. Adipocyte functions are modulated by cell size change: Potential involvement of an integrin/erk signalling pathway. *Int. J. Obes. Relat. Metab. Disord.* **2003**, *27*, 1178–1186.
31. Mittelman, S.D.; van Citters, G.W.; Kirkman, E.L.; Bergman, R.N. Extreme insulin resistance of the central adipose depot *in vivo*. *Diabetes* **2002**, *51*, 755–761.
32. Nguyen, M.T.; Favelyukis, S.; Nguyen, A.K.; Reichart, D.; Scott, P.A.; Jenn, A.; Liu-Bryan, R.; Glass, C.K.; Neels, J.G.; Olefsky, J.M. A subpopulation of macrophages infiltrates hypertrophic adipose tissue and is activated by free fatty acids via toll-like receptors 2 and 4 and JNK-dependent pathways. *J. Biol. Chem.* **2007**, *282*, 35279–35292.
33. Elnakish, M.T.; Hassanain, H.H.; Janssen, P.M.; Angelos, M.G.; Khan, M. Emerging role of oxidative stress in metabolic syndrome and cardiovascular diseases: Important role of rac/nadph oxidase. *J. Pathol.* **2013**, *231*, 290–300.
34. Ford, E.S.; Mokdad, A.H.; Giles, W.H.; Brown, D.W. The metabolic syndrome and antioxidant concentrations: Findings from the third national health and nutrition examination survey. *Diabetes* **2003**, *52*, 2346–2352.
35. Lissner, L.; Lindroos, A.K.; Sjostrom, L. Swedish obese subjects (SOS): An obesity intervention study with a nutritional perspective. *Eur. J. Clin. Nutr.* **1998**, *52*, 316–322.
36. Del Mar Bibiloni, M.; Maffeis, C.; Llompart, I.; Pons, A.; Tur, J.A. Dietary factors associated with subclinical inflammation among girls. *Eur. J. Clin. Nutr.* **2013**, *67*, 1264–1270.
37. Rose, F.J.; Webster, J.; Barry, J.B.; Phillips, L.K.; Richards, A.A.; Whitehead, J.P. Synergistic effects of ascorbic acid and thiazolidinedione on secretion of high molecular weight adiponectin from human adipocytes. *Diabetes Obes. Metab.* **2010**, *12*, 1084–1089.
38. Afkhami-Ardekani, M.; Shojaoddiny-Ardekani, A. Effect of vitamin C on blood glucose, serum lipids & serum insulin in type 2 diabetes patients. *Indian J. Med. Res.* **2007**, *126*, 471–474.
39. Soares, A.F.; Guichardant, M.; Cozzone, D.; Bernoud-Hubac, N.; Bouzaidi-Tiali, N.; Lagarde, M.; Geloen, A. Effects of oxidative stress on adiponectin secretion and lactate production in 3T3-L1 adipocytes. *Free Radic. Biol. Med.* **2005**, *38*, 882–889.
40. Hui, J.M.; Hodge, A.; Farrell, G.C.; Kench, J.G.; Kriketos, A.; George, J. Beyond insulin resistance in NASH: TNF-α or adiponectin? *Hepatology* **2004**, *40*, 46–54.

41. Chalasani, N.; Younossi, Z.; Lavine, J.E.; Diehl, A.M.; Brunt, E.M.; Cusi, K.; Charlton, M.; Sanyal, A.J. The diagnosis and management of non-alcoholic fatty liver disease: Practice guideline by the american gastroenterological association, american association for the study of liver diseases, and american college of gastroenterology. *Gastroenterology* **2012**, *142*, 1592–1609.
42. Bechmann, L.P.; Hannivoort, R.A.; Gerken, G.; Hotamisligil, G.S.; Trauner, M.; Canbay, A. The interaction of hepatic lipid and glucose metabolism in liver diseases. *J. Hepatol.* **2012**, *56*, 952–964.
43. Hebbard, L.; George, J. Animal models of nonalcoholic fatty liver disease. *Nat. Rev. Gastroenterol. Hepatol.* **2011**, *8*, 35–44.
44. Adams, L.A.; Sanderson, S.; Lindor, K.D.; Angulo, P. The histological course of nonalcoholic fatty liver disease: A longitudinal study of 103 patients with sequential liver biopsies. *J. Hepatol.* **2005**, *42*, 132–138.
45. Ekstedt, M.; Franzen, L.E.; Mathiesen, U.L.; Thorelius, L.; Holmqvist, M.; Bodemar, G.; Kechagias, S. Long-term follow-up of patients with NAFLD and elevated liver enzymes. *Hepatology* **2006**, *44*, 865–873.
46. Bugianesi, E.; Leone, N.; Vanni, E.; Marchesini, G.; Brunello, F.; Carucci, P.; Musso, A.; de Paolis, P.; Capussotti, L.; Salizzoni, M.; *et al.* Expanding the natural history of nonalcoholic steatohepatitis: From cryptogenic cirrhosis to hepatocellular carcinoma. *Gastroenterology* **2002**, *123*, 134–140.
47. Angelico, F.; del Ben, M.; Conti, R.; Francioso, S.; Feole, K.; Fiorello, S.; Cavallo, M.G.; Zalunardo, B.; Lirussi, F.; Alessandri, C.; *et al.* Insulin resistance, the metabolic syndrome, and nonalcoholic fatty liver disease. *J. Clin. Endocrinol. Metab.* **2005**, *90*, 1578–1582.
48. Marchesini, G.; Bugianesi, E.; Forlani, G.; Cerrelli, F.; Lenzi, M.; Manini, R.; Natale, S.; Vanni, E.; Villanova, N.; Melchionda, N.; *et al.* Nonalcoholic fatty liver, steatohepatitis, and the metabolic syndrome. *Hepatology* **2003**, *37*, 917–923.
49. Luyckx, F.H.; Desaive, C.; Thiry, A.; Dewe, W.; Scheen, A.J.; Gielen, J.E.; Lefebvre, P.J. Liver abnormalities in severely obese subjects: Effect of drastic weight loss after gastroplasty. *Int. J. Obes. Relat. Metab. Disord.* **1998**, *22*, 222–226.
50. Mohan, V.; Farooq, S.; Deepa, M.; Ravikumar, R.; Pitchumoni, C.S. Prevalence of non-alcoholic fatty liver disease in urban south indians in relation to different grades of glucose intolerance and metabolic syndrome. *Diabetes Res. Clin. Pract.* **2009**, *84*, 84–91.
51. Abdelmalek, M.F.; Diehl, A.M. Nonalcoholic fatty liver disease as a complication of insulin resistance. *Med. Clin. N. Am.* **2007**, *91*, 1125–1149.
52. Gaggini, M.; Morelli, M.; Buzzigoli, E.; deFronzo, R.A.; Bugianesi, E.; Gastaldelli, A. Non-alcoholic fatty liver disease (NAFLD) and its connection with insulin resistance, dyslipidemia, atherosclerosis and coronary heart disease. *Nutrients* **2013**, *5*, 1544–1560.
53. Donnelly, K.L.; Smith, C.I.; Schwarzenberg, S.J.; Jessurun, J.; Boldt, M.D.; Parks, E.J. Sources of fatty acids stored in liver and secreted via lipoproteins in patients with nonalcoholic fatty liver disease. *J. Clin. Investig.* **2005**, *115*, 1343–1351.
54. Bardini, G.; Rotella, C.M.; Giannini, S. Dyslipidemia and diabetes: Reciprocal impact of impaired lipid metabolism and beta-cell dysfunction on micro- and macrovascular complications. *Rev. Diabet. Stud.* **2012**, *9*, 82–93.

55. McRae, M.P. Vitamin C supplementation lowers serum low-density lipoprotein cholesterol and triglycerides: A meta-analysis of 13 randomized controlled trials. *J. Chiropr. Med.* **2008**, *7*, 48–58.
56. Moschen, A.R.; Molnar, C.; Geiger, S.; Graziadei, I.; Ebenbichler, C.F.; Weiss, H.; Kaser, S.; Kaser, A.; Tilg, H. Anti-inflammatory effects of excessive weight loss: Potent suppression of adipose interleukin 6 and tumour necrosis factor alpha expression. *Gut* **2010**, *59*, 1259–1264.
57. Kamada, Y.; Tamura, S.; Kiso, S.; Matsumoto, H.; Saji, Y.; Yoshida, Y.; Fukui, K.; Maeda, N.; Nishizawa, H.; Nagaretani, H.; *et al.* Enhanced carbon tetrachloride-induced liver fibrosis in mice lacking adiponectin. *Gastroenterology* **2003**, *125*, 1796–1807.
58. Finelli, C.; Tarantino, G. What is the role of adiponectin in obesity related non-alcoholic fatty liver disease? *World J. Gastroenterol.* **2013**, *19*, 802–812.
59. Kim, J.Y.; van de Wall, E.; Laplante, M.; Azzara, A.; Trujillo, M.E.; Hofmann, S.M.; Schraw, T.; Durand, J.L.; Li, H.; Li, G.; *et al.* Obesity-associated improvements in metabolic profile through expansion of adipose tissue. *J. Clin. Investig.* **2007**, *117*, 2621–2637.
60. Park, E.J.; Lee, J.H.; Yu, G.Y.; He, G.; Ali, S.R.; Holzer, R.G.; Osterreicher, C.H.; Takahashi, H.; Karin, M. Dietary and genetic obesity promote liver inflammation and tumorigenesis by enhancing Il-6 and TNF expression. *Cell* **2010**, *140*, 197–208.
61. Tappy, L.; Le, K.A. Does fructose consumption contribute to non-alcoholic fatty liver disease? *Clin. Res. Hepatol. Gastroenterol.* **2012**, *36*, 554–560.
62. Podszun, M.C.; Grebenstein, N.; Spruss, A.; Schlueter, T.; Kremoser, C.; Bergheim, I.; Frank, J. Dietary α-tocopherol and atorvastatin reduce high-fat-induced lipid accumulation and down-regulate cd36 protein in the liver of guinea pigs. *J. Nutr. Biochem.* **2014**, *25*, 573–579.
63. Ye, P.; Cheah, I.K.; Halliwell, B. A high-fat and cholesterol diet causes fatty liver in guinea pigs. The role of iron and oxidative damage. *Free Radic. Res.* **2013**, *47*, 602–613.
64. Coban, J.; Evran, B.; Ozkan, F.; Cevik, A.; Dogru-Abbasoglu, S.; Uysal, M. Effect of blueberry feeding on lipids and oxidative stress in the serum, liver and aorta of guinea pigs fed on a high-cholesterol diet. *Biosci. Biotechnol. Biochem.* **2013**, *77*, 389–391.
65. Kim, J.E.; Clark, R.M.; Park, Y.; Lee, J.; Fernandez, M.L. Lutein decreases oxidative stress and inflammation in liver and eyes of guinea pigs fed a hypercholesterolemic diet. *Nutr. Res. Pract.* **2012**, *6*, 113–119.
66. Mari, M.; Caballero, F.; Colell, A.; Morales, A.; Caballeria, J.; Fernandez, A.; Enrich, C.; Fernandez-Checa, J.C.; Garcia-Ruiz, C. Mitochondrial free cholesterol loading sensitizes to TNF- and FAS-mediated steatohepatitis. *Cell Metab.* **2006**, *4*, 185–198.
67. Feldstein, A.E.; Werneburg, N.W.; Canbay, A.; Guicciardi, M.E.; Bronk, S.F.; Rydzewski, R.; Burgart, L.J.; Gores, G.J. Free fatty acids promote hepatic lipotoxicity by stimulating TNF-α expression via a lysosomal pathway. *Hepatology* **2004**, *40*, 185–194.
68. Basaranoglu, M.; Basaranoglu, G.; Senturk, H. From fatty liver to fibrosis: A tale of "second hit". *World J. Gastroenterol.* **2013**, *19*, 1158–1165.
69. Pessayre, D. Role of mitochondria in non-alcoholic fatty liver disease. *J. Gastroenterol. Hepatol.* **2007**, *22*, S20–S27.

70. Wei, Y.; Wang, D.; Topczewski, F.; Pagliassotti, M.J. Saturated fatty acids induce endoplasmic reticulum stress and apoptosis independently of ceramide in liver cells. *Am. J. Physiol. Endocrinol. Metab.* **2006**, *291*, E275–E281.
71. Van Rooyen, D.M.; Larter, C.Z.; Yeh, M.M.; Haigh, W.G.; Teoh, N.; Farrell, G.C. Ezetimibe and atorvastatin ameliorate liver injury in foz/foz mice with NASH. *J. Gastroenterol. Hepatol.* **2011**, *26*, 2–14.
72. Fujii, H.; Kawada, N. Inflammation and fibrogenesis in steatohepatitis. *J. Gastroenterol.* **2012**, *47*, 215–225.
73. Laurent, A.; Nicco, C.; Tran van Nhieu, J.; Borderie, D.; Chereau, C.; Conti, F.; Jaffray, P.; Soubrane, O.; Calmus, Y.; Weill, B.; *et al.* Pivotal role of superoxide anion and beneficial effect of antioxidant molecules in murine steatohepatitis. *Hepatology* **2004**, *39*, 1277–1285.
74. Farrell, G.C.; van Rooyen, D.; Gan, L.; Chitturi, S. Nash is an inflammatory disorder: Pathogenic, prognostic and therapeutic implications. *Gut Liver* **2012**, *6*, 149–171.
75. Narasimhan, S.; Gokulakrishnan, K.; Sampathkumar, R.; Farooq, S.; Ravikumar, R.; Mohan, V.; Balasubramanyam, M. Oxidative stress is independently associated with non-alcoholic fatty liver disease (NAFLD) in subjects with and without type 2 diabetes. *Clin. Biochem.* **2010**, *43*, 815–821.
76. Valdecantos, M.P.; Perez-Matute, P.; Quintero, P.; Martinez, J.A. Vitamin C, resveratrol and lipoic acid actions on isolated rat liver mitochondria: All antioxidants but different. *Redox Rep.* **2010**, *15*, 207–216.
77. Musso, G.; Gambino, R.; de Michieli, F.; Cassader, M.; Rizzetto, M.; Durazzo, M.; Faga, E.; Silli, B.; Pagano, G. Dietary habits and their relations to insulin resistance and postprandial lipemia in nonalcoholic steatohepatitis. *Hepatology* **2003**, *37*, 909–916.
78. Ferolla, S.M.; Ferrari, T.C.; Lima, M.L.; Reis, T.O.; Tavares, W.C., Jr.; Couto, O.F.; Vidigal, P.V.; Fausto, M.A.; Couto, C.A. Dietary patterns in brazilian patients with nonalcoholic fatty liver disease: A cross-sectional study. *Clinics* **2013**, *68*, 11–17.
79. Koruk, M.; Taysi, S.; Savas, M.C.; Yilmaz, O.; Akcay, F.; Karakok, M. Oxidative stress and enzymatic antioxidant status in patients with nonalcoholic steatohepatitis. *Ann. Clin. Lab. Sci.* **2004**, *34*, 57–62.
80. Videla, L.A.; Rodrigo, R.; Orellana, M.; Fernandez, V.; Tapia, G.; Quinones, L.; Varela, N.; Contreras, J.; Lazarte, R.; Csendes, A.; *et al.* Oxidative stress-related parameters in the liver of non-alcoholic fatty liver disease patients. *Clin. Sci.* **2004**, *106*, 261–268.
81. Frikke-Schmidt, H.; Lykkesfeldt, J. Role of marginal vitamin C deficiency in atherogenesis: *In vivo* models and clinical studies. *Basic Clin. Pharmacol. Toxicol.* **2009**, *104*, 419–433.
82. Roomi, M.W. Association between hyperlipidemia and hepatic cytochrome p-450 in guinea pigs. *Res. Commun. Mol. Pathol. Pharmacol.* **1997**, *97*, 139–150.
83. Montano, C.E.; Fernandez, M.L.; McNamara, D.J. Regulation of apolipoprotein B-containing lipoproteins by vitamin C level and dietary fat saturation in guinea pigs. *Metabolism* **1998**, *47*, 883–891.
84. Ginter, E.; Cerven, J.; Nemec, R.; Mikus, L. Lowered cholesterol catabolism in guinea pigs with chronic ascorbic acid deficiency. *Am. J. Clin. Nutr.* **1971**, *24*, 1238–1245.
85. Ginter, E. Ascorbic acid in cholesterol and bile acid metabolism. *Ann. N. Y. Acad. Sci.* **1975**, *258*, 410–421.

86. Sharma, P.; Pramod, J.; Sharma, P.K.; Sapra, M.; Manorma; Kothari, L.K. Effect of vitamin C deficiency and excess on the liver: A histopathological and biochemical study in guinea pigs fed normal or high cholesterol diet. *Indian J. Pathol. Microbiol.* **1990**, *33*, 307–313.
87. Frikke-Schmidt, H.; Tveden-Nyborg, P.; Birck, M.M.; Lykkesfeldt, J. High dietary fat and cholesterol exacerbates chronic vitamin C deficiency in guinea pigs. *Br. J. Nutr.* **2011**, *105*, 54–61.
88. Horio, F.; Ozaki, K.; Oda, H.; Makino, S.; Hayashi, Y.; Yoshida, A. Effect of dietary ascorbic acid, cholesterol and PCB on cholesterol concentrations in serum and liver in a rat mutant unable to synthesize ascorbic acid. *J. Nutr.* **1987**, *117*, 1036–1044.
89. Uchida, K.; Nomura, Y.; Takase, H.; Tasaki, T.; Seo, S.; Hayashi, Y.; Takeuchi, N. Effect of vitamin C depletion on serum cholesterol and lipoprotein levels in ODS (od/od) rats unable to synthesize ascorbic acid. *J. Nutr.* **1990**, *120*, 1140–1147.
90. Fernandez, M.L. Guinea pigs as models for cholesterol and lipoprotein metabolism. *J. Nutr.* **2001**, *131*, 10–20.
91. Yang, R.; Guo, P.; Song, X.; Liu, F.; Gao, N. Hyperlipidemic guinea pig model: Mechanisms of triglyceride metabolism disorder and comparison to rat. *Biol. Pharm. Bull.* **2011**, *34*, 1046–1051.
92. Barja, G.; Lopez-Torres, M.; Perez-Campo, R.; Rojas, C.; Cadenas, S.; Prat, J.; Pamplona, R. Dietary vitamin C decreases endogenous protein oxidative damage, malondialdehyde, and lipid peroxidation and maintains fatty acid unsaturation in the guinea pig liver. *Free Radic. Biol. Med.* **1994**, *17*, 105–115.
93. Mori, T.; Kitamura, R.; Imaoka, S.; Funae, Y.; Kitada, M.; Kamataki, T. Examination for lipid peroxidation in liver microsomes of guinea pigs as a causal factor in the decrease in the content of cytochrome p-450 due to ascorbic acid deficiency. *Res. Commun. Chem. Pathol. Pharmacol.* **1992**, *75*, 209–219.
94. Amano, A.; Sato, Y.; Kishimoto, Y.; Takahashi, K.; Handa, S.; Aigaki, T.; Maruyama, N.; Ishigami, A. Effects of ascorbic acid deficiency on protein and lipid oxidation in livers from SMP30/GNL knockout mice. *J. Nutr. Sci. Vitaminol.* **2013**, *59*, 489–495.
95. Pierce, M.R.; Diasio, D.L.; Rodrigues, L.M.; Harrison, F.E.; May, J.M. Combined vitamin C and E deficiency induces motor defects in gulo($^{-/-}$)/SVCT2($^{+/-}$) mice. *Nutr. Neurosci.* **2013**, *16*, 160–173.
96. Harrison, F.E.; Meredith, M.E.; Dawes, S.M.; Saskowski, J.L.; May, J.M. Low ascorbic acid and increased oxidative stress in gulo($^{-/-}$) mice during development. *Brain Res.* **2010**, *1349*, 143–152.
97. Horio, F.; Kiyama, K.; Kobayashi, M.; Kawai, K.; Tsuda, T. Ascorbic acid deficiency stimulates hepatic expression of inflammatory chemokine, cytokine-induced neutrophil chemoattractant-1, in scurvy-prone ODS rats. *J. Nutr. Sci. Vitaminol.* **2006**, *52*, 28–32.
98. Al-Serri, A.; Anstee, Q.M.; Valenti, L.; Nobili, V.; Leathart, J.B.; Dongiovanni, P.; Patch, J.; Fracanzani, A.; Fargion, S.; Day, C.P.; *et al.* The SOD2 C47T polymorphism influences NAFLD fibrosis severity: Evidence from case-control and intra-familial allele association studies. *J. Hepatol.* **2012**, *56*, 448–454.
99. Seki, S.; Kitada, T.; Yamada, T.; Sakaguchi, H.; Nakatani, K.; Wakasa, K. *In situ* detection of lipid peroxidation and oxidative DNA damage in non-alcoholic fatty liver diseases. *J. Hepatol.* **2002**, *37*, 56–62.

100. Rezazadeh, A.; Yazdanparast, R.; Molaei, M. Amelioration of diet-induced nonalcoholic steatohepatitis in rats by Mn-salen complexes via reduction of oxidative stress. *J. Biomed. Sci.* **2012**, *19*, 26.
101. Rezazadeh, A.; Yazdanparast, R. Prevention of nonalcoholic steatohepatitis in rats by two manganese-salen complexes. *Iran. Biomed. J.* **2014**, *18*, 41–48.
102. Oliveira, C.P.; Gayotto, L.C.; Tatai, C.; Della Nina, B.I.; Lima, E.S.; Abdalla, D.S.; Lopasso, F.P.; Laurindo, F.R.; Carrilho, F.J. Vitamin C and vitamin E in prevention of nonalcoholic fatty liver disease (NAFLD) in choline deficient diet fed rats. *Nutr. J.* **2003**, *2*, 9.
103. Nambisan, B.; Kurup, P.A. Ascorbic acid and glycosaminoglycan and lipid metabolism in guinea pigs fed normal and atherogenic diets. *Atherosclerosis* **1975**, *22*, 447–461.
104. Hathcock, J.N.; Azzi, A.; Blumberg, J.; Bray, T.; Dickinson, A.; Frei, B.; Jialal, I.; Johnston, C.S.; Kelly, F.J.; Kraemer, K.; *et al.* Vitamins E and C are safe across a broad range of intakes. *Am. J. Clin. Nutr.* **2005**, *81*, 736–745.
105. The National Academies. Institute of Medicine. *Dietary Reference Intakes for Vitamin C, Vitamin E, Selenium, and Carotenoids*; The National Academies Press: Washington, DC, USA, 2000.
106. Monsen, E.R. Dietary reference intakes for the antioxidant nutrients: Vitamin C, vitamin E, selenium, and carotenoids. *J. Am. Diet. Assoc.* **2000**, *100*, 637–640.
107. Johnson, R.K. Dietary intake—How do we measure what people are really eating? *Obes. Res.* **2002**, *10*, 63s–68s.
108. Han, J.M.; Jo, A.N.; Lee, S.M.; Bae, H.S.; Jun, D.W.; Cho, Y.K.; Suk, K.T.; Yoon, J.H.; Ahn, S.B.; Cho, Y.J.; *et al.* Associations between intakes of individual nutrients or whole food groups and non-alcoholic fatty liver disease among korean adults. *J. Gastroenterol. Hepatol.* **2014**, *29*, 1265–1272.
109. Vos, M.B.; Colvin, R.; Belt, P.; Molleston, J.P.; Murray, K.F.; Rosenthal, P.; Schwimmer, J.B.; Tonascia, J.; Unalp, A.; Lavine, J.E. Correlation of vitamin E, uric acid, and diet composition with histologic features of pediatric NAFLD. *J. Pediatr. Gastroenterol. Nutr.* **2012**, *54*, 90–96.
110. Mager, D.R.; Patterson, C.; So, S.; Rogenstein, C.D.; Wykes, L.J.; Roberts, E.A. Dietary and physical activity patterns in children with fatty liver. *Eur. J. Clin. Nutr.* **2010**, *64*, 628–635.
111. Da Silva, H.E.; Arendt, B.M.; Noureldin, S.A.; Therapondos, G.; Guindi, M.; Allard, J.P. A cross-sectional study assessing dietary intake and physical activity in canadian patients with nonalcoholic fatty liver disease *vs.* healthy controls. *J. Acad. Nutr. Diet.* **2014**, *114*, 1181–1194.
112. Madan, K.; Bhardwaj, P.; Thareja, S.; Gupta, S.D.; Saraya, A. Oxidant stress and antioxidant status among patients with nonalcoholic fatty liver disease (NAFLD). *J. Clin. Gastroenterol.* **2006**, *40*, 930–935.
113. Canbakan, B.; Senturk, H.; Tahan, V.; Hatemi, I.; Balci, H.; Toptas, T.; Sonsuz, A.; Velet, M.; Aydin, S.; Dirican, A.; *et al.* Clinical, biochemical and histological correlations in a group of non-drinker subjects with non-alcoholic fatty liver disease. *Acta Gastro-Enterol. Belgica* **2007**, *70*, 277–284.
114. Dehghan, M.; Akhtar-Danesh, N.; McMillan, C.R.; Thabane, L. Is plasma vitamin C an appropriate biomarker of vitamin C intake? A systematic review and meta-analysis. *Nutr. J.* **2007**, *6*, 41.

115. Levine, M.; Conry-Cantilena, C.; Wang, Y.; Welch, R.W.; Washko, P.W.; Dhariwal, K.R.; Park, J.B.; Lazarev, A.; Graumlich, J.F.; King, J.; *et al.* Vitamin C pharmacokinetics in healthy volunteers: Evidence for a recommended dietary allowance. *Proc. Natl. Acad. Sci. USA* **1996**, *93*, 3704–3709.
116. Pfister, R.; Sharp, S.J.; Luben, R.; Wareham, N.J.; Khaw, K.T. Plasma vitamin C predicts incident heart failure in men and women in european prospective investigation into cancer and nutrition-norfolk prospective study. *Am. Heart J.* **2011**, *162*, 246–253.
117. Nobili, V.; Manco, M.; Devito, R.; Ciampalini, P.; Piemonte, F.; Marcellini, M. Effect of vitamin E on aminotransferase levels and insulin resistance in children with non-alcoholic fatty liver disease. *Aliment. Pharmacol. Ther.* **2006**, *24*, 1553–1561.
118. Nobili, V.; Manco, M.; Devito, R.; di Ciommo, V.; Comparcola, D.; Sartorelli, M.R.; Piemonte, F.; Marcellini, M.; Angulo, P. Lifestyle intervention and antioxidant therapy in children with nonalcoholic fatty liver disease: A randomized, controlled trial. *Hepatology* **2008**, *48*, 119–128.
119. Harrison, S.A.; Torgerson, S.; Hayashi, P.; Ward, J.; Schenker, S. Vitamin E and vitamin C treatment improves fibrosis in patients with nonalcoholic steatohepatitis. *Am. J. Gastroenterol.* **2003**, *98*, 2485–2490.
120. Adams, L.A.; Angulo, P. Vitamins E and C for the treatment of NASH: Duplication of results but lack of demonstration of efficacy. *Am. J. Gastroenterol.* **2003**, *98*, 2348–2350.
121. Piñeiro-Carrero, V.M.; Piñeiro, E.O. Liver. *Pediatrics* **2004**, *113*, 1097–1106.
122. Papandreou, D.; Rousso, I.; Mavromichalis, I. Update on non-alcoholic fatty liver disease in children. *Clin. Nutr.* **2007**, *26*, 409–415.
123. Kawanaka, M.; Nishino, K.; Nakamura, J.; Suehiro, M.; Goto, D.; Urata, N.; Oka, T.; Kawamoto, H.; Nakamura, H.; Yodoi, J.; *et al.* Treatment of nonalcoholic steatohepatitis with vitamins E and C: A pilot study. *Hepat. Med.* **2013**, *5*, 11–16.
124. Ersöz, G.; Gunsar, F.; Karasu, Z.; Akay, S.; Batur, Y.; Akarca, U.S. Management of fatty liver disease with vitamin E and C compared to ursodeoxycholic acid treatment. *Turkish J. Gastroenterol.* **2005**, *16*, 124–128.
125. Foster, T.; Budoff, M.J.; Saab, S.; Ahmadi, N.; Gordon, C.; Guerci, A.D. Atorvastatin and antioxidants for the treatment of nonalcoholic fatty liver disease: The St. Francis Heart Study randomized clinical trial. *Am. J. Gastroenterol.* **2011**, *106*, 71–77.
126. Targher, G.; Bertolini, L.; Rodella, S.; Lippi, G.; Franchini, M.; Zoppini, G.; Muggeo, M.; Day, C.P. Nash predicts plasma inflammatory biomarkers independently of visceral fat in men. *Obesity* **2008**, *16*, 1394–1399.
127. Speliotes, E.K.; Massaro, J.M.; Hoffmann, U.; Vasan, R.S.; Meigs, J.B.; Sahani, D.V.; Hirschhorn, J.N.; O'Donnell, C.J.; Fox, C.S. Fatty liver is associated with dyslipidemia and dysglycemia independent of visceral fat: The framingham heart study. *Hepatology* **2010**, *51*, 1979–1987.
128. Hatzitolios, A.; Savopoulos, C.; Lazaraki, G.; Sidiropoulos, I.; Haritanti, P.; Lefkopoulos, A.; Karagiannopoulou, G.; Tzioufa, V.; Dimitrios, K. Efficacy of omega-3 fatty acids, atorvastatin and orlistat in non-alcoholic fatty liver disease with dyslipidemia. *Indian J. Gastroenterol.* **2004**, *23*, 131–134.

129. Saadeh, S.; Younossi, Z.M.; Remer, E.M.; Gramlich, T.; Ong, J.P.; Hurley, M.; Mullen, K.D.; Cooper, J.N.; Sheridan, M.J. The utility of radiological imaging in nonalcoholic fatty liver disease. *Gastroenterology* **2002**, *123*, 745–750.

2

Effects of Pulsed Electric Fields (PEF) on Vitamin C and its Antioxidant Properties

Zhi-Hong Zhang [1], Xin-An Zeng [1,*], Charles S. Brennan [1,2,*], Margaret Brennan [2], Zhong Han [1] and Xia-Yu Xiong [1]

[1] College of Light Industry and Food Science, South China University of Technology, Guangzhou 510640, China; E-Mails: zhihong1942@foxmail.com (Z.-H.Z.); fezhonghan@scut.edu.cn (Z.H.); hsiungxiayu@163.com (X.-Y.X.)

[2] Centre for Food Research and Innovation, Department of Wine, Food and Molecular Biosciences, Lincoln University, Lincoln 85084, New Zealand; E-Mail: margaret.brennan@lincoln.ac.nz

* Authors to whom correspondence should be addressed;
E-Mails: xazeng@scut.edu.cn (X.-A.Z.); charles.brennan@lincoln.ac.nz (C.S.B.);

Academic Editor: Maurizio Battino

Abstract: In this study, pulsed electric fields (PEF) treatments and their effects on the structure of vitamin C (VIT-C) were estimated by fluorescence and Fourier transform infrared (FT-IR) spectroscopy, the relative content of VIT-C was measured by HPLC and the antioxidant properties of treated VIT-C by DPPH radical scavenging as well as reducing power tests. The fluorescence intensity of treated VIT-C increased slightly compared to the untreated VIT-C. Moreover, the effect of PEF on the structure of VIT-C was observed using the FT-IR spectra. These phenomena indicated that the PEF affected the conformation of VIT-C, which promoted the VIT-C isomer transformed enol-form into keto-form. In addition, the PEF treatments did not suffer the damage to VIT-C and could slow down the oxidation process in involving of experimental conditions by HPLC. The antioxidant properties of the treated VIT-C were enhanced, which was proved by radical scavenging and also the reducing power tests.

Keywords: vitamin C; PEF; fluorescence; FTIR; HPLC; antioxidant properties

1. Introduction

Vitamins are a diverse group of essential organic compounds that participate in normal growth, metabolism and maintenance of life [1,2]. In order to maintain an adequate intake of vitamins, humans must eat a wide variety of food products, either naturally high or, enriched with vitamins or alternatively supplement with multivitamin drugs, because the human body cannot synthesize them or the synthetic amount may not satisfy the bodily needs. Vitamin C (VIT-C) or L-ascorbic acid (AA) is an essential water-soluble vitamin in humans [3,4]. Humans lack the final enzyme (L-gulono-1,4-lactone oxidase) in the VIT-C biosynthesis pathway, thus, humans are dependent on fruits and vegetables (such as orange, sweet potato, and carrot) in their diet to provide VIT-C [5,6]. Vitamin C is beneficial for its antioxidant capacity and stimulation of immune system [7–9].

Although most vegetables and fruits contain certain amount of VIT-C, various storage conditions and processing methods can significantly affect VIT-C content [10], because VIT-C is a thermally sensitive bioactive nutrient when in the presence of oxygen [11–16]. Some advanced non-thermal methods, therefore are used in fruit and vegetable processing in order to maintain nutrition, such as ultra-high pressure processing (UHP) [17,18], pulsed electric fields (PEF) [19–21].

PEF technology involves the application of very short pulses (1–10 μs) of high electric intensity (10–100 kV/cm) to treat food products placed between two electrodes without substantially heating the product [22,23]. Nowadays, it is one of the hot points regarding the effect of PEF technology on nutrient, especially, vitamins and polyphenols [11–13,24]. Ade-Omowaye *et al.* [25] showed that the VIT-C retention of red bell pepper immediately after PEF treatment (50 pulses at 2 kV/cm, pulse duration 400 ms) ranged from 89.6% to 96.5%. Odriozola-Serrano *et al.* [20] observed that the VIT-C retention of strawberry juice was 98% after High Intensity Pulse Electric Field (HIPEF) (35 kV/cm, 1000 μs, and monopole mode). Moreover, they found that VIT-C retention was related to some parameters in terms of frequency, electric field intensity, pulsed width and polarity mode by a response surface methodology. In addition, many studies have proven that the retention of VIT-C was higher after PEF treatments than after thermal treatments [20,21,26]. In previous studies, it has been reported that the PEF-processing resulted in increased VIT-C retention when compared to other thermal treatments [20,21,27].

As mentioned above, there are some ambiguous results in effect of PEF treatment on VIT-C properties in previous studies. In addition, the complex food structures of fabricated foods have made it difficult to determine the effect of PEF treatment on the VIT-C. Relatively few studies mentioned that the PEF treatment directly affected the VIT-C. To solve the problem, systematically characterizing the effect of PEF treatment involved in different electric field strength and treatment time on the structure of VIT-C by fluorescence and Fourier transform infrared (FT-IR) spectroscopy is attempted. Moreover, the effect of PEF treatment on relative content of VIT-C was determined by high performance liquid chromatography (HPLC) and the antioxidant properties were measured by DPPH radical scavenging and the reducing power test.

2. Results and Discussion

2.1. Fluorescence of VIT-C

The effects of different electric field strength and treatment time on fluorescence of VIT-C are shown in Figures 1 and 2, respectively. Previously researchers have illustrated that the condensation product emits strong fluorescence and that the detection limit is very low (0.006 μg/mL) [28]. Therefore, fluorescence of VIT-C was determined based on the condensation reaction between VIT-C and *o*-phenylenediamine. This method can not only determine the content of VIT-C, but also observe the effects of PEF on the structure of VIT-C. It was observed that the fluorescence intensity of PEF treated VIT-C was higher than untreated VIT-C at 405 nm, and showed a tendency that the higher electric field strength was corresponding to the stronger fluorescence intensity. Moreover, the PEF treatment time also affected the fluorescence intensity of VIT-C. The fluorescence intensity of VIT-C treated by 3, 9, 15, 21 and 27 min (the effective PEF treatment was 0.8, 2.4, 4.0, 5.6, and 7.2 ms) were higher than the untreated (0 ms) sample at 405 nm, and the fluorescence intensity gradually increased with the treatment time. This phenomenon indicated that the PEF treatment could exert influence on the condensation reaction process of VIT-C and *o*-phenylenediamine, which is due to the type of VIT-C isomer present.

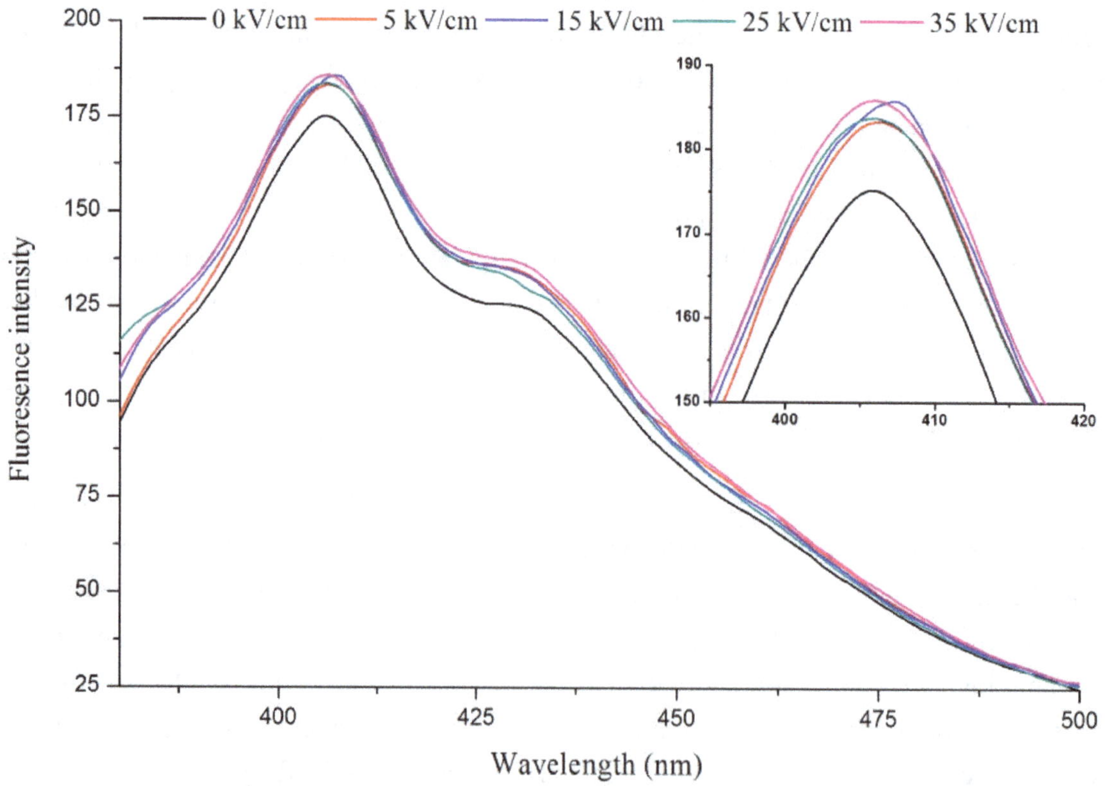

Figure 1. The effect of different electric field strength at 9 min on fluorescence of vitamin C (VIT-C).

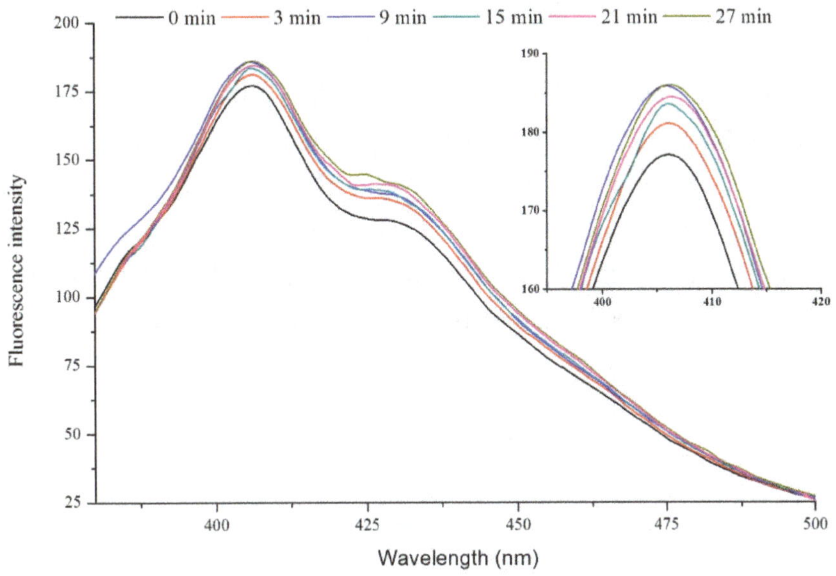

Figure 2. The effect of different pulsed electric fields (PEF) treatment time at 35 kV/cm electric field strength on fluorescence of VIT-C.

Wu *et al.* (2003) [28] reported that hydroxyl ion (–OH) could promote the conversion of VIT-C isomer from enol-form to keto-form in the range of pH 9.3–9.5, which proved that alkaline condition was conducive to the condensation reaction. In this study, the reaction system was under acidic conditions (pH < 7.0), but the fluorescence intensity was increased by PEF treatment, which indicated that PEF treatment promoted the conversion of VIT-C isomer. It has been reported that the water molecule was easily polarized by PEF and was dissociated into ions at high field strength [29]. The presence of polar groups can react with the interior macromolecules or active ingredients. Zhang *et al.* [30] reported that the PEF processing generated hydrogen radicals in phosphate buffer and oleic acid emulsion, they also illustrated that the electric field strength had a significant effect on H_2O_2 concentrations ($p < 0.5$) when estimated using electron spin resonance (ESR) techniques. Thus, it was believed that the free radicals generated by PEF treatment attacked the hydroxyl, which belonged to the VIT-C second carbon atom to complete the conversion of configuration. The possible mechanism is illustrated in Figure 3. This theory was consistent with the experimental phenomenon of VIT-C degradation by PEF processing in previous studies [21,31]. Moreover, some previous studies reported that the PEF treatment could influence the structure of amino acids, proteins and polysaccharides, which mainly related to the weak bonds such as hydrogen bonds, disulfide bonds and hydrophobic bonds [32–34].

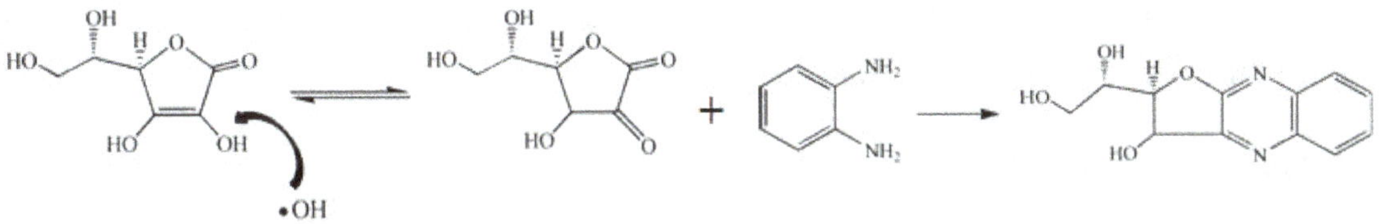

Figure 3. The possible mechanism of condensation reactions of VIT-C with *o*-phenylenediamine by PEF treatments.

2.2. FT-IR Analysis

The FT-IR spectra of PEF treated VIT-C solution are shown in Figure 4. The infrared spectroscopy characteristic absorption band of the VIT-C mainly appeared in wavenumber as follows. The band at 1600 cm^{-1} is contributes to vibration of C=C bonds. The band at 1680 cm^{-1} causes vibration of the C=O area present in the lactone ring system. Data presented in this manuscript illustrates that the stretching vibration of C=C and C=O, respectively, appeared at about 1700 and 1660 cm^{-1} by FT-IR spectra recorded in KBr pellets, this is consistent with previous studies when the effect of the solvent is taken into consideration [35,36].

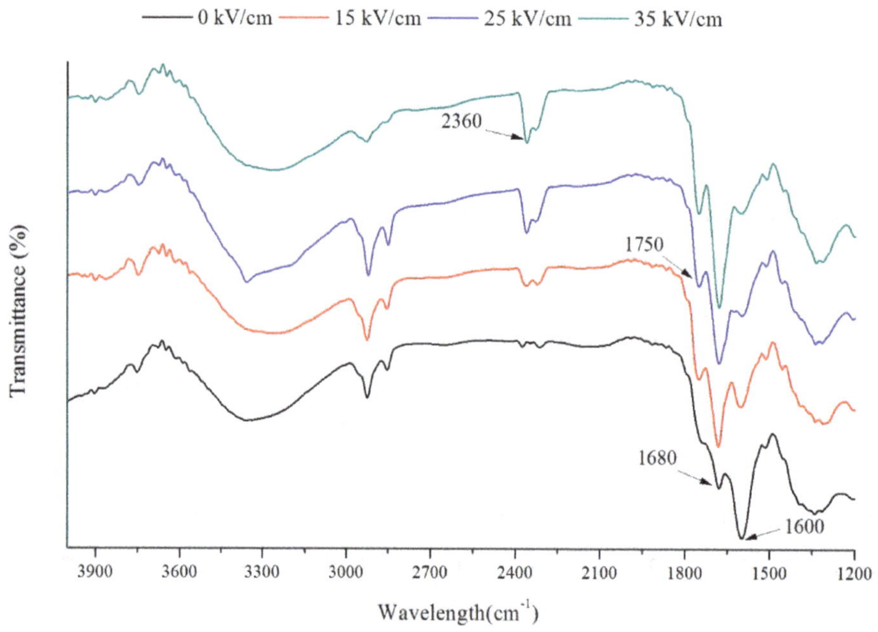

Figure 4. Fourier transform infrared (FTIR) spectra of VIT-C solution by PEF treatments.

The characteristic absorption band of the VIT-C showed some changes due to PEF treatment from the FT-IR spectra. When the electric field strength increased, the intensity of the band at 1600 cm^{-1} decreased, while the intensity of the band at 1680 cm^{-1} increased compared with untreated VIT-C. This phenomenon indicated that the structure of VIT-C has been transformed from the enol-form to keto-form by PEF treatment. Moreover, an obvious absorption peak was located at the band of 2360 cm^{-1}, which was attributed to the O–H stretching vibration. It indicates that the hydrogen atom from the O–H on third carbon was generated with carbonyl on second carbon atom bonded to a five membered ring system. Thus, it is believed that the PEF treatment could influence the structure of VIT-C from the FT-IR spectra. In addition, other previous studies also identified that the PEF could affect the structures of the protein and chitosan [37,38].

2.3. The Relative Content of VIT-C

When the PEF treatment affects the VIT-C content it is reflected through a change in the peak area of VIT-C by HPLC. The effect of PEF treatment on the relative content of VIT-C measured by HPLC is shown in Table 1. The relative content of PEF treated VIT-C was 97.56, 97.98, 93.60

and 95.28 mg/L at 5, 15, 25 and 35 kV/cm for 3 min, which was apparently higher than the untreated VIT-C of 93.96 mg/L. The results also showed that the VIT-C content of PEF treated samples was higher than the untreated VIT-C samples, also the untreated samples decreased in VIT-C over the increasing treatment time. This result was in agreement with the findings of Odriozola-Serrano *et al.* [21], who reported that the PEF treatment exhibited higher VIT-C retention than heat treatments in different fruits and vegetables juice. Moreover, some other studies showed that the 35 kV/cm of PEF treatment exhibited higher effectiveness on the retention of VIT-C than other selected electric field strengths [20] or thermal treatments [39,40]. The results showed that the content of VIT-C decreased with the increasing treatment time under 5 and 15 kV/cm, which was in agreement with the finding of Elez-Martinez and Martin-Belloso [41]. Meanwhile, a very interesting phenomenon was noted at 35 kV/cm and that was that the relative content of VIT-C increased from 95.28 to 98.14 mg/L as time increased from 3 to 27 min. A previous study reported that the ascorbic acid of orange-carrot juice decreased from 25.07 ± 0.68 to 22.53 ± 1.192 mg/100 mL with an increase in treatment time from 90 to 200 μs at 35 kV/cm [31]. The reason for this phenomenon may be due to the difference of the reaction conditions such as pH, electrical conductivity and temperature. These results indicate that whether using PEF treatment or not, the content of VIT-C could reduce as a consequence of extending the processing time which can be due to the natural oxidation of VIT-C. Moreover, the PEF treatments did not cause the damage to VIT-C and were able to retard the oxidation process under the experimental conditions created.

Table 1. The effect of PEF treatment on the relative content of VIT-C as detected by HPLC.

Relative Content (mg/L)	0 kV/cm	5 kV/cm	15 kV/cm	25 kV/cm	35 kV/cm
3 min	93.69 ± 0.12 $^{A a}$	97.56 ±0.10 $^{BC a}$	97.98 ± 0.38 $^{C a}$	93.60 ± 0.81 $^{A a}$	95.28 ± 0.24 $^{D a}$
9 min	92.85 ± 0.23 $^{A b}$	98.12 ± 0.31 $^{B ab}$	97.96 ± 0.50 $^{B a}$	96.77 ± 0.24 $^{C b}$	96.30 ± 0.56 $^{C a}$
15 min	91.72 ± 0.41 $^{A c}$	98.53 ± 0.27 $^{B b}$	97.77 ± 0.43 $^{B a}$	98.45 ± 0.62 $^{B c}$	96.50 ± 0.70 $^{C a}$
21 min	91.51 ± 0.15 $^{A c}$	97.43 ± 0.42 $^{B a}$	97.59 ± 0.41 $^{B a}$	98.33 ± 0.47 $^{B c}$	98.19 ± 0.53 $^{B b}$
27 min	91.38 ± 0.22 $^{A c}$	95.12 ± 0.51 $^{B c}$	97.32 ± 0.35 $^{C a}$	98.01 ± 0.53 $^{C bc}$	98.14 ± 0.42 $^{C b}$

PEF: pulsed electric fields; VIT-C: vitamin C. Values with different letters in the column (a–c) and in the row (A–D) mean significant difference ($p < 0.05$).

2.4. 1,1-Diphenyl-2-picrylhydrazyl (DDPH) Radical Scavenging Activity

Figure 5 illustrates that the 1,1-diphenyl-2-picrylhydrazyl (DDPH) radical scavenging ability of PEF treated VIT-C increased compared to untreated VIT-C. The DDPH radical scavenging of VIT-C was 87.84%, 91.89%, 89.99% and 89.32%, respectively, with 5, 15, 25 and 35 kV/cm of PEF treatment for 15 min; these were all a significant increase compared with untreated VIT-C, which had a DDPH radical scavenging activity of 83.28% ($p < 0.05$). However, the DPPH radical scavenging activity that was treated for 3 min with different electric field strengths was not significantly different at 15–35 kV/cm. This result indicated that the treatment time was obvious influence on the DPPH radical scavenging activity. As treatment time increased, the DPPH radical scavenging activity of non-treated VIT-C was obviously decreased, but the PEF treatment of VIT-C caused DPPH radical scavenging activity to show a trend of either no reduction or some increase. These results illustrated that the PEF treatment at appropriate electric field strength and treatment time could effectively maintain the activity of VIT-C.

Similar results were found in a previous study by Wang and coworkers [38]. In this context, the antioxidant activity of glutathione (GSH) treated with different electric field intensities from 10 to 30 kV/cm were significantly increased, especially at the electric field strength of 10 kV/cm. Other previous studies have also indicated that under certain electric field strengths, the structure of protein showed some changes, such as the molecular weight, the quaternary structure, and polarization of the proteins molecule, which caused the increase or decrease of the DDPH radical inhibition [42,43]. It can be shown that the PEF treatment influenced the structure of VIT-C in Sections 3.1 and 3.2, which may be one of the reasons for the increasing DPPH radical scavenging activity. In addition, the PEF treated solutions could exhibit the higher VIT-C retention (95.12–98.53 mg/L), which may be one of the reasons for enhancing the DPPH radical scavenging.

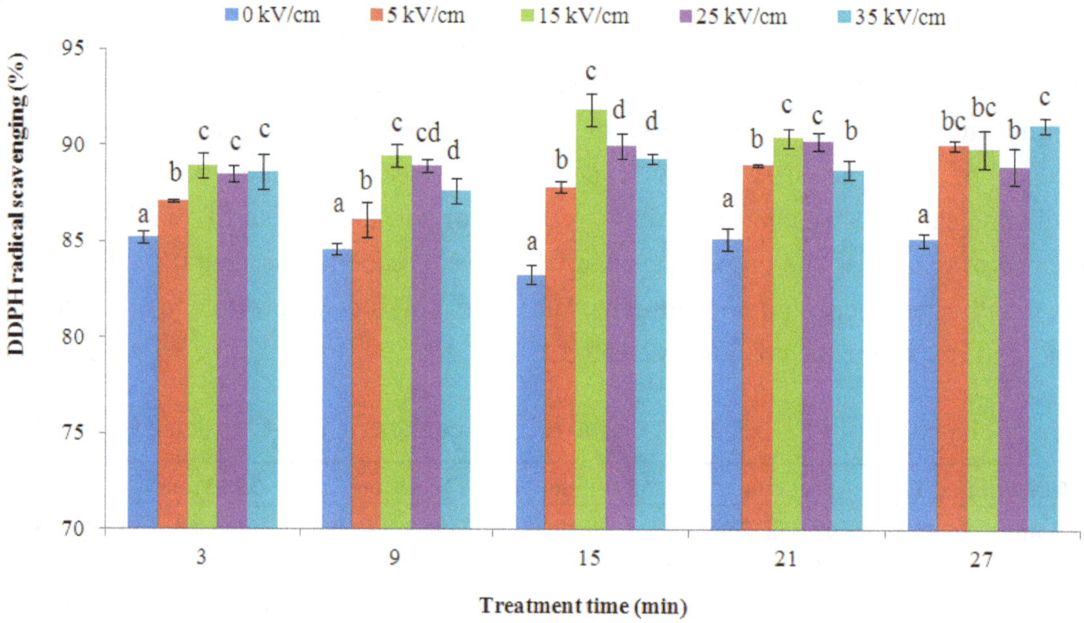

Figure 5. 1,1-diphenyl-2-picrylhydrazyl (DDPH) radical scavenging activity of VIT-C by PEF treatments. Values in columns followed by different letters mean significant difference ($p < 0.05$).

2.5. Reducing Power Ability

The reducing power activity of PEF treated VIT-C using the potassium ferricyanide reduction method is shown in Figure 6. The results were expressed as absorbance at 700 nm. It is shown that the reducing power ability, by different electric field strengths based on 3 min treatment of PEF treated VIT-C, significantly increased as compared with non-treated VIT-C ($p < 0.05$), reducing power increased by 13.50%, 10.24%, 11.42%, and 15.28% at 5, 15, 25 and 35 kV/cm, respectively. Among the different electric field strengths, however, there was no significant difference. At other processing times, the PEF treated VIT-C also showed a tendency for the reducing power ability to increase as compared to non-treated VIT-C. These results indicate that the reducing power of PEF treated VIT-C can be increased compared with non-treatment. The reason for this phenomenon was that the PEF treatment altered the structure and polarization of VIT-C. As a result, it is easier for the VIT-C to provide electrons, thereby the antioxidant capacity was enhanced; similar results were found in the previous study [44].

In this study, the treatment time was extended and the reducing power of peptides derived from egg white was increased by treatment with 10 kV/cm PEF. Notably, the reducing power was increased by 0.118 after a 5 h PEF treatment compared to an untreated sample of 0.646. This result showed that the PEF treatment time could significantly increase the antioxidant activity of the peptides. It was believed that PEF treatment could activate the antioxidant activity of peptides derived from egg white by polarization of peptide molecules, and destroy the non-covalent bonds, by hydrophobic interactions, electrostatic interactions and creating hydrogen bonds [44]. In addition, a previous study observed the effects of different electrode materials on antioxidant capacity and other characteristics of cyaniding-3-glucoside (Cy-3-glc) and cyaniding-3-sophoroside (Cy-3-sop) during 10 kV/cm of PEF treatment. The results showed that the antioxidant of Cy-3-glc and Cy-3-sop was increased, regardless of the method used (FRAP, DDPH and ORAC), which was due to the higher retention of Cy-3-sop and Cy-3-glc, the electrochemical reaction and forming of anthocyanin–metal complexes that have higher antioxidant capacity [45].

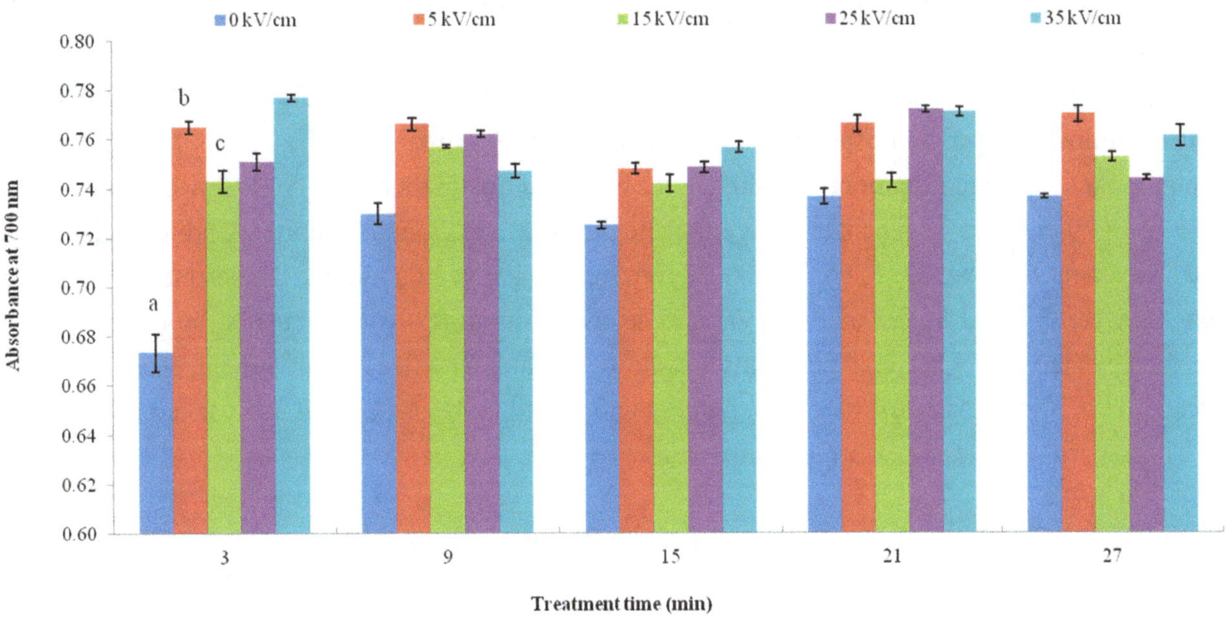

Figure 6. Reduce power activity of VIT-C by PEF treatments. Values in columns followed by different letters mean significant difference ($p < 0.05$).

3. Materials and Methods

3.1. Materials

Vitamin C and ethanol were purchased from Sinopharm Chemical Reagent Co., Ltd. (Shanghai, China). Potassium ferricyanide purchased from Tianjin Fuchen Chemical Reagent Factory (Tianjin, China). *O*-phenylenediamine was obtained from Tianjin Kemiou Chemical Reagent Co., Ltd. (Tianjin, China). Methanol was obtained from ANPEL Laboratory Technologies Inc. (Shanghai, China). 1,1-Diphenyl-2-picrylhydrazyl (DDPH radical) was obtained from Sigma-Aldrich, Chemie GmbH (St. Louis, MO, USA). All other reagents and chemicals used were of analytical grade. All reagents were prepared with deionized water (conductivity 0.3 μS/cm).

3.2. PEF Treatment System

The continuous PEF system was designed and manufactured by South China University of Technology PEF team (SY-Z-500; Guangzhou, China). The structure of the equipment has been reported in previous studies [46,47]. The main parameters of this equipment were as follows: frequency of 1 kHz, pulse width of 40 μs, unipolar square-wave. A two channel digital storage oscilloscope (DST1102B, Tekway Technologies Co., Ltd., Nanjing, China) was used to monitor the power supply of PEF system during the treatment. The treatment chamber was made of Teflon. The parameters of chamber were as follows: the volume of 0.02 mL, the distance between two parallel titanium-based alloy electrodes of 0.3 cm. The sample flow was controlled by a peristaltic pump (323 E/D, Watson Marlow, NC, USA). The sample temperature was measured by thermocouple (EW-981, Ewelly, Guangzhou, China) and was maintained by a cooling circulator (DLSK 3/10, Ketai Laboratory Equipment Co., Ltd., Zhengzhou, China). The scheme of the PEF treatment system used in the experiment is shown in Figure 7. In this study, 100 mg/L of VIT-C solution was prepared by ethanol-aqueous (volume ratio of 1:1) in a 1 L volumetric flask. The bubbles were removed by vacuum pump before the treatment. The pH of VIT-C solution was 4.47 and conductivity value was 10.0 mS/cm (20 ± 1 °C). The flow rate of sample was set at 60 mL/min by a peristaltic pump and the temperature was maintained at 20 ± 1 °C by cooling circulator. According to Equations (1) and (2), the effective treatment time (t) of PEF were calculated to be 0.8, 2.4, 4.0, 5.6 and 7.2 ms inthe different cycle times (1, 3, 5, 7, and 9), corresponding to the sample actual treatment time was 3, 9, 15, 21 and 27 min, respectively. In addition, the selected electric field strengths were 0, 0.5, 12.5, 25 and 35 kV/cm. The energy input (Q) was calculated by Equation (3) as described by Han *et al.* [32], and the results are shown in Table 2. After PEF treatment, each sample was collected in a 10 mL glass test tube with stopper and stored at 4 ± 1 °C until analysis could be carried out. The experiments were performed three times.

$$t = N_t \times W_p \times n \tag{1}$$

$$N_t = \frac{f \times V}{S} \tag{2}$$

where N_t is pulse number, W_p represents pulse width (μs), n denotes sample cycles, f represents pulse repetition rates, V is the volume of the chamber (mL) and S is the flow rate (mL/s).

$$Q = E^2 \times t \times \delta \tag{3}$$

where Q is the energy input (J/m^3), E is the electric field strength (V/m), t is the treatment time and δ is the conductivity of the sample (S/m).

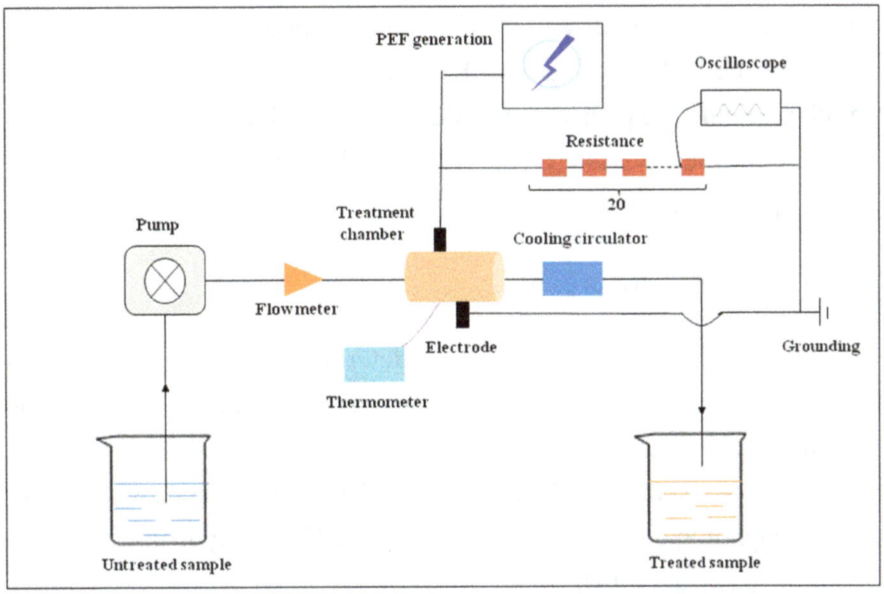

Figure 7. The scheme of the PEF treatment system used in the experiment.

Table 2. The energy input (Q, kJ/cm^3) of PEF in the different treatment condition.

Electric Field Strength (kV/cm)	Treatment Time (ms)				
	0.8	**2.4**	**4.0**	**5.6**	**7.2**
5	0.05	0.15	0.25	0.35	0.45
15	0.45	1.35	2.25	3.15	4.05
25	1.25	3.75	6.25	8.75	11.25
35	2.45	7.35	12.25	17.15	22.05

3.3. Fluorescence Measurement

The determination of VIT-C was performed as described by Wu *et al.* [28] with some modifications. The VIT-C content was determined by a spectrofluorometer (Perkin–Elmer LS55, Beaconsfield, Bucks, UK). Briefly, 0.5 mL of sample was added to 4.5 mL of ethanol-aqueous (volume ratio of 1:1), and then mixed with 0.5 mL *o*-phenylenediamine solution (0.2 g/L). The mixture was placed in dark and allowed to stand for 30 min. Fluorescence intensities of samples were determined in a 1 cm quartz cell (excitation and emission wavelengths of 355 and 405 nm, respectively). Width of excitation and emission slit were both set at 10 nm, and the relative fluorescence was determined.

3.4. FT-IR Analysis

Spectrometry analysis of the VIT-C solutions by PEF treatment was carried out to observe the structure by using an FT-IR spectrometer (Vector33, Bruker, Ettlingen, Germany). The samples were fixed in the CaF_2 window and FTIR spectra were collected in the range of 1100–4000 cm^{-1}.

3.5. Determination of VIT-C by HPLC

The relative content of VIT-C was determined using Waters 1525 Binary HPLC (Waters Corp., Milford, MA, USA) equipped with a C_{18} column (250 × 4.0 mm, 5 μm, SunFire, Waters, Milford, MA,

USA), an autosampler (2707, Waters, Milford, MA, USA) and a photodiode array detector (2998, Waters, Singapore). The method described by Klimczak and Gliszczyńska-Świgło [48] with some modifications. A gradient of mobile phase composed of water (solvent A) and methanol (solvent B) was used 10% A in 15 min with the flow rate of 0.8 mL/min. The eluate was detected by UV detection at 245 nm. The injection volume was 20 μL.

3.6. DDPH Radical Scavenging Activity

The antioxidant activity of VIT-C solutions was determined by a stable capacity DDPH radical following the method described by *Gu et al.* [49] with some modifications. Sample (200 mL) was mixed with 3.5 mL of 0.1 mmol/L DPPH solution (DPPH was dissolved in ethanol) and vortexed for mixing before leaving the samples to stand for 20 min in the dark. Absorbance values were determined at 517 nm using a spectrophotometer (UV-1800, SHIMADZU, Tokyo, Japan). DPPH activity was calculated by the following Equation (4).

$$SA(\%) = (1 - \frac{A_1 - A_2}{A_3}) \times 100 \tag{4}$$

where SA is the scavenging activity DDPH radical. A_1 is the absorbance of the sample. A_2 is the absorbance of the blank. A_3 is the absorbance of the control.

3.7. Reducing Power Ability

The reducing power of sample was determined by the method of Yen *et al.* [50] with some modifications. The sample solutions were mixed with 2.5 mL of 0.2 mol/L phosphate buffer (pH 6.6) and 2.5 mL of 1% potassium ferricyanide. Each sample solution was incubated for 20 min at 50 °C and then cooled to room temperature. Trichloroacetic acid (2.5 mL) was added to each sample, followed by vigorous mixing. An aliquot of 2.5 mL of each sample was mixed 0.5 mL of 1 g/L ferric chloride and the absorbance of the resultant solution was measured at 700 nm. Higher absorbance of the reaction mixture indicated greater reducing power.

3.8. Statistical Analysis

All results were reported as mean ± standard deviation ($n = 3$) using SPSS 16.0 software (IBM, New York, NY, USA). Variance analysis and graphs were obtained by Origin 8.0 software (OriginLab, Massachusetts, MA, USA) to determine the different treatment variations. Significance testing was performed by Tukey's multiple-comparison test and the differences were statistically significant. The significance level was 5% ($p < 0.05$) unless otherwise stated.

4. Conclusions

The effects of PEF treatment on VIT-C structure, and its relative content and antioxidant properties were investigated in this study. The fluorescence intensity increased by PEF treatment as compared to the non-treated VIT-C using the fluorescence measurement. This result indicated that the PEF treatment could modify the molecular conformation of VIT-C (from enol-form to keto-form). FT-IR spectra proved the changes of VIT-C structure by PEF treatment. Moreover, the PEF treatments did not damage the VIT-C and could slow down the oxidation process in involving of experimental conditions. In addition, PEF treatment could enhance the antioxidant properties through the DPPH radical scavenging and reducing power test, which could be due to the structure changes of VIT-C. The antioxidant properties showed that the DPPH radical scavenging was significantly increased by 4.56%, 8.61%, 6.71%, and 6.04%, respectively, which were corresponding to 5, 15, 25, and 35 kV/cm under 3 min processing time compared to the non-treated VIT-C ($p < 0.05$).

Acknowledgments

This research was supported by "863 project" (2011AA100801), National Natural Science Foundation of China (21376094 and 31301559) and Science and Technology Projects of Guangdong Province (2012A020200002, 2012A020100005 and 2013B020311008). The authors are also grateful to the Guangdong Province Government (China) for support through the program of "Leading Talent of Guangdong Province (Da-Wen Sun)".

Author Contributions

Zhi-Hong Zhang carried out most of the theoretical analysis and drafted the manuscript, while Xin-An Zeng, Charles S. Brennan and Zhong Han carried out some of the theoretical analyses; Xia-Yu Xiong carried on the Statistical Analysis; Xin-An Zeng, Charles S. Brennan and Margaret Brennan revised the paper. All authors read and approved the final manuscript.

References

1. Engel, R.; Stefanovits-Bányai, É.; Abrankó, L. LC simultaneous determination of the free forms of B group vitamins and vitamin C in various fortified food products. *Chromatographia* **2010**, *71*, 1069–1074.
2. Reis, S.F.; Rai, D.K.; Abu-Ghannam, N. Apple pomace as a potential ingredient for the development of new functional foods. *Int. J. Food Sci. Technol.* **2014**, *49*, 1743–1750.
3. Carr, A.C.; Vissers, M. Synthetic or food-derived vitamin C–Are they equally bioavailable? *Nutrients* **2013**, *5*, 4284–4304.
4. Gallie, D.R. Increasing vitamin C content in plant foods to improve their nutritional value—Successes and challenges. *Nutrients* **2011**, *5*, 3424–3446.
5. Fenoll, J.; Martínez, A.; Hellín, P.; Flores, P. Simultaneous determination of ascorbic and dehydroascorbic acids in vegetables and fruits by liquid chromatography with tandem-mass spectrometry. *Food Chem.* **2011**, *127*, 340–344.
6. Shashirekha, M.N.; Mallikarjuna, S.E.; Rajarathnam, S. Status of bioactive compounds in foods, with focus on fruits and vegetables. *Crit. Rev. Food Sci.* **2015**, *55*, 1324–1339.

7. Cui, J.; Yuan, X.; Wang, L.; Jones, G.; Zhang, S. Recent loss of vitamin C biosynthesis ability in bats. *PLoS ONE* **2011**, *6*, e27114.
8. Davey, M.W.; Montagu, M.V.; Inzé, D.; Sanmartin, M.; Kanellis, A.; Smirnoff, N.; Benzie, I.J.J.; Strain, J.J.; Favell, D.; Fletcher, J. Plant L-ascorbic acid: Chemistry, function, metabolism, bioavailability and effects of processing. *J. Sci. Food Agric.* **2000**, *80*, 825–860.
9. Valente, A.; Albuquerque, T.G.; Sanches-Silva, A.; Costa, H.S. Ascorbic acid content in exotic fruits: A contribution to produce quality data for food composition databases. *Food Res. Int.* **2011**, *44*, 2237–2242.
10. Spínola, V.; Mendes, B.; Câmara, J.S.; Castilho, P.C. Effect of time and temperature on vitamin C stability in horticultural extracts. UHPLC-PDA *vs.* iodometric titration as analytical methods. *LWT-Food Sci. Technol.* **2013**, *50*, 489–495.
11. Roohinejad, S.; Everett, D.W.; Oey, I. Effect of pulsed electric field processing on carotenoid extractability of carrot purée. *Int. J. Food Sci. Technol.* **2014**, *49*, 2120–2127.
12. Pedras, M.M.; Tribst, A.A.L.; Cristianini, M. Effects of high-pressure homogenisation on physicochemical characteristics of partially skimmed milk. *Int. J. Food Sci. Technol.* **2014**, *49*, 861–866.
13. Jabbar, S.; Abid, M.; Hu, B.; Hashim, M.M.; Saeeduddin, M.; Lei, S.; Wu, T.; Zeng, X. Influence of sonication and high hydrostatic pressure on the quality of carrot juice. *Int. J. Food Sci. Technol.* **2014**, *49*, 2449–2457.
14. Unni, L.E.; Chauhan, O.P.; Raju, P.S. High pressure processing of garlic paste: Effect on the quality attributes. *Int. J. Food Sci. Technol.* **2014**, *49*, 1579–1585.
15. Lafuente, M.T.; Ballester, A.R.; Calejero, J.; González-Candelas, L. Effect of high-temperature-conditioning treatments on quality, flavonoid composition and vitamin C of cold stored "Fortune" mandarins. *Food Chem.* **2011**, *128*, 1080–1086.
16. Polydera, A.; Stoforos, N.; Taoukis, P. Comparative shelf life study and vitamin C loss kinetics in pasteurised and high pressure processed reconstituted orange juice. *J. Food Eng.* **2003**, *60*, 21–29.
17. Patras, A.; Brunton, N.P.; da Pieve, S.; Butler, F. Impact of high pressure processing on total antioxidant activity, phenolic, ascorbic acid, anthocyanin content and colour of strawberry and blackberry purées. *Innov. Food Sci. Emerg. Technol.* **2009**, *10*, 308–313.
18. Suárez-Jacobo, Á.; Rüfer, C.E.; Gervilla, R.; Guamis, B.; Roig-Sagués, A.X.; Saldo, J. Influence of ultra-high pressure homogenisation on antioxidant capacity, polyphenol and vitamin content of clear apple juice. *Food Chem.* **2011**, *127*, 447–454.
19. Barba, F.; Jäger, H.; Meneses, N.; Esteve, M.; Frígola, A.; Knorr, D. Evaluation of quality changes of blueberry juice during refrigerated storage after high-pressure and pulsed electric fields processing. *Innov. Food Sci. Emerg. Technol.* **2012**, *14*, 18–24.
20. Odriozola-Serrano, I.; Soliva-Fortuny, R.; Martín-Belloso, O. Impact of high-intensity pulsed electric fields variables on vitamin C, anthocyanins and antioxidant capacity of strawberry juice. *LWT-Food Sci. Technol.* **2009**, *42*, 93–100.
21. Odriozola-Serrano, I.; Aguilo-Aguayo, I.; Soliva-Fortuny, R.; Martin-Belloso, O. Pulsed electric fields processing effects on quality and health-related constituents of plant-based foods. *Trends Food Sci. Technol.* **2013**, *29*, 98–107.

22. Meneses, N.; Jaeger, H.; Knorr, D. pH-changes during pulsed electric field treatments—Numerical simulation and in situ impact on polyphenoloxidase inactivation. *Innov. Food Sci. Emerg. Technol.* **2011**, *12*, 499–504.
23. Siemer, C.; Toepfl, S.; Heinz, V. Inactivation of *Bacillus subtilis* spores by pulsed electric fields (PEF) in combination with thermal energy—I. Influence of process- and product parameters. *Food Control* **2014**, *39*, 163–171.
24. Oms-Oliu, G.; Odriozola-Serrano, I.; Soliva-Fortuny, R.; Elez-Martinez, P.; Martin-Belloso, O. Stability of health-related compounds in plant foods through the application of non thermal processes. *Trends Food Sci. Technol.* **2012**, *23*, 111–123.
25. Ade-Omowaye, B.; Taiwo, K.; Eshtiaghi, N.; Angersbach, A.; Knorr, D. Comparative evaluation of the effects of pulsed electric field and freezing on cell membrane permeabilisation and mass transfer during dehydration of red bell peppers. *Innov. Food Sci. Emerg. Technol.* **2003**, *4*, 177–188.
26. Marsellés-Fontanet, Á.R.; Puig-Pujol, A.; Olmos, P.; Mínguez-Sanz, S.; Martín-Belloso, O. A comparison of the effects of pulsed electric field and thermal treatments on grape juice. *Food Bioprocess Technol.* **2013**, *6*, 978–987.
27. Quitão-Teixeira, L.J.; Odriozola-Serrano, I.; Soliva-Fortuny, R.; Mota-Ramos, A.; Martín-Belloso, O. Comparative study on antioxidant properties of carrot juice stabilised by high-intensity pulsed electric fields or heat treatments. *J. Sci. Food Agric.* **2009**, *89*, 2636–2642.
28. Wu, X.; Diao, Y.; Sun, C.; Yang, J.; Wang, Y.; Sun, S. Fluorimetric determination of ascorbic acid with *o*-phenylenediamine. *Talanta* **2003**, *59*, 95–99.
29. Boussetta, N.; Soichi, E.; Lanoisellé, J.-L.; Vorobiev, E. Valorization of oilseed residues: Extraction of polyphenols from flaxseed hulls by pulsed electric fields. *Ind. Crop. Prod.* **2014**, *52*, 347–353.
30. Zhang, S.; Yang, R.; Zhao, W.; Liang, Q.; Zhang, Z. The first ESR observation of radical species generated under pulsed electric fields processing. *LWT-Food Sci. Technol.* **2011**, *44*, 1233–1235.
31. Torregrosa, F.; Esteve, M.J.; Frígola, A.; Cortés, C. Ascorbic acid stability during refrigerated storage of orange-carrot juice treated by high pulsed electric field and comparison with pasteurized juice. *J. Food Eng.* **2006**, *73*, 339–345.
32. Han, Z.; Zeng, X.A.; Fu, N.; Yu, S.J.; Chen, X.D.; Kennedy, J.F. Effects of pulsed electric field treatments on some properties of tapioca starch. *Carbohydr. Polym.* **2012**, *89*, 1012–1017.
33. Liu, Y.Y.; Zeng, X. A.; Deng, Z.; Yu, S.J.; Yamasaki, S. Effect of pulsed electric field on the secondary structure and thermal properties of soy protein isolate. *Eur. Food Res. Technol.* **2011**, *233*, 841–850.
34. Perez, O.E.; Pilosof, A.M. Pulsed electric fields effects on the molecular structure and gelation of β-lactoglobulin concentrate and egg white. *Food Res. Int.* **2004**, *37*, 102–110.
35. Dabbagh, H.A.; Azami, F.; Farrokhpour, H.; Chermahini, A.N. UV-vis, NMR and FT-IR spectra of tautomers of vitamin C. Experimental and DFT calculations. *J. Chil. Chem. Soc.* **2014**, *59*, 2588–2594.
36. Panicker, C.Y.; Varghese, H.T.; Philip, D. FT-IR, FT-Raman and SERS spectra of vitamin C. *Spectrochim. Acta Part A: Mol. Biomol. Spectrosc.* **2006**, *65*, 802–804.
37. Luo, W.B.; Han, Z.; Zeng, X.A.; Yu, S.J.; Kennedy, J.F. Study on the degradation of chitosan by pulsed electric fields treatment. *Innov. Food Sci. Emerg. Technol.* **2010**, *11*, 587–591.

38. Wang, J.; Wang, K.; Wang, Y.; Lin, S.; Zhao, P.; Jones, G. A novel application of pulsed electric field (PEF) processing for improving glutathione (GSH) antioxidant activity. *Food Chem.* **2014**, *161*, 361–366.
39. Plaza, L.; Sánchez-Moreno, C.; Elez-Martínez, P.; de Ancos, B.; Martín-Belloso, O.; Cano, M.P. Effect of refrigerated storage on vitamin C and antioxidant activity of orange juice processed by high-pressure or pulsed electric fields with regard to low pasteurization. *Eur. Food Res. Technol.* **2006**, *223*, 487–493.
40. Yeom, H.W.; Streaker, C.B.; Zhang, Q.H.; Min, D.B. Effects of pulsed electric fields on the quality of orange juice and comparison with heat pasteurization. *J. Agric. Food Chem.* **2000**, *48*, 4597–4605.
41. Elez-Martinez, P.; Martin-Belloso, O. Effects of high intensity pulsed electric field processing conditions on vitamin C and antioxidant capacity of orange juice and gazpacho, a cold vegetable soup. *Food Chem.* **2007**, *102*, 201–209.
42. Lin, S.; Guo, Y.; You, Q.; Yin, Y.; Liu, J. Preparation of antioxidant peptide from egg white protein and improvement of its activities assisted by high-intensity pulsed electric field. *J. Sci. Food Agric.* **2012**, *92*, 1554–1561.
43. Wang, K.; Wang, J.; Zhao, P.; Lin, S.Y.; Liu, B.L.; Liu, J.B.; Jones, G.; Huang, H.C. Optimized PEF treatment for antioxidant polypeptides with MW 10–30 kDa and preliminary analysis of structure change. *Int. J. Biol. Macromol.* **2012**, *51*, 819–825.
44. Lin, S.Y.; Jin, Y.; Liu, M.Y.; Yang, Y.; Zhang, M.S.; Guo, Y.; Jones, G.; Liu, J.B.; Yin, Y.G. Research on the preparation of antioxidant peptides derived from egg white with assisting of high-intensity pulsed electric field. *Food Chem.* **2013**, *139*, 300–306.
45. Sun, J.; Bai, W.; Zhang, Y.; Liao, X.; Hu, X. Effects of electrode materials on the degradation, spectral characteristics, visual colour, and antioxidant capacity of cyanidin-3-glucoside and cyanidin-3-sophoroside during pulsed electric field (PEF) treatment. *Food Chem.* **2011**, *128*, 742–747.
46. Liu, Z.W.; Zeng, X.A.; Sun, D.W.; Han, Z. Effects of pulsed electric fields on the permeabilization of calcein-filled soybean lecithin vesicles. *J. Food Eng.* **2014**, *131*, 26–32.
47. Wang, M.S.; Zeng, X.A.; Sun, D.W.; Han, Z. Quantitative analysis of sublethally injured Saccharomyces cerevisiae cells induced by pulsed electric fields. *LWT-Food Sci. Technol.* **2015**, *60*, 672–677.
48. Klimczak, I.; Gliszczyńska-Świgło, A. Comparison of UPLC and HPLC methods for determination of vitamin C. *Food Chem.* **2015**, *175*, 100–105.
49. Gu, F.; Kim, J.M.; Hayat, K.; Xia, S.; Feng, B.; Zhang, X. Characteristics and antioxidant activity of ultrafiltrated Maillard reaction products from a casein-glucose model system. *Food Chem.* **2009**, *117*, 48–54.
50. Yen, W.J.; Wang, B.S.; Chang, L.W.; Duh, P.D. Antioxidant properties of roasted coffee residues. *J. Agric. Food Chem.* **2005**, *53*, 2658–2663.

3

Increasing Vitamin C Content in Plant Foods to Improve their Nutritional Value—Successes and Challenges

Daniel R. Gallie

Department of Biochemistry, University of California, Riverside, CA 92521-0129, USA;
E-Mail: drgallie@citrus.ucr.edu

Abstract: Vitamin C serves as a cofactor in the synthesis of collagen needed to support cardiovascular function, maintenance of cartilage, bones, and teeth, as well as being required in wound healing. Although vitamin C is essential, humans are one of the few mammalian species unable to synthesize the vitamin and must obtain it through dietary sources. Only low levels of the vitamin are required to prevent scurvy but subclinical vitamin C deficiency can cause less obvious symptoms such as cardiovascular impairment. Up to a third of the adult population in the U.S. obtains less than the recommended amount of vitamin C from dietary sources of which plant-based foods constitute the major source. Consequently, strategies to increase vitamin C content in plants have been developed over the last decade and include increasing its synthesis as well as its recycling, *i.e.*, the reduction of the oxidized form of ascorbic acid that is produced in reactions back into its reduced form. Increasing vitamin C levels in plants, however, is not without consequences. This review provides an overview of the approaches used to increase vitamin C content in plants and the successes achieved. Also discussed are some of the potential limitations of increasing vitamin C and how these may be overcome.

Keywords: L-ascorbic acid; ascorbate; photosynthesis; DHAR; MDAR; reactive oxygen species

---

Abbreviations:

ABA, abscisic acid;
AO, ascorbate oxidase;
APX, ascorbate peroxidase;

Asc, ascorbate;
CaMV, cauliflower mosaic virus;
CAT, catalase;
chl, chlorophyll;
DHA, dehydroascorbate;
DHAR, dehydroascorbate reductase;
ETR, electron transport rate;
Fd, ferredoxin;
GalLDH, L-galactono-1,4-lactone dehydrogenase;
GulLO, L-gulono-1,4-lactone oxidase;
GalUR, D-galacturonic acid reductase;
GR, glutathione reductase;
GSH, glutathione;
GST, glutathione-S-transferase;
MDA, monodehydroascorbate reductase;
MDAR, monodehydroascorbate reductase;
NPQ, non-photochemical quenching;
φPSII, quantum yield of PSII;
qE, energy-dependent NPQ;
qI, photoinhibition;
RbcL, ribulose bisphosphate carboxylase/oxygenase large subunit;
QC, quiescent center;
PSI, photosystem I;
PSII, photosystem II;
ROS, reactive oxygen species;
SOD, superoxide dismutase;
TBARS, thiobarbituric acid reactive substance;
VDE, violaxanthin de-epoxidase

1. Introduction

In addition to its roles in cardiovascular function, immune cell development, and iron utilization, vitamin C (L-ascorbic acid) serves as a water-soluble antioxidant in animals [1–3]. Despite the fact that most mammals can synthesize ascorbic acid (Asc), humans are an exception as a result of a mutation to L-gulono-1,4-lactone oxidase, the last enzyme in the animal Asc biosynthetic pathway [4]. Because Asc is water-soluble, it is not stored and is readily excreted from the body. Therefore, Asc must be obtained regularly from dietary sources. The National Academy of Sciences has recommend 90 mg/day of the vitamin for adult males and 75 mg/day for adult females. Although vitamin C can be obtained from the consumption of fresh meat, it is destroyed by heating and is more typically obtained from plant sources. Asc is present in high amounts generally in fruits and leafy vegetables whereas grains typically have much lower levels of the vitamin, particularly in dried grain. Moreover, the diet of a significant portion of the global population consists largely of plant-based foods. Although post-harvest reductions in Asc can occur, particularly in leafy vegetables, increasing Asc content would help to preserve the nutritional quality of stored foods. As a result, much research has focused on developing strategies to increase vitamin C content in plant foods to improve their nutritional value including strategies to increase the biosynthetic capacity of plants and to increase the recycling of Asc once it has been used in a reaction [5–7].

Figure 1. Plants and animals employ distinct pathways for the synthesis of L-ascorbic acid. The pathway in animals is represented by reactions 1-8 whereas the pathways in plants are represented by reactions 9–24. Enzymes catalyzing the reactions are: 1, phosphoglucomutase; 2, UDP-glucose pyrophosphorylase; 3, UDP-glucose dehydrogenase; 4, glucuronate-1-phosphate uridylyltransferase; 5, glucuronate 1-kinase; 6, glucuronate reductase; 7, aldonolactonase (gluconolactonase); 8, gulono-1,4-lactone oxidase or dehydrogenase; 9, glucose-6-phosphate isomerase; 10, mannose-6-phosphate isomerase; 11, phosphomannose mutase; 12, GDP-mannose pyrophosphorylase (mannose-1-phosphate guanylyltransferase) (*VTC1*); 13, GDP-mannose-3′,5′-epimerase; 14, GDP-L-galactose phosphorylase (*VTC2* and *VTC5*); 15, L-galactose-1-phosphate phosphatase (*VTC4*); 16, L-galactose dehydrogenase; 17, L-galactono-1,4-lactone dehydrogenase; 18, methylesterase; 19, D-galacturonate reductase; 20, aldonolactonase; 21, phosphodiesterase; 22, sugar phosphatase; 23, L-gulose dehydrogenase; 24, *myo*-inositol oxygenase.

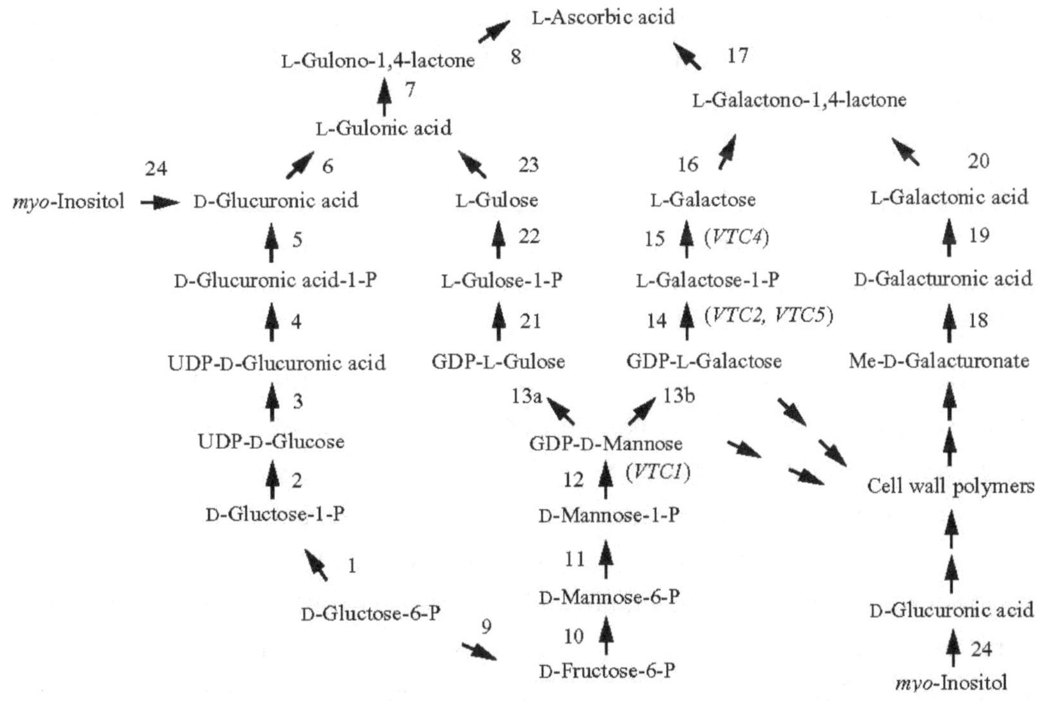

2. Increasing Vitamin C Content through Improved Biosynthesis

The pathway of vitamin C synthesis in mammals begins with D-glucose and proceeds through D-glucose-1-P, UDP-glucose, UDP-D-glucuronic acid, UDP-D-glucuronic acid-1-P, D-glucuronic acid, L-gulonic acid, and finally gulono-1,4-lactone (Figure 1). Gulono-1,4-lactone oxidase then converts gulono-1,4-lactone into 2-keto-gulono-γ-lactone which spontaneously converts to L-ascorbic acid [8].

In contrast to this single pathway, there are at least four biosynthetic pathways suggested to date in plants. The first discovered was the Smirnoff-Wheeler pathway in which Asc synthesis originates with L-galactose [9] (Figure 1). L-Galactose is produced from mannose-1-phosphate through the intermediates guanosine diphosphate (GDP)-mannose and GDP-L-galactose [10]. L-Galactose then undergoes oxidation to L-galactono-1,4-lactone catalyzed by the NAD-dependent L-galactose dehydrogenase followed by oxidation to L-ascorbic acid by the mitochondrial-localized L-galactono-1,4-lactone dehydrogenase [11,12].

Feeding experiments provided support for the Smirnoff-Wheeler pathway. For example, feeding leaf tissue with the Asc precursors L-galactose or L-galactono-1,4-lactone resulted in their conversion to Asc and therefore increased Asc content [9,13,14]. In another study, exogenous application of L-galactono-1,4-lactone to *Arabidopsis* or *Medicago sativa* leaves increased foliar Asc content up to 8-fold and was proportional to the amount applied [15]. Application of L-galactono-1,4-lactone or L-galactose to source potato leaves also increased the Asc content of these leaves as well as in sink organs, e.g., flowers and developing tubers [16].

Arabidopsis mutants affected at different steps in the Smirnoff-Wheeler pathway resulted in substantial reductions in Asc content, supporting the conclusion that this pathway is responsible for much of the Asc biosynthetic capacity in this species. For example, the *vtc1* mutant lacks GDP-mannose pyrophosphorylase expression whereas the *vtc2* and *vtc5* mutants lack GDP-L-galactose phosphorylase expression. The *vtc1* mutant exhibits a 70%–75% reduction in Asc content while the *vtc2* mutant contains just 10%–20% of the wild-type level of Asc, *vtc5* contains 80% of the wild-type level, and the *vtc2*/*vtc5* double mutant bleaches in the absence of exogenous Asc or L-galactose which overcomes the block in the pathway [13,17,18]. The *vtc4* mutant results from a mutation in L-galactose-1-P phosphatase [19,20].

Attempts to increase Asc content through increasing its biosynthesis have achieved some success. Overexpression of GDP-L-galactose phosphorylase from kiwifruit (*Actinidia chinensis*) increased Asc content in tobacco leaves by more than 3-fold with an accompanying 50-fold increase in enzyme activity [21]. Although the agroinfection approach employed resulted in only a transient increase in enzyme expression, up to a 4-fold increase in Asc content was observed in stably-transformed *Arabidopsis* where the enzyme was overexpressed [21,22]. Stable transformation of GDP-L-galactose phosphorylase into potato, tomato, and strawberry resulted in up to a 3, 6, and 2-fold increase in Asc, respectively, in tubers and fruits, although some loss of seed and the jelly of locular tissue surrounding the seed were observed in tomato and an increase in polyphenolic content was observed in strawberry and tomato [23]. A combinatorial approach in which kiwifruit GDP-L-galactose phosphorylase and GDP-mannose-3′,5′-epimerase were transiently overexpressed in agroinfected tobacco leaves increased Asc content up to 7-fold [22]. Overexpression of L-galactose dehydrogenase, which catalyzes the conversion of L-galactose to L-galactono-1,4-lactone (Figure 1), however, failed to increase foliar Asc content in tobacco despite a 3.5-fold increase in the activity of the enzyme [24], suggesting that the endogenous level of L-galactose dehydrogenase is not rate-limiting. Transformation of *Arabidopsis with* GDP-galactose guanylyltransferase resulted in a 2.9-fold increase in Asc and co-transformation with either L-galactose-1-phosphate phosphatase or L-galactono-1,4-lactone dehydrogenase increased Asc content up to 4.1-fold [25]. Overexpressing multiple enzymes within the Smirnoff–Wheeler pathway, particularly those whose endogenous level is closest to being rate-limiting, may offer more promise to achieving substantial increases in Asc rather than the overexpression of any one enzyme. The choice of which enzymes to overexpress may be species-dependent as the level of expression for each enzyme in the pathway may differ among species.

Evidence for other biosynthetic pathways has suggested three alternative routes for the synthesis of Asc. In the first of these alternative pathways, D-galacturonic acid, generated from the breakdown of pectin during fruit ripening, serves as the starting point for Asc synthesis and is reduced to L-galactonic acid as catalyzed by the NADPH-dependent D-galacturonic acid reductase (GalUR) [26] (Figure 1). L-Galactonic acid spontaneously converts to L-galactono-1,4 lactone which L-galactono-1,4-lactone dehydrogenase converts to Asc [26]. Early support for this pathway came from the observation that D-galacturonic acid-1-^{14}C was metabolized to L-ascorbic acid-6-^{14}C through an inversion pathway in detached ripening strawberry fruit [27]. Supplying a methyl ester of D-galacturonic acid to cress seedlings and *Arabidopsis* cell cultures also increased Asc [28,29], suggesting that GalUR expression was not confined to fruits. Expression of the GalUR gene from strawberry increased whole-plant Asc content 2- to 3-fold in *Arabidopsis* [30], supporting the existence of this pathway. Demonstration that GalUR can increase foliar Asc biosynthesis through D-galactonic acid and D-galacturonic acid suggests that the substrates for this pathway are present in leaves. The potential for manipulating this pathway to achieve increased Asc content will depend on whether the enzymes of the pathway are expressed and whether D-galacturonic acid is present, e.g., following pectin degradation.

An example of the contingent basis of this pathway was observed in developing tomato fruit. Feeding tomato plants with D-galacturonate failed to increase Asc content in immature green tomato fruit while feeding with L-galactose, representing the D-mannose/L-galactose (or Smirnoff–Wheeler) pathway, did increase Asc content [31]. In contrast, feeding of either precursor increased Asc content of red ripened fruits, correlating with the increase in activity of D-galacturonate reductase and aldonolactonase, the last two enzymes of the D-galacturonate pathway in ripe fruits [31]. These observations suggest that the D-galacturonate pathway is not operative prior to ripening during which pectin is degraded. Thus, the contribution that the D-galacturonate pathway makes to Asc biosynthesis in tomato fruit may be limited to the ripening stage while the Smirnoff-Wheeler pathway is operative throughout fruit development (e.g., [23]). In addition, tracer studies have suggested that the D-galacturonate pathway may contribute only moderately to fruit Asc content [32] while its contribution in other organs has not been examined. In the second alternative pathway, GDP-mannose 3′,5′-epimerase, which catalyzes conversion of GDP-D-mannose to GDP-L-galactose in the L-galactose pathway [10], also catalyzes the 5′-epimerization of GDP-D-mannose to produce GDP-L-gulose [33] (Figure 1). Conversion of GDP-L-gulose to L-gulonic acid allows Asc synthesis essentially as described in the animal pathway although evidence for this is still lacking. The presence of L-gulonic acid and L-gulono-1,4-lactone dehydrogenase activity [33,34] supports the existence of this pathway in plants. The expression of L-gulono-1,4-lactone oxidase (GulLO) from rat in lettuce and tobacco increased Asc content up to 7-fold [35] and reversed the reduction in Asc content in *Arabidopsis* mutants affected in the Smirnoff–Wheeler pathway [36] although it is not known whether L-gulono-1,4-lactone or L-galactono-1,4-lactone served as the substrate as the possibility that L-galactono-1,4-lactone served as the substrate was not examined. Although feeding with L-gulono-1,4-lactone did not increase the Asc content of tomato fruit at any developmental stage [31], its conversion to Asc has been reported for several plant species [28,37,38], supporting the presence of this pathway in plants. Expression of a foreign gene, however, can result in the ectopic expression of a pathway or the introduction of a novel pathway. Therefore, the degree to which this pathway functions in plants remains to be determined. Demonstrating that a labeled precursor directly labels Asc or that mutating a specific enzyme decreases Asc would provide more compelling evidence for such pathways.

The third alternative pathway involves D-glucuronic acid, an intermediate of the animal pathway which in plants can be generated by *myo*-inositol oxygenase (Figure 1). Support for this pathway in plants comes from the observation that overexpressing an *Arabidopsis* gene having homology to a porcine *myo*-inositol oxygenase increased Asc content [39]. As *myo*-inositol does not function as a precursor of Asc in strawberry fruit or in parsley leaves [32], this raises the question of the extent to which this pathway contributes to Asc content in plants. Nevertheless, the ability to increase Asc through the overexpression of this putative *myo*-inositol oxygenase gene may provide another strategy for increasing Asc biosynthesis.

Although multiple Asc biosynthetic pathways may exist in plants, the observation that mutants affected in the Smirnoff–Wheeler pathway result in substantial reductions in Asc content does indicate that the alternative pathways are unable to compensate for the loss in Asc biosynthetic capacity in Smirnoff–Wheeler pathway mutants. Thus, these alternative pathways may make only minor contributions to Asc biosynthesis and strategies focusing on these other pathways may be limited to increasing Asc in specific organs or at specific developmental stages.

3. Increasing Vitamin C Content through Improved Asc Recycling

3.1. Targeting MDAR Expression to Increase Ascorbic Acid

Once used in enzymatic or non-enzymatic reactions, Asc is oxidized to monodehydroascorbate (MDHA). Asc can be regenerated from MDHA through reduction by several means. If MDHA is produced in the chloroplast stroma, it can be recycled to Asc by ferredoxin (Fd), which is part of the photosynthetic electron transport chain, or by monodehydroascorbate reductase (MDAR) in the stroma [40]. Other MDAR isoforms are present in the cytosol, peroxisome, and mitochondria which reduce MDHA produced in those compartments. As no MDAR isoform is in the thylakoid lumen, MDHA cannot be reduced by MDAR or by Fd, which lies on the stromal side of the thylakoid membrane. As a result, this short-lived radical spontaneously disproportionates rapidly to Asc and DHA, particularly when the pH of the thylakoid lumen is low which occurs during the light driven transport of protons across the thylakoid membrane from the stroma into the lumen [40,41]. Under these conditions, the high pH of the stroma slows the disproportionation of MDHA and it undergoes reduction primarily through Fd or MDAR. Once photoreduced by PsaC in the PSI complex, Fd reduces MDHA directly or alternatively reduces $NADP^+$ to NADPH as catalyzed by Fd-$NADP^+$

reductase (FNR) which MDAR uses (or NADH instead of NADPH) to reduce MDHA to Asc [42,43]. Fd reduces MDHA at a rate that is 34-fold greater than the rate of photoreduction of $NADP^+$ so that MDHA is likely reduced through Fd as part of the thylakoid scavenging system rather than by stromal MDAR when it is produced proximal to the thylakoid membrane [42]. MDAR, however, is available to reduce any stromal MDHA produced distal to the thylakoid membrane as part of the stromal scavenging system.

The multiple isoforms of MDAR are encoded by a five member nuclear gene family in *Arabidopsis* (referred to as *AtMDAR1* through *AtMDAR5*) that are targeted to the cytosol, chloroplast, mitochondria, and peroxisomes [44]. Dual targeting of MDAR to chloroplasts and mitochondria results from the use of at least two transcription start sites which produce a seven amino acid extension in the mitochondrial-targeted form of the protein [45]. The 47-kDa AtMDAR1 and 54-kDa AtMDAR4 isoforms contain a *C*-terminal sequence that targets them to the peroxisomal matrix (PTS1) and peroxisomal membrane, respectively [46]. MDAR isoforms targeted to peroxisomes, chloroplasts, or mitochondria typically function together with ascorbate peroxidase (APX) to scavenge H_2O_2 [47] through the transfer of electrons from two molecules of Asc to H_2O_2 to form water and two molecules of MDHA. Disproportionation of H_2O_2 is also catalyzed by catalase (CAT) when present, e.g., in the peroxisome.

Increasing Asc content by targeting MDAR expression has achieved only limited success. Expression of a cytosolic tomato MDAR from a constitutive promoter in tomato (var. Micro-Tom) resulted in a reduction in Asc in mature green tomato fruits but unaltered foliar Asc content [48] although it may improve the chilling tolerance of fruit [49]. Improved tolerance against salt and osmotic stresses was also observed following an increase in MDAR expression in tobacco [50]. Increasing expression of a tomato chloroplast-targeted MDAR in tomato increased Asc marginally (1.2-fold) but was accompanied by a decrease in DHA, resulting in an approximate doubling of the Asc redox state [51]. Similar results were obtained following the expression of an *Arabidopsis* cytosolic MDAR in tobacco [52]. The little work that has been reported to date suggests that increasing MDAR expression may achieve only minor increases in Asc content.

3.2. Targeting DHAR Expression to Increase Ascorbic Acid

If MDHA is not enzymatically reduced by Fd or MDAR, it will undergo spontaneous disproportionation to Asc and DHA, the rate of which is dependent on the pH, such as in the thylakoid lumen where Fd and MDAR are absent and the pH is low during light exposure. Disproportionation of MDHA can also occur in other cellular compartments if not enzymatically reduced. The DHA produced can be reduced to Asc by dehydroascorbate reductase (DHAR) using glutathione (GSH) as the reductant [53,54] (Figure 2). If it is not rapidly reduced, DHA undergoes irreversible hydrolysis to 2,3-diketogulonic acid and, as this is unable to be converted to Asc, it is lost to the Asc pool. Increasing the level of DHAR activity, therefore, limits DHA degradation by improving its recycling back into Asc before it is lost. As DHAR activity determines the relative levels of DHA and Asc and the enzyme is expressed in rate-limiting amounts in plants, it serves as a major regulator of the Asc redox state [5,55–57].

Figure 2. L-Ascorbic acid recycling through DHAR and MDAR. Following Asc synthesis from L-galactono-1,4-lactone by L-galactono-1,4-lactone dehydrogenase (GLDH) and oxidization to monodehydroascorbate (MDHA), monodehydroascorbate reductase (MDAR) can reduce MDHA to Asc. Alternatively, two MDHA molecules can disproportionate non-enzymatically to Asc and dehydroascorbate (DHA). Dehydroascorbate reductase (DHAR) can reduce DHA to Asc using glutathione (GSH) as the reductant. Oxidized glutathione (GSSG) is reduced by glutathione reductase (GR) to GSH using NADPH as the reductant. DHA will spontaneously hydrolyze to 2,3-diketogulonic acid if not reduced by DHAR.

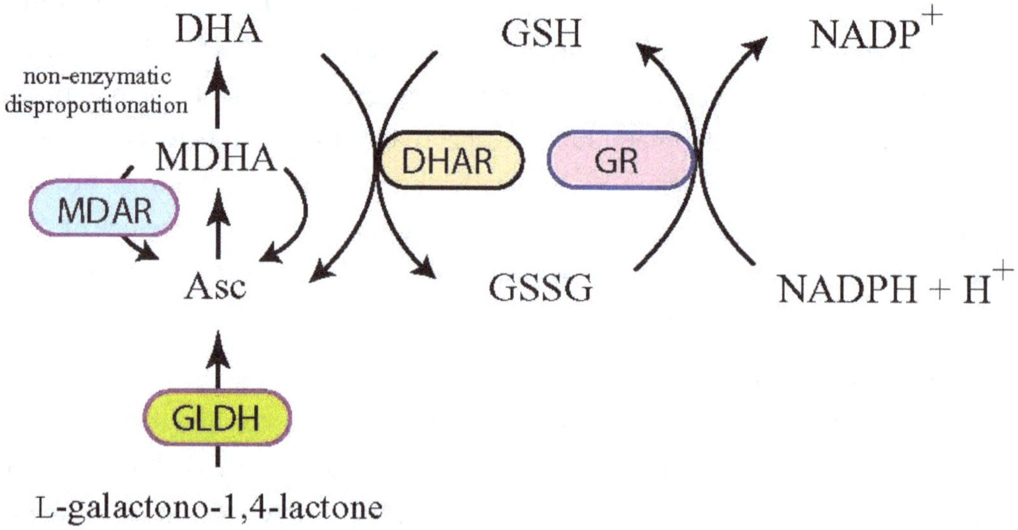

DHAR is encoded by three gene members in *Arabidopsis*: (*AtDHAR1*; At5g16710), (*AtDHAR3*; At1g75270), and (*AtDHAR5*; At1g19570) [44]. Microarray expression analysis suggests another gene, At5g36270 (*AtDHAR2*), is likely a pseudogene as it may not be expressed [44]. A fifth gene, At1g19550 (*AtDHAR4*), is smaller than other DHAR paralogs due to multiple deletions throughout the polypeptide. AtDHAR3 is likely cytoplasmic while AtDHAR5 and AtDHAR1 are targeted to the mitochondria and chloroplast, respectively [58]. No DHAR isoform is transported to the apoplast. Consequently, any Asc transported to the apoplast is quickly oxidized, disproportionates, and the resulting DHA is either degraded or transported to the cytoplasm for recycling into Asc.

Because DHAR is a major recycler of Asc, a number of studies have focused on increasing the expression of this enzyme as a means to increase Asc content in plants, which has achieved success in several species. Although ectopic expression of a human DHAR in tobacco chloroplasts failed to increase Asc despite a 2-fold increase in DHAR activity [59,60], expression of a cytosolic wheat DHAR in tobacco did increase Asc content up to 4-fold as well as the redox state (*i.e.*, an increase in the Asc to DHA ratio) with a simultaneous increase in Asc and a decrease in DHA [5]. Similar results were obtained when this cytosolic wheat DHAR was expressed in leaves and developing kernels of maize [5], demonstrating that changes in Asc can be made in photosynthetic and non-photosynthetic organs. Because Asc is transported from the cytoplasm to the apoplast and apoplastic DHA is transported back to the cytoplasm, expression of the cytosolic wheat DHAR not only increased the Asc content of the cytosol but the apoplast as well when measured from the apoplastic fluid [55], demonstrating that cytosolic DHAR regulates the symplastic and apoplastic Asc pool size and redox state. No change in Asc biosynthesis was observed following the increase in DHAR expression indicating that the synthesis of Asc and its recycling are independently controlled. The increase in DHAR expression and Asc recycling was accompanied by an increase in the GSH pool size and redox state [5]. As GSH is used by DHAR as the reductant, this suggests that the GSH pool size is affected by changes in DHAR activity. The extent to which the increase in GSH contributed to any physiological changes in these plants was not examined.

As the Asc pool size is determined by the rate of its synthesis and decay, the ability of DHAR to increase Asc content is a consequence of its recycling function that reduces DHA before it is lost through decay. As increasing DHAR expression results in improved Asc recycling and higher Asc levels, the endogenous level of DHAR is likely rate-limiting. Whether this is generally true throughout plant species is unknown. Consequently, the potential to increase Asc through increased DHAR expression will be greatest for species in which DHAR expression is rate-limiting. The strategy of increasing Asc content through increased DHAR expression, however, has been validated by subsequent studies that increased DHAR expression in the cytosol or in the chloroplast of a variety of species. Two studies that expressed a cytosolic DHAR from *Arabidopsis* in tobacco reported increases in Asc content by nearly 2-fold [52,61] whereas expression of an *Arabidopsis* cytosolic DHAR in *Arabidopsis* increased foliar Asc by 2 to 4.25-fold [62]. Expression of a rice cytosolic DHAR in *Arabidopsis* resulted in a slight increase in Asc content [63] as did expression of a rice DHAR in transformed tobacco chloroplasts [64]. Further increases in Asc content were observed when chloroplasts were transformed with glutathione reductase (GR) and DHAR [64].

Grains represent the most important food group supporting the global population either directly or indirectly as use in animal feed. Improving the nutritional value of grains offers the greatest potential for improving the diet of many and recent research has focused on engineering increasing multiple vitamins and micronutrients in grains as an efficient delivery mechanism for those whose diets are deficient in several vitamins. Although Asc content in grains is typically low, it is present during grain development but undergoes progressive oxidation during late development and is largely present as DHA by maturity [65]. The relationship between increased DHAR expression and increased Asc content in cereals was first shown in developing maize grain [5]. This was followed by a combinatorial approach to increase the levels of Asc, folate and β-carotene in maize grain using a barley D-hordein promoter to drive expression of a rice DHAR and an *E. coli* GTP cyclohydrolase (*folE*) to increase the level of Asc and folate, respectively, and a wheat LMW glutenin promoter to drive expression of maize phytoene synthase (*psy1*) and the D-hordein promoter to drive expression of *Pantoea ananatis* carotene desaturase (*crtI*) in order to increase β-carotene content [7]. These transgenes resulted in a 6-fold increase in Asc, a 2-fold increase in folate, and a 169-fold increase in β-carotene [7], demonstrating that an increase in Asc content can be combined with increases in the level of other vitamins to improve substantially the nutritional value of a fundamentally important staple. Increasing Asc content in other important, non-grain foods has been reported. Expression of a potato cytosolic DHAR from the CaMV 35S promoter increased foliar Asc content by more than 1.6-fold and in tubers by more than 1.2-fold which correlated with its expression where it is expressed higher in tubers than in leaves [66]. Expression of a chloroplast-localized potato DHAR increased foliar Asc content up to 1.5-fold but not in tubers which also correlated with its expression in leaves but a lack of expression in tubers [66]. Therefore, the strategy of increasing Asc content through increased Asc recycling through chloroplast-targeting of DHAR expression is likely to be limited to photosynthetically active tissues whereas increasing Asc content in non-photosynthetic organs will likely require expression of a cytosolic isoform of DHAR. Supporting this conclusion were results from the expression of a sesame DHAR under the control of a patatin promoter in potato. Just as the patatin promoter is active in tubers but not in leaves, expression of the sesame DHAR increased Asc 1.1 to 1.3-fold in tubers but no increase was observed in leaves. In contrast, expression of sesame DHAR under the constitutively active CaMV 35S promoter increased Asc content in leaves by 1.5-fold and 1.6-fold in tubers [67]. Overexpressing a cytosolic tomato DHAR from a constitutive promoter in tomato (var. Micro-Tom) increased Asc content in mature green and red ripe fruit by 1.6-fold in plants grown under low light [48]. In this example, however, no increase in foliar Asc was observed. The increase in Asc and GSH observed during the initial phases of embryogeny in Norway spruce following overexpression of the class I homeobox of knox 3 gene, HBK3, was attributed to increased activities of DHAR, GR, and ascorbate free radical reductase [68], suggesting that DHAR may also contribute to regulating Asc content in gymnosperm species.

4. Consequences of Increasing Asc Content in Plants

4.1. Effects on Other Antioxidants and ROS-Detoxifying Enzymes

As a major antioxidant in plants, changes in Asc content may well affect other antioxidant pools. Moreover, different approaches used for increasing Asc might be expected to affect specific antioxidants disproportionately. For example, increasing Asc by increasing biosynthetic activity would impact different antioxidant pools than would increasing Asc through improved Asc recycling which requires GSH and NADPH (or NADH) for the reduction of DHA or MDHA by DHAR or MDAR, respectively. Although most reports have observed increases in Asc content and/or in the Asc redox state following an increase in DHAR expression, the impact of this increase of DHAR activity on other antioxidants is less clear. Increases in GSH were observed in tobacco and maize expressing wheat DHAR with no change in glutathione reductase (GR), superoxide dismutase (SOD), APX, or CAT activities [5], suggesting coordinate regulation between DHAR and GSH. A similar increase in GSH content was reported for *Arabidopsis* overexpressing DHAR [62]. In contrast, expression of human DHAR in tobacco chloroplasts resulted in a reduction in GSH that was accompanied by a 1.43-fold increase in GR activity [59]. Whether this was a consequence of expression of DHAR in chloroplasts remains to be determined.

4.2. Increasing Ascorbic Acid Improves Tolerance to Many Environmental Stresses

Although oxygen is essential to plants, it can be highly damaging, particularly as singlet oxygen ($^1O_2$) or in its reactive forms such as the superoxide anion ($O_2^{\bullet-}$), hydroxyl radical ($^{\bullet}OH$), or hydrogen peroxide (H_2O_2). ROS are detoxified through the action of antioxidants such as Asc and GSH either directly or in reactions catalyzed by SOD, APX, and CAT [69,70]. Under conditions of excess light, $O_2^{\bullet-}$ is produced during photosynthesis and is converted by SOD to H_2O_2 which is reduced to H_2O by APX as one means to maintain electron flow through the photosystems [71]. Abiotic stresses such as cold, drought, or high light increase ROS production by creating conditions of light stress at lower light levels. H_2O_2 rapidly inactivates APX if Asc is limiting [72] and inhibits CO_2 assimilation by inhibiting several Calvin cycle enzymes [40]. ROS can invade a plant in the form of environmental pollutants, e.g., ozone [73,74], which damages cell membranes or induces programmed cell death [75–77]. As a defense mechanism, H_2O_2 produced from ozone functions as a signaling intermediate in guard cells to promote stomatal closure thus limiting ozone entry into the leaf interior [78,79].

As an antioxidant, Asc would be expected to affect tolerance to environmental stress. This was first demonstrated using *vtc* mutants of *Arabidopsis* in which their reduced Asc content correlated with a reduction in tolerance to environmental ROS. With 70%–75% less Asc, the *vtc1* mutant is hypersensitive to ozone and sulfur dioxide [13,19,80] and contains a higher oxidative load relative to wild-type plants when exposed to stress conditions such as salt despite its increased GSH content [81]. The expression level of regulators of Asc biosynthesis can also affect the degree of ozone tolerance. Knockout mutants of AMR1 (for ascorbic acid mannose pathway regulator 1) resulted in up to 3-fold greater foliar Asc content in *Arabidopsis* and increased ozone tolerance [82]. In contrast, plants with increased expression of AMR1 through activation-tagging exhibited a 60% reduction in Asc and greater ozone sensitivity [82]. As AMR1 coordinately regulates transcript expression of six Smirnoff–Wheeler pathway enzyme genes to negatively regulate Asc biosynthesis, targeting regulators of biosynthetic pathways offers yet another promising approach to alter Asc content. In a second study, overexpression of the *Arabidopsis* ethylene response factor gene AtERF98 increased Asc content up to approximately 1.6-fold which was attributed primarily to an increase in the expression of genes in the Smirnoff–Wheeler pathway [83]. As AtERF98 binds to the promoter of *VTC1*, AtERF98 likely functions as a transcriptional activator of one or more genes in the Smirnoff–Wheeler pathway [83]. Increasing AtERF98 expression resulted in enhanced salt tolerance, demonstrating that increasing Asc biosynthesis improves tolerance to this abiotic stress [83].

That the endogenous level of apoplastic Asc is important in detoxifying ozone was shown in tobacco in which the level of apoplastic Asc was specifically altered [84]. Overexpressing an apoplastic-localized cucumber ascorbate oxidase (AO), which oxidizes apoplastic Asc, increased the ozone sensitivity of transgenic tobacco, correlating with the conversion of virtually all apoplastic Asc to DHA and depriving the apoplast of its ability to detoxify ozone entering the leaf interior [84]. A decrease in the cytosolic Asc redox state was also observed which would compromise the ability of a cell to detoxify ozone entering the cytosol.

Increased sensitivity to ozone following a reduction in Asc recycling was observed following loss of cytosolic DHAR expression in the *Arabidopsis AtDHAR3* mutant [58]. The lower redox state but not pool size of Asc in this mutant indicates that Asc recycling is important in preventing oxidative damage. Consistent with its role in ozone tolerance, *AtDHAR3* expression is induced by ozone [58].

If decreasing Asc content reduces tolerance to environmental ROS, increasing Asc content would be predicted to have the opposite effect, a notion supported by several studies published to date. Increasing Asc content in tobacco by increasing DHAR expression increased the Asc content of the apoplast and symplast and thus increased tolerance to ozone by reducing the oxidative load of the plant (*i.e.*, a lower level of foliar and apoplastic H_2O_2) which was accompanied by a lower induction of antioxidant-related enzyme activities, more chlorophyll, and a higher level of photosynthetic activity following ozone exposure [56]. This increase in tolerance occurred despite the guard cells being less responsive to ozone as a consequence of their higher Asc content which reduces H_2O_2 levels [73,85]. Thus, increasing Asc content throughout a plant reduces guard cell responsiveness which permits more ozone to enter the leaf interior. The increased ozone tolerance can be understood, however, by the increased ability of every cell to detoxify ozone invading the leaf interior. Consistent with these findings, increasing Asc content 2-fold in tobacco through the expression of a cytosolic *Arabidopsis* DHAR enhanced its tolerance to ozone as well as drought, salt, or polyethylene glycol [61].

Conversely, a reduction in Asc recycling through the suppression of DHAR expression increased the responsiveness of guard cells to ozone thereby limiting ozone diffusion into the leaf interior [56]. At the same time, however, the decrease in DHAR activity lowered the Asc content of leaf cells and thus reduced their ability to detoxify any ozone that did invade [56]. Thus, increasing Asc content provides greater protection against environmental oxidative damage without compromising photosynthetic activity than does increasing guard cell responsiveness through decreasing Asc which reduces ozone entry but also reduces photosynthetic activity.

In addition to ozone, increasing Asc content provides greater tolerance to other environmental stresses. *Arabidopsis* with increased Asc content and redox state resulting from an increase in DHAR expression retained more Asc and chlorophyll with less membrane damage following exposure to high light and temperature or following treatment with paraquat [62]. *Arabidopsis* expressing a rice DHAR had greater tolerance to salt stress despite the small increases in DHAR activity and Asc achieved although no difference in cold tolerance was observed [63]. Although tobacco expressing a chloroplast-targeted human DHAR failed to increase Asc, it did increase the Asc redox state and the plants experienced less membrane damage following exposure to methyl viologen or H_2O_2 and had improved tolerance to low temperature and salt [60]. Combining expression of a chloroplast-localized DHAR with the expression of a chloroplast-localized CuZnSOD and APX increased the Asc and GSH redox states and the plants exhibited greater tolerance to paraquat and salt [86]. Greater tolerance to salt and cold was also observed in tobacco following the simultaneous expression of two pairs of chloroplast-localized enzymes, *i.e.*, an *E. coli* GR with either an *E. coli* glutathione-S-transferase (GST) or a rice DHAR, that increased Asc and GSH content and their redox states [64].

Because fewer studies on increasing Asc through MDAR expression have been reported and those that have been carried out have observed smaller increases in Asc content, much less is known about the effects of MDAR-mediated increases in Asc on plant growth and plant responses. However, the results to date suggest that increasing Asc through MDAR expression has similar effects to those following an increase in DHAR expression. The slight increase in Asc content and decrease in DHA content that resulted in an approximate doubling of the Asc redox state in tomato seedlings overexpressing a chloroplast-targeted tomato MDAR resulted in a reduced oxidative load (as measured by H_2O_2), lower thiobarbituric acid reactive substance (TBARS) content (a measure of membrane damage), a higher net photosynthetic rate, higher maximal photochemical efficiency of PSII and greater fresh weight when subjected to low or high temperature stress [51]. Reducing Asc and its redox state through the suppression of MDAR expression resulted in largely opposite phenotypes [51]. In agreement with these results, greater tolerance to ozone, reduced H_2O_2 levels, and increased photosynthetic activity were observed in tobacco expressing an *Arabidopsis* MDAR following salt stress [50].

ROS can also be generated during development. For example, H_2O_2 is produced in the peroxisome of oilseeds as a by-product of fatty acid β-oxidation during lipid catabolism that accompanies seedling growth [87,88]. Catalase in the peroxisomal matrix detoxifies H_2O_2 and a membrane-bound APX3 and MDAR4, encoded by *SUGAR-DEPENDENT2* (*SDP2*), together detoxify H_2O_2 using Asc [87,89–91]. Loss of MDAR4 expression in the *Arabidopsis sdp2* mutant is conditionally seedling-lethal as MDAR activity is needed to reduce leakage of H_2O_2 from peroxisomes that protects *SDP1*-encoded triacylglycerol (TAG) lipase activity and storage oil hydrolysis in the closely associated oil bodies during seedling growth [92]. Loss of MDAR4 activity results in inactivation of TAG lipase by H_2O_2 and a reduced ability to catabolize storage oil needed to support seedling growth [92]. Whether increasing Asc through increasing MDAR4 expression might improve seedling growth has not been examined. However, increasing APX3 expression increases tolerance against oxidative stress [93], suggesting an increase in Asc and the peroxisomal-associated APX3 and MDAR4 that use and recycle Asc may improve seedling tolerance against oxidative stress.

4.3. Increasing Ascorbic Acid Improves Tolerance to High Light

As mentioned above, in addition to environmental sources, ROS is generated during exposure to high light. Excess light energy can generate triplet state chlorophyll (^{3}Chl) which transfers its energy to ground-state O_2 to produce $^1O_2$. Photosystem over reduction also produces ROS such as $O_2^{\bullet-}$ and H_2O_2 [94] which can damage proteins, membranes, and pigments of photosystem I (PSI) and photosystem II (PSII), resulting in the inactivation of reaction centers as well as compromise their repair [95,96]. An increase in DHAR expression in tobacco resulted in less photoinhibition following exposure to high light that was likely due to an increase in the foliar levels of xanthophyll pigments and chlorophyll as well as in the electron transport rate (ETR) and CO_2 assimilation, particularly at high light intensities, while ROS were reduced [97]. Thus, an increase in Asc maintains photosynthetic functioning by limiting ROS-mediated damage. Conversely, reducing Asc through suppression of DHAR results in elevated ROS and photoinhibition that is accompanied by reductions in the quantum yield of PSII and ETR [97].

4.4. Increasing Ascorbic Acid Decreases Tolerance to Drought Stress

While ROS are generally detrimental they also serve as important signaling cues about the external environment, e.g., the role of H_2O_2 in guard cells in regulating gas exchange and transpiration in response to water availability [98]. Abscisic acid (ABA) can promote H_2O_2 production during periods of water limitation which signals for stomatal closure [99]. Although tobacco overexpressing DHAR grew normally under well-watered conditions, the higher Asc content in guard cells not only reduced their responsiveness to ozone but also their responsiveness to the onset of water stress which normally triggers stomatal closure to prevent further water loss [55]. The reduction in responsiveness can be understood through the role of Asc as a scavenger of H_2O_2 and the balance between H_2O_2 production and Asc establishes whether H_2O_2 rises to a level that triggers stomatal closure. As a consequence, increasing Asc in DHAR-overexpressing tobacco maintains H_2O_2 at a lower level which delays stomatal closure upon onset of water stress, resulting in greater open stomatal area, increased transpiration and water loss, and ultimately decreased tolerance to water stress [55]. Reducing Asc content through suppressing DHAR expression results in an elevated accumulation of H_2O_2 in guard cells and a greater degree of stomatal closure even under non-stress conditions [55]. This hyperresponsiveness enables such plants to reduce transpiration during drought conditions resulting in up to 30% less water loss [55]. Thus, increasing Asc content throughout a plant confers protection against environmental ROS while reducing drought tolerance whereas reducing Asc content reduces CO_2 assimilation under normal growth conditions as a consequence of the reduction in the open stomatal area but also reduces water loss resulting in improved drought tolerance. A strategy to increase foliar Asc content while maintaining normal levels of Asc in guard cells may improve nutritional value and tolerance to environmental ROS without increasing sensitivity to drought conditions.

4.5. Increasing Ascorbic Acid Prolongs Leaf Function

Increasing Asc through increasing DHAR expression resulted in higher levels of ribulose bisphosphate carboxylase/oxygenase large subunit (RbcL), chlorophyll, and CO_2 assimilation but this had no effect on plant growth under normal conditions [57]. In contrast, reducing Asc content through reduced biosynthesis resulted in slower shoot growth, smaller leaves, and reduced shoot fresh weight and dry weight [80] while plants with lower Asc content following suppression of DHAR expression exhibited a slower rate of leaf expansion, slower shoot growth, delayed flowering time, and reduced foliar dry weight [57]. These phenotypes correlated with reduced leaf function as measured by a disproportionate loss in chlorophyll a, a reduction in RbcL, and a lower rate of CO_2 assimilation [57]. The lower rate of CO_2 assimilation was not due to a limitation in CO_2 diffusion into DHAR-suppressed leaves as the sub-stomatal CO_2 concentration was actually higher [57]. Rather, the reduced growth likely resulted from a premature loss of leaf function and early onset of senescence in mature leaves that may have reduced photosynthate available to young leaves.

4.6. Increasing Ascorbic Acid Can Alter Pathogen Defense Responses

The role of Asc in pathogen defense has received only limited attention. In an early study, the reduced Asc content of *Arabidopsis vtc1* or *vtc2* mutants resulted in reduced growth of the bacterial pathogen *Pseudomonas syringae* pv *maculicola* ES4326 and hyphal growth of the fungal pathogen *Peronospora parasitica* pv *Noco* [100]. The reduction in growth of *P. syringae* in *vtc1* plants correlated with a greater induction of the pathogenesis-related proteins PR-1 and PR-5, increased expression from some senescence-associated gene (SAG) genes and higher levels of salicylic acid. The reduced Asc content in these mutants resulted in the premature senescence of uninfected plants with an accompanying increase in salicylic acid [100]. These observations suggest that reducing Asc content predisposed *Arabidopsis* to induce defense responses faster upon pathogen attack. Whether an increase in Asc content would have had the opposite effect on these pathogens was not examined in this study. Quite different results were observed in a more recent study that also employed the same mutants. In this study, *Arabidopsis vtc1* and *vtc2* were more susceptible to the pathogenic ascomycete *Alternaria brassicicola* and Asc strongly inhibited growth of fungal cultures [101]. Asc levels decreased following *A. brassicicola* infection with an increase in DHA, suggesting that Asc is being consumed during infection [101]. Given the limited number of studies focusing on the relationship between Asc content and pathogen defense, it is not possible at this point to conclude how increasing Asc content will affect defense responses. These two studies do suggest, however, that changes in Asc content may affect defense responses in a very pathogen-specific manner.

4.7. Increasing Ascorbic Acid Induces Twinning

In addition to being an antioxidant, Asc regulates the cell cycle by promoting G_1 to S progression of cells, e.g., in the quiescent center of onion roots [102–106]. Repression of L-galactono-1,4-lactone dehydrogenase (GalLDH) expression in tobacco BY-2 cell lines resulted in 30% less Asc and a reduction in the rate of cell division and growth [107]. The ability of Asc to promote cell division had dramatic consequences when its level was elevated during early embryo development. Embryo development initiates with a transverse zygotic division to produce an apical, proembryo cell and a basal cell that gives rise to the suspensor and in most species, a single embryo develops in each seed. Increasing Asc content in tobacco by increasing DHAR expression, however, resulted in monozygotic twinning and polycotyly [108]. The twin zygotes resulted from a longitudinal instead of transverse cell division and these twin zygotes developed into embryos of equal size. Direct injection of Asc into tobacco ovaries was sufficient to induce twinning but only if delivered within the first two days after pollination during which the zygote undergoes its first division. The twinning can be understood as an Asc-induced alteration in the normal transverse division of the zygote that results in a loss of the positional cues needed for the normal differentiation of the apical cell into the embryo and the basal cell into the suspensor.

Polycotyly (*i.e.*, the development of more than two cotelydons) was also induced by Asc, either following an increase in DHAR expression or when Asc was injected at the globular stage of embryo development prior to the initiation of cotyledon development [108]. As in zygotic division, an Asc-induced alteration in cell division during the specification of cotyledon-forming fields likely is responsible for the observed polycotyly. Although Asc likely affects cell division in other tissues [102–106], the lack of a readily observable phenotype may make the effect of increased Asc content in other aspects of plant development less apparent.

5. Conclusions

From its role as an antioxidant essential for photosynthesis and for detoxifying ROS from endogenous and exogenous sources, to its role in regulating cell division and flowering, to its function as a co-factor in multiple enzymatic reactions, ascorbic acid has fundamentally enabled the colonization of land by plant species. This is likely due to the challenge that the rise in atmospheric oxygen during Earth's past presented to multicellular organisms, which required limiting the harmful consequences of increased exposure to oxygen that a land-based existence entails. Vitamin C is critical to plants as it is unlikely they could tolerate a single day of exposure to sunlight without ascorbic acid detoxifying the ROS generated by photosynthetic activity. In contrast, animals unable to synthesize ascorbic acid, such as humans, can survive the absence of the vitamin for weeks or even months before succumbing to disease and death. Despite the importance of its role in detoxifying

ROS, ascorbic acid's functions are now so integrated into plant growth and development that its importance cannot be underestimated. Because of the complexity of its many roles, any attempts to engineer changes in ascorbic acid content in plants that improves one aspect, such as nutritional content, will require close examination of how such changes impact the overall health and performance of the plant under field conditions. In addition to the engineering approaches described above, genetic diversity within plants offers another means to increase Asc content through standard breeding approaches [109], although whether changes in Asc content through these means may limit any deleterious effects on plant growth and development is unknown at this time. The most successful strategies will undoubtedly involve highly targeted approaches to alter ascorbic acid content in specific cell types or tissues to achieve a desired end while limiting possible unintended consequences in other aspects of growth, development, and responses to biotic and abiotic stresses.

Acknowledgments

The author thanks the United States Department of Agriculture (NRICGP 02-35100-12469) and the University of California Agricultural Experiment Station for support of his work cited.

References

1. Sies, H.; Stahl, W. Vitamins E and C, β-carotene, and other carotenoids as antioxidants. *Am. J. Clin. Nutr.* **1995**, *62*, 1315S–1321S.
2. Levine, M. New concepts in the biology and biochemisty of ascorbic acid. *N. Engl. J. Med.* **1986**, *314*, 892–902.
3. Levine, M.; Cantilena, C.C.; Dhariwal, K.R. Determination of optimal vitamin C requirements in humans. *Am. J. Clin. Nutr.* **1995**, *62*, 1347S–1356S.
4. Chatterjee, I.B. Evolution and the biosynthesis of ascorbic acid. *Science* **1973**, *182*, 1271–1272.
5. Chen, Z.; Young, T.E.; Ling, J.; Chang, S.-C.; Gallie, D.R. Increasing vitamin C content of plants through enhanced ascorbate recycling. *Proc. Natl. Acad. Sci. USA* **2003**, *100*, 3525–3530.
6. Hancock, R.D.; Viola, R. Improving the nutritional value of crops through enhancement of L-ascorbic acid (vitamin C) content: Rationale and biotechnological opportunities. *J. Agric. Food Chem.* **2005**, *53*, 5248–5257.
7. Naqvi, S.; Zhu, C.; Farre, G.; Ramessar, K.; Bassie, L.; Breitenbach, J.; Perez Conesa, D.; Ros, G.; Sandmann, G.; Capell, T.; *et al.* Transgenic multivitamin corn through biofortification of endosperm with three vitamins representing three distinct metabolic pathways. *Proc. Natl. Acad. Sci. USA* **2009**, *106*, 7762–7767.
8. Burns, J.J. Ascorbic Acid. In *Metabolic Pathways*, 3rd ed.; Greenberg, D.M., Ed.; Academic Press: New York, NY, USA, 1967; pp. 394–411.
9. Wheeler, G.L.; Jones, M.A.; Smirnoff, N. The biosynthetic pathway of vitamin C in higher plants. *Nature* **1998**, *393*, 365–369.

10. Wolucka, B.A.; Persiau, G.; van Doorsselaere, J.; Davey, M.W.; Demol, H.; Vandekerckhove, J.; van Montagu, M.; Zabeau, M.; Boerjan, W. Partial purification and identification of GDP-mannose 3′,5′-epimerase of *Arabidopsis thaliana*, a key enzyme of the plant vitamin C pathway. *Proc. Natl. Acad. Sci. USA* **2001**, *98*, 14843–14848.
11. Siendones, E.; González-Reyes, J.A.; Santos-Ocaña Navas, P.; Córdoba, F. Biosynthesis of ascorbic acid in kidney bean. L-Galactono-γ-lactone dehydrogenase is an intrinsic protein located at the mitochondrial inner membrane. *Plant Physiol.* **1999**, *120*, 907–912.
12. Bartoli, C.G.; Pastori, G.M.; Foyer, C.H. Ascorbate biosynthesis in mitochondria is linked to the electron transport chain between complexes III and IV. *Plant Physiol.* **2000**, *123*, 335–343.
13. Conklin, P.L.; Williams, E.H.; Last, R.L. Environmental stress sensitivity of an ascorbic acid-deficient Arabidopsis mutant. *Proc. Natl. Acad. Sci. USA* **1996**, *93*, 9970–9974.
14. Conklin, P.L.; Pallanca, J.E.; Last, R.L.; Smirnoff, N. L-Ascorbic acid metabolism in the ascorbate-deficient Arabidopsis mutant *vtc1*. Plant Physiol. **1997**, *115*, 1277–1285.
15. Franceschi, V.R.; Tarlyn, N.N. L-Ascorbic acid is accumulated in source leaf phloem and transported to sink tissues in plants. *Plant Physiol.* **2002**, *130*, 649–656.
16. Tedone, L.; Hancock, R.D.; Alberino, S.; Haupt, S.; Viola, R. Long-distance transport of L-ascorbic acid in potato. BMC Plant Biol. **2004**, *4*, 16.
17. Conklin, P.L.; Saracco, S.A.; Norrism, S.R.; Last, R.L. Identification of ascorbic acid-deficient *Arabidopsis thaliana* mutants. *Genetics* **2000**, *154*, 847–856.
18. Dowdle, J.; Ishikawa, T.; Gatzek, S.; Rolinski, S.; Smirnoff, N. Two genes in *Arabidopsis thaliana* encoding GDP-L-galactose phosphorylase are required for ascorbate biosynthesis and seedling viability. Plant J. **2007**, *52*, 673–689.
19. Conklin, P.L.; Norris, S.R.; Wheeler, G.L.; Williams, E.H.; Smirnoff, N.; Last, R.L. Genetic evidence for the role of GDP-mannose in plant ascorbic acid (vitamin C) biosynthesis. *Proc. Natl. Acad. Sci. USA* **1999**, *96*, 4198–4203.
20. Conklin, P.L.; Gatzek, S.; Wheeler, G.L; Dowdle, J.; Raymond, M.J.; Rolinski, S.; Isupov, M.; Littlechild, J.A.; Smirnoff, N. *Arabidopsis thaliana VTC4* encodes L-galactose-1-P phosphatase, a plant ascorbic acid biosynthetic enzyme. *J. Biol. Chem.* **2006**, *281*, 15662–15670.
21. Laing, W.A.; Wright, M.A.; Cooney, J.; Bulley, S.M. The missing step of the L-galactose pathway of ascorbate biosynthesis in plants, an L-galactose guanyltransferase, increases leaf ascorbate content. *Proc. Natl. Acad. Sci. USA* **2007**, *104*, 9534–9539.
22. Bulley, S.M.; Rassam, M.; Hoser, D.; Otto, W.; Schünemann, N.; Wright, M.; MacRae, E.; Gleave, A.; Laing, W. Gene expression studies in kiwifruit and gene over-expression in Arabidopsis indicates that GDP-L-galactose guanyltransferase is a major control point of vitamin C biosynthesis. *J. Exp. Bot.* **2009**, *60*, 765–778.
23. Bulley, S.; Wright, M.; Rommens, C.; Yan, H.; Rassam, M.; Lin-Wang, K.; Andre, C.; Brewster, D.; Karunairetnam, S.; Allan, A.C.; *et al*. Enhancing ascorbate in fruits and tubers through over-expression of the L-galactose pathway gene GDP-L-galactose phosphorylase. *Plant Biotechnol. J.* **2012**, *10*, 390–397.
24. Gatzek, S.; Wheeler, G.L.; Smirnoff, N. Antisense suppression of L-galactose dehydrogenase in *Arabidopsis thaliana* provides evidence for its role in ascorbate synthesis and reveals light modulated L-galactose synthesis. *Plant J.* **2002**, *30*, 541–553.

25. Zhou, Y.; Tao, Q.C.; Wang, Z.N.; Fan, R.; Li, Y.; Sun, X.F.; Tang, K.X. Engineering ascorbic acid biosynthetic pathway in *Arabidopsis* leaves by single and double gene transformation. *Biol. Plant.* **2012**, *56*, 451–457.
26. Valpuesta, V.; Botella, M.A. Biosynthesis of L-ascorbic acid in plants: New pathways for an old antioxidant. *Trends Plant Sci.* **2004**, *9*, 573–577.
27. Loewus, F.A.; Kelly, S. The metabolism of D-galacturonic acid and its methyl ester in the detached ripening strawberry. *Arch. Biochem. Biophys.* **1961**, *95*, 483–493.
28. Isherwood, F.A.; Chen, Y.T.; Mapson, L.W. Synthesis of L-ascorbic acid in plants and animals. *Biochem. J.* **1954**, *56*, 1–15.
29. Davey, M.W.; Gilot, C.; Persiau, G.; Østergaard, J.; Han, Y.; Bauw, G.C.; van Montagu, M.C. Ascorbate biosynthesis in *Arabidopsis* cell suspension culture. *Plant Physiol.* **1999**, *121*, 535–543.
30. Agius, F.; Gonzalez-Lamothe, R.; Caballero, J.L.; Munoz-Blanco, J.; Botella, M.A.; Valpuesta, V. Engineering increased vitamin C levels in plants by overexpression of a D-galacturonic acid reductase. *Nat. Biotechnol.* **2003**, *21*, 177–181.
31. Badejo, A.A.; Wada, K.; Gao, Y.; Maruta, T.; Sawa, Y.; Shigeoka, S.; Ishikawa, T. Translocation and the alternative D-galacturonate pathway contribute to increasing the ascorbate level in ripening tomato fruits together with the D-mannose/L-galactose pathway. *J. Exp. Bot.* **2012**, *63*, 229–239.
32. Loewus, F.A. Tracer studies on ascorbic acid formation in plants. *Phytochemistry* **1963**, *2*, 109–128.
33. Wolucka, B.A.; van Montagu, M. GDP-mannose 3′,5′-epimerase forms GDP-L-gulose, a putative intermediate for the de novo biosynthesis of vitamin C in plants. *J. Biol. Chem.* **2003**, *278*, 47483–47490.
34. Wagner, C.; Sefkow, M.; Kopka, J. Construction and application of a mass spectral and retention time index database generated from plant GC/EI-TOF-MS metabolite profile. *Phytochemistry* **2003**, *62*, 887–900.
35. Jain, A.K.; Nessler, C.L. Metabolic engineering of an alternative pathway for ascorbic acid biosynthesis in plants. *Mol. Breed.* **2000**, *6*, 73–78.
36. Radzio, J.A.; Lorence, A.; Chevone, B.I.; Nessler, C.L. L-Gulono-1,4-lactone oxidase expression rescues vitamin C-deficient *Arabidopsis* (*vtc*) mutants. *Plant Mol. Biol.* **2004**, *53*, 837–844.
37. Baig, M.M.; Kelly, S.; Loewus, F. L-Ascorbic acid biosynthesis in higher plants from L-gulono-1,4-lactone and L-galactono-1,4-lactone. *Plant Physiol.* **1970**, *46*, 277–280.
38. Oba, K.; Fukui, M.; Imai, Y.; Iriyama, S.; Nogami, K. L-Galactono-γ-lactone dehydrogenase: Partial characterization, induction of activity and role in the synthesis of ascorbic acid in wounded white potato tuber tissue. *Plant Cell Physiol.* **1994**, *35*, 473–478.
39. Lorence, A.; Chevone, B.I.; Mendes, P.; Nessler, C.L. *myo*-Inositol oxygenase offers a possible entry point into plant ascorbate biosynthesis. *Plant Physiol.* **2004**, *134*, 1200–1205.
40. Asada, K. The water-water cycle in chloroplasts: Scavenging of active oxygens and dissipation of excess photons. *Annu. Rev. Plant Physiol. Plant Mol. Biol.* **1999**, *50*, 601–639.

41. Mano, J.; Hideg, E.; Asada, K. Ascorbate in thylakoid lumen functions as an alternative electron donor to photosystem II and photosystem I. *Arch. Biochem. Biophys*. **2004**, *429*, 71–80.
42. Miyake, C.; Asada, K. Ferredoxin dependent photoreduction of monodehydroascorbate radical in spinach thylakoids. *Plant Cell Physiol*. **1994**, *34*, 539–549.
43. Sano, S.; Miyake, C.; Mikami, B.; Asada, K. Molecular characterization of monodehydroascorbate radical reductase from cucumber overproduced in *Escherichia coli*. *J. Biol. Chem.* **1995**, *270*, 21354–21361.
44. Mittler, R.; Vanderauwera, S.; Gollery, M.; van Breusegem, F. Reactive oxygen gene network of plants. *Trends Plant Sci.* **2004**, *9*, 490–498.
45. Obara, K.; Sumi, K.; Fukuda, H. The use of multiple transcription starts causes the dual targeting of *Arabidopsis* putative monodehydroascorbate reductase to both mitochondria and chloroplasts. *Plant Cell Physiol.* **2002**, *43*, 697–705.
46. Lisenbee, C.S.; Lingard, M.J.; Trelease, R.N. Arabidopsis peroxisomes possess functionally redundant membrane and matrix isoforms of monodehydroascorbate reductase. *Plant J.* **2005**, *43*, 900–914.
47. Jimenez, A.; Hernandez, J.A.; del Reo, L.A.; Sevilla, F. Evidence for the presence of the ascorbate-glutathione cycle in mitochondria and peroxisomes of pea leaves. *Plant Physiol.* **1997**, *114*, 272–284.
48. Haroldsen, V.M.; Chi-Ham, C.L.; Kulkarni, S.; Lorence, A.; Bennett, A.B. Constitutively expressed DHAR and MDHAR influence fruit, but not foliar ascorbate levels in tomato. *Plant Physiol. Biochem.* **2011**, *49*, 1244–1249.
49. Stevens, R.; Page, D.; Gouble, B.; Garchery, C.; Zamir, D.; Causse, M. Tomato fruit ascorbic acid content is linked with monodehydroascorbate reductase activity and tolerance to chilling stress. *Plant Cell Environ.* **2008**, *31*, 1086–1096.
50. Eltayeb, A.E.; Kawano, N.; Badawi, G.H.; Kaminaka, H.; Sanekata, T.; Shibahara, T.; Inanaga, S.; Tanaka, K. Overexpression of monodehydroascorbate reductase in transgenic tobacco confers enhanced tolerance to ozone, salt and polyethylene glycol stresses. *Planta* **2007**, *225*, 1255–1264.
51. Li, F.; Wu, Q.Y.; Sun, Y.L.; Wang, L.Y.; Yang, X.H.; Meng, Q.W. Overexpression of chloroplastic monodehydroascorbate reductase enhanced tolerance to temperature and methyl viologen-mediated oxidative stresses. *Physiol. Plant* **2010**, *139*, 421–434.
52. Yin, L.; Wang, S.; Eltayeb, A.E.; Uddin, M.I.; Yamamoto, Y.; Tsuji, W.; Takeuchi, Y.; Tanaka, K. Overexpression of dehydroascorbate reductase, but not monodehydroascorbate reductase, confers tolerance to aluminum stress in transgenic tobacco. *Planta* **2010**, *231*, 609–621.
53. Smirnoff, N.; Conklin, P.L.; Loewus, F.A. Biosynthesis of ascorbic acid in plants: A Renaissance. *Annu. Rev. Plant Physiol. Plant Mol. Biol.* **2001**, *52*, 437–467.
54. Noctor, G.; Foyer, C.H. Ascorbate and glutathione: Keeping active oxygen under control. *Ann. Rev. Plant Physiol. Plant Mol. Biol.* **1998**, *49*, 249–279.
55. Chen, Z.; Gallie, D.R. The ascorbic acid redox state controls guard cell signaling and stomatal movement. *Plant Cell* **2004**, *16*, 1143–1162.

56. Chen, Z.; Gallie, D.R. Increasing tolerance to ozone by elevating foliar ascorbic acid confers greater protection against ozone than increasing avoidance. *Plant Physiol.* **2005**, *138*, 1673–1689.
57. Chen, Z.; Gallie, D.R. Dehydroascorbate reductase affects leaf growth, development, and function. *Plant Physiol.* **2006**, *142*, 775–787.
58. Yoshida, S.; Tamaoki, M.; Shikano, T.; Nakajima, N.; Ogawa, D.; Ioki, M.; Aono, M.; Kubo, A.; Kamada, H.; Inoue, Y.; *et al.* Cytosolic dehydroascorbate reductase is important for ozone tolerance in *Arabidopsis thaliana*. *Plant Cell Physiol.* **2006**, *47*, 304–308.
59. Kwon, S.Y.; Ahn, Y.O.; Lee, H.S.; Kwak, S.S. Biochemical characterization of transgenic tobacco plants expressing a human dehydroascorbate reductase gene. *J. Biochem. Mol. Biol.* **2001**, *34*, 316–321.
60. Kwon, S.Y.; Choi ,S.M.; Ahn, Y.O.; Lee, H.S.; Lee, H.B.; Park, Y.M.; Kwak, S.S. Enhanced stress-tolerance of transgenic tobacco plants expressing a human dehydroascorbate reductase gene. *J. Plant Physiol.* **2003**, *160*, 347–353.
61. Eltayeb, A.E.; Kawano, N.; Badawi, G.H.; Kaminaka, H.; Sanekata, T.; Morishima, I.; Shibahara, T.; Inanaga, S.; Tanaka, K. Enhanced tolerance to ozone and drought stresses in transgenic tobacco overexpressing dehydroascorbate reductase in cytosol. *Physiol. Plant* **2006**, *127*, 57–65.
62. Wang, Z.; Xiao, Y.; Chen, W.; Tang, K.; Zhang, L. Increased vitamin C content accompanied by an enhanced recycling pathway confers oxidative stress tolerance in *Arabidopsis*. *J. Integr. Plant Biol.* **2010**, *52*, 400–409.
63. Ushimaru, T.; Nakagawa, T.; Fujioka, Y.; Daicho, K.; Naito, M.; Yamauchi, Y.; Nonaka, H.; Amako, K.; Yamawaki, K.; Murata, N. Transgenic *Arabidopsis* plants expressing the rice dehydroascorbate reductase gene are resistant to salt stress. *J. Plant Physiol.* **2006**, *163*, 1179–1184.
64. Le Martret, B.; Poage, M.; Shiel, K.; Nugent, G.D.; Dix, P.J. Tobacco chloroplast transformants expressing genes encoding dehydroascorbate reductase, glutathione reductase, and glutathione-S-transferase, exhibit altered anti-oxidant metabolism and improved abiotic stress tolerance. *Plant Biotechnol. J.* **2011**, *9*, 661–673.
65. Arrigoni, O.; De Gara, L.; Tommasi, F.; Liso, R. Changes in the ascorbate system during seed development of *Vicia faba* L. *Plant Physiol.* **1992**, *99*, 235–238.
66. Qin, A.; Shi, Q.; Yu, X. Ascorbic acid contents in transgenic potato plants overexpressing two dehydroascorbate reductase genes. *Mol. Biol. Rep.* **2011**, *38*, 1557–1566.
67. Goo, Y.M.; Chun, H.; Kim, T.W.; Lee, C.H.; Ahn, M.J.; Bae, S.C.; Cho, K.J.; Chun, J.A.; Chung, C.H.; Lee, S.W. Expressional characterization of dehydroascorbate reductase cDNA in transgenic potato plants. *J. Plant Biol.* **2008**, *51*, 35–41.
68. Belmonte, M.F.; Stasolla, C. Altered HBK3 expression affects glutathione and ascorbate metabolism during the early phases of Norway spruce (*Picea abies*) somatic embryogenesis. *Plant Physiol. Biochem.* **2009**, *47*, 904–911.
69. Halliwell, B.; Gutteridge, J.M.C. *Free Radicals in Biology and Medicine*; Oxford University Press: New York, NY, USA, 2000.

70. Foyer, C.H. Oxygen Metabolism and Electron Transport in Photosynthesis. *In Oxidative Stress and the Molecular Biology of Antioxidant Defenses*; Scandalios, J.G., Ed.; Cold Spring Harbor Laboratory Press: Cold Spring Harbor, NY, USA, 1997; pp. 587–621.
71. Asada, K. The water-water cycle as alternative photon and electron sinks. *Philos. Trans. R. Soc. Lond. B* **2000**, *355*, 1419–1431.
72. Nakano, Y.; Asada, K. Spinach chloroplasts scavenge hydrogen peroxide on illumination. *Plant Cell Physiol.* **1980**, *21*, 1295–1307.
73. Mudd, J.B. Biochemical Basis for the Toxicity of Ozone. In *Plant Response to Air Pollution*; Yunus, M., Iqba, M., Eds.; Wiley & Sons: New York, NY, USA, 1997; pp. 267–284.
74. Schraudner, M.; Moeder, W.; Wiese, C.; van Camp, W.; Inze, D.; Langebartels, C.; Sandermann, H., Jr. Ozone-induced oxidative burst in the ozone biomonitor plant, tobacco Bel W3. *Plant J.* **1998**, *16*, 235–245.
75. Rao, M.V.; Koch, J.R.; Davis, K.R. Ozone: A tool for probing programmed cell death in plants. *Plant Mol. Biol.* **2000**, *44*, 345–358.
76. Koch, J.R.; Creelman, R.A.; Eshita, S.M.; Seskar, M.; Mullet, J.E.; Davis, K.R. Ozone sensitivity in hybrid poplar correlates with insensitivity to both salicylic acid and jasmonic acid. The role of programmed cell death in lesion formation. *Plant Physiol.* **2000**, *123*, 487–496.
77. Pasqualini, S.; Piccioni, C.; Reale, L.; Ederli, L.; Della Torre, G.; Ferranti, F. Ozone-induced cell death in tobacco cultivar bel w3 plants. The role of programmed cell death in lesion formation. *Plant Physiol.* **2003**, *133*, 1122–1134.
78. Pei, Z.M.; Murata, Y.; Benning, G.; Thomine, S.; Klusener, B.; Allen, G.J.; Grill, E.; Schroeder, J.I. Calcium channels activated by hydrogen peroxide mediate abscisic acid signaling in guard cells. *Nature* **2000**, *406*, 731–734.
79. Zhang, X.; Zhang, L.; Dong, F.; Gao, J.; Galbraith, D.W.; Song, C.P. Hydrogen peroxide is involved in abscisic acid-induced stomatal closure in *vicia faba*. *Plant Physiol.* **2001**, *126*, 1438–1448.
80. Veljovic-Jovanovic, S.D.; Pignocchi, C.; Noctor, G.; Foyer, C.H. Low ascorbic acid in the *vtc-1* mutant of Arabidopsis is associated with decreased growth and intracellular redistribution of the antioxidant system. *Plant Physiol.* **2001**, *127*, 426–435.
81. Huang, C.; He, W.; Guo, J.; Chang, X.; Su, P.; Zhang, L. Increased sensitivity to salt stress in an ascorbate-deficient *Arabidopsis* mutant. *J. Exp. Bot.* **2005**, *56*, 3041–3049.
82. Zhang, W.; Lorence, A.; Gruszewski, H.A.; Chevone, B.I.; Nessler, C.L. AMR1, an Arabidopsis gene that coordinately and negatively regulates the mannose/L-galactose ascorbic acid biosynthetic pathway. *Plant Physiol.* **2009**, *150*, 942–950.
83. Zhang, Z.; Wang, J.; Zhang, R.; Huang, R. The ethylene response factor Aterf98 enhances tolerance to salt through the transcriptional activation of ascorbic acid synthesis in Arabidopsis. *Plant J.* **2012**, *71*, 273–287.
84. Sanmartin, M.; Drogoudi, P.A.; Lyons, T.; Pateraki, I.; Barnes, J.; Kanellis, A.K. Over-expression of ascorbate oxidase in the apoplast of transgenic tobacco results in altered ascorbate and glutathione redox states and increased sensitivity to ozone. *Planta* **2003**, *216*, 918–928.

85. Grimes, H.D.; Perkins, K.K.; Boss, W.F. Ozone degrades into hydroxyl radical under physiological conditions: A spin trapping study. *Plant Physiol.* **1983**, *72*, 1016–1020.
86. Lee, Y.P.; Kim, S.H.; Bang, J.W.; Lee, H.S.; Kwak, S.S.; Kwon, S.Y. Enhanced tolerance to oxidative stress in transgenic tobacco plants expressing three antioxidant enzymes in chloroplasts. *Plant Cell Rep.* **2007**, *26*, 591–598.
87. Mullen, R.T.; Trelease, R.N. Biogenesis and membrane properties of peroxisomes: Does the boundary membrane serve and protect? *Trends Plant Sci.* **1996**, *1*, 389–394.
88. Graham, I.A.; Eastmond, P.J. Pathways of straight and branched chain fatty acid catabolism in higher plants. *Prog. Lipid Res.* **2002**, *41*, 156–181.
89. Yamaguchi, K.; Mori, H.; Nishimura, M. A novel isoenzyme of ascorbate peroxidase localized on glyoxysomal and leaf peroxisomal membranes in pumpkin. *Plant Cell Physiol.* **1995**, *36*, 1157–1162.
90. Bunkelmann, J.R.; Trelease, R.N. Ascorbate peroxidase: A promenent membrane protein in oilseed glyoxysomes. *Plant Physiol.* **1996**, *110*, 589–598.
91. Karyotou, K.; Donaldson, R.P. Ascorbate peroxidase, a scavenger of hydrogen peroxide in glyoxysomal membranes. *Arch. Biochem. Biophys.* **2005**, *434*, 248–257.
92. Eastmond, P.J. MONODEHYROASCORBATE REDUCTASE4 is required for seed storage oil hydrolysis and postgerminative growth in *Arabidopsis*. *Plant Cell* **2007**, *19*, 1376–1387.
93. Wang, J.; Zhang, H.; Allen, R.D. Overexpression of an Arabidopsis peroxisomal ascorbate peroxidase gene in tobacco increases protection against oxidative stress. *Plant Cell Physiol.* **1999**, *40*, 725–732.
94. Asada, K.; Takahashi, M. Production and Scavenging of Active Oxygen in Photosynthesis. In *Photoinhibition*; Kyle, D.J., Osmond, C.B., Arntzen, C.J., Eds.; Elsevier: Amsterdam, The Netherlands, 1987; pp. 227–287.
95. Aro, E.M.; Virgin, I.; Andersson, B. Photoinhibition of photosystem II. Inactivation, protein damage and turnover. *Biochim. Biophys. Acta* **1993**, *1143*, 113–134.
96. Nishiyama, Y.; Allakhverdiev, S.I.; Murata, N. A new paradigm for the action of reactive oxygen species in the photoinhibition of photosystem II. *Biochim. Biophys. Acta* **2006**, *7157*, 742–749.
97. Chen, Z.; Gallie, D.R. Dehydroascorbate reductase affects non-photochemical quenching and photosynthetic performance. *J. Biol. Chem.* **2008**, *283*, 21347–21361.
98. Assmann, S.M.; Wang, X.Q. From milliseconds to millions of years: Guard cells and environmental responses. *Curr. Opin. Plant Biol.* **2001**, *4*, 421–428.
99. Schroeder, J.I.; Allen, G.J.; Hugouvieux, V.; Kwak, J.M.; Waner, D. Guard cell signal transduction. *Annu. Rev. Plant Physiol. Plant Mol. Biol.* **2001**, *52*, 627–658.
100. Barth, C.; Moeder, W.; Klessig, D.F.; Conklin, P.L. The timing of senescence and response to pathogens is altered in the ascorbate-deficient Arabidopsis mutant *vitamin c-1*. *Plant Physiol.* **2004**, *134*, 1784–1792.
101. Botanga, C.J.; Bethke, G.; Chen, Z.; Gallie, D.R.; Fiehn, O.; Glazebrook, J. Metabolite profiling of *Arabidopsis* inoculated with *Alternaria brassicicola* reveals that ascorbate reduces disease severity. *Mol. Plant Microbe Interact.* **2012**, *25*, 1628–1638.

102. Liso, R.; Calabrese, G.; Bitonti, M.B.; Arrigoni, O. Relationship between ascorbic acid and cell division. *Exp. Cell Res.* **1984**, *150*, 314–320.

103. Arrigoni, O.; Bitonti, M.B.; Cozza, R.; Innocenti, A.M.; Liso, R.; Veltri, R. Ascorbic acid effect on pericycle cell line in *Allium cepa* root. *Caryologia* **1989**, *42*, 213–216.

104. Innocenti, A.M.; Bitonti, M.B.; Arrigoni, O.; Liso, R. The size of quiescent centre in roots of *Allium Cepa* L. grown with ascorbic acid. *New Phytol.* **1990**, *110*, 507–509.

105. Arrigoni, O. Ascorbate system in plant development. *J. Bioenerg. Biomembr.* **1994**, *26*, 407-419.

106. Citterio, S.; Sgorbati, S.; Scippa, S.; Sparvoli, E. Ascorbic acid effect on the onset of cell proliferation in pea root. *Physiol. Plant* **1994**, *92*, 601–607.

107. Tabata, K.; Oba, K.; Suzuki, K.; Esaka, M. Generation and properties of ascorbic acid-deficient transgenic tobacco cells expressing antisense RNA for L-galactono-1,4-lactone dehydrogenase. *Plant J.* **2001**, *27*, 139–148.

108. Chen, Z.; Gallie, D.R. Induction of monozygotic twinning by ascorbic acid in tobacco. *PLoS One* **2012**, *7*, e39147.

109. Gest, N.; Gautier, H.; Stevens, R. Ascorbate as seen through plant evolution: The rise of a successful molecule? *J. Exp. Bot.* **2013**, *64*, 33–53.

4

A Randomised Cross-Over Pharmacokinetic Bioavailability Study of Synthetic *versus* Kiwifruit-Derived Vitamin C

Anitra C. Carr *, Stephanie M. Bozonet and Margreet C. M. Vissers

Centre for Free Radical Research, Department of Pathology & Biomedical Science, University of Otago, Christchurch, P.O. Box 4345, Christchurch 8140, New Zealand; E-Mails: stephanie.bozonet@otago.ac.nz (S.M.B.); margreet.vissers@otago.ac.nz (M.C.M.V.)

* Author to whom correspondence should be addressed; E-Mail: anitra.carr@otago.ac.nz;

Abstract: Kiwifruit are a rich source of vitamin C and also contain numerous phytochemicals, such as flavonoids, which may influence the bioavailability of kiwifruit-derived vitamin C. The aim of this study was to compare the relative bioavailability of synthetic *versus* kiwifruit-derived vitamin C using a randomised cross-over pharmacokinetic study design. Nine non-smoking males (aged 18–35 years) received either a chewable tablet (200 mg vitamin C) or the equivalent dose from gold kiwifruit (*Actinidia chinensis* var. *Sungold*). Fasting blood and urine were collected half hourly to hourly over the eight hours following intervention. The ascorbate content of the plasma and urine was determined using HPLC with electrochemical detection. Plasma ascorbate levels increased from 0.5 h after the intervention ($P = 0.008$). No significant differences in the plasma time-concentration curves were observed between the two interventions ($P = 0.645$). An estimate of the total increase in plasma ascorbate indicated complete uptake of the ingested vitamin C tablet and kiwifruit-derived vitamin C. There was an increase in urinary ascorbate excretion, relative to urinary creatinine, from two hours post intervention ($P < 0.001$). There was also a significant difference between the two interventions, with enhanced ascorbate excretion observed in the kiwifruit group ($P = 0.016$). Urinary excretion was calculated as ~40% and ~50% of the ingested dose from the vitamin C tablet and kiwifruit arms, respectively. Overall, our pharmacokinetic study has shown comparable relative bioavailability of kiwifruit-derived vitamin C and synthetic vitamin C.

Keywords: human; ascorbic acid; ascorbate; plasma; urine; kiwi fruit

1. Introduction

In contrast to most mammals, humans cannot synthesis vitamin C (ascorbate) due to mutation of the terminal biosynthetic enzyme [1]. Thus, the micronutrient must be obtained from dietary sources in order to prevent hypovitaminosis C and the potentially fatal deficiency disease scurvy [1]. Vitamin C was first isolated from fruit and vegetables and the adrenal glands of animals in the early 1930s and was chemically synthesized in 1933 [2]. Although synthetic and food-derived vitamin C is chemically identical, fruit and vegetables contain numerous nutrients and phytochemicals, e.g., flavonoids, which may affect the bioavailability of food-derived vitamin C. Flavonoids can act as antioxidants via direct scavenging of free radicals [3] and/or chelation of redox-active metal ions [4,5]. Thus, it has been proposed that food-derived flavonoids may "spare" vitamin C and thus increase its bioavailability.

Due to the low bioavailability of flavonoids [6] and tight sequestration of metal ions *in vivo* [7], this vitamin C "sparing" mechanism may be expected to occur primarily in the intestinal lumen. Vitamin C is actively transported through the intestinal epithelium via the sodium-dependent vitamin C transporter 1 (SVCT1) [8]. This transporter is also responsible for renal reabsorption of vitamin C, which helps to maintain whole body homeostasis [9]. SVCT1 has a higher capacity, but lower affinity, for vitamin C than the SCVT2 isoform, which is found in most other metabolically active cells and tissues [9].

Although food matrix interactions can influence the bioavailability of some nutrients, such as carotenoids [10], the bioavailability of vitamin C does not appear to be influenced by the food matrix. Kamp *et al.* [11] found no difference in vitamin C bioavailability from a micronutrient supplement administered in the absence or presence of a corn-based porridge. Mangels *et al.* [12] also found no difference between vitamin C bioavailability from oranges compared with orange juice, and although there was a difference in bioavailability between raw and cooked broccoli, this was likely due to differences in mechanical homogenization (chewing), a similar effect to that observed for carotenoid absorption from raw *versus* cooked carrots.

Vitamin C bioavailability can be determined using either steady-state or pharmacokinetic study designs. The former monitors ascorbate levels in blood, cells, tissues and/or urine following a number of weeks of supplementation, while the latter monitors transient changes in plasma levels and/or urinary excretion over the hours following ingestion of the test substance. We have carried out a steady state bioavailability study comparing synthetic with kiwifruit-derived vitamin C in healthy non-smoking males supplemented with a vitamin C tablet or the equivalent dose of vitamin C from gold kiwifruit [13]. No differences in steady state bioavailability were observed in plasma, urine, semen, leukocytes, or muscle tissue following six weeks of supplementation, despite significant differences being observed in our earlier animal model study [14].

Transient differences between synthetic vitamin C and that from different fruit juices have been observed using pharmacokinetic models [15–18]. Therefore, the aim of the current study was to compare the relative bioavailability of synthetic *versus* kiwifruit-derived vitamin C using a randomised cross-over pharmacokinetic study design to determine whether there are any transient differences between the two interventions. Uptake of vitamin C exhibits sigmoidal steady state kinetics between doses of 30–400 mg/day, with plasma uptake decreasing at doses of >200 mg/day and urinary excretion increasing at doses ≥100 mg/day [19]. Therefore, we chose a dose of 200 mg vitamin C and the comparable dose derived from gold kiwifruit (*Actinidia chinensis* var. *Sungold*). Our study participants were young non-smoking men with "healthy" (*i.e.*, >50 μmol/L) baseline levels of plasma vitamin C.

2. Study Design and Methods

2.1. Participants

All procedures involving human participants were approved by the New Zealand Health and Disability Ethics Committee (#URA/11/02/003). Non-smoking males aged 18–35 years were recruited from our previous vitamin C study databases, and were primarily from local tertiary institutes. Exclusion criteria included: recent smoker (within previous year), low plasma vitamin C (<50 μmol/L), allergy/intolerance to kiwifruit, taking prescription medication (within past three months), and fainting due to fear of needles. Anthropometric measurements were carried out to determine body mass index (BMI) and a fasting venous blood sample was drawn to determine plasma ascorbate levels as described below. Nine participants with above average plasma ascorbate levels were enrolled for the study and provided written informed consent.

Figure 1. Pharmacokinetic study design. Participants received either 1.5 *Sungold* kiwifruit (containing ~200 mg vitamin C) or chewable vitamin C tablets (total of 200 mg vitamin C) in a randomised cross-over design with a three week washout period between the two clinic days.

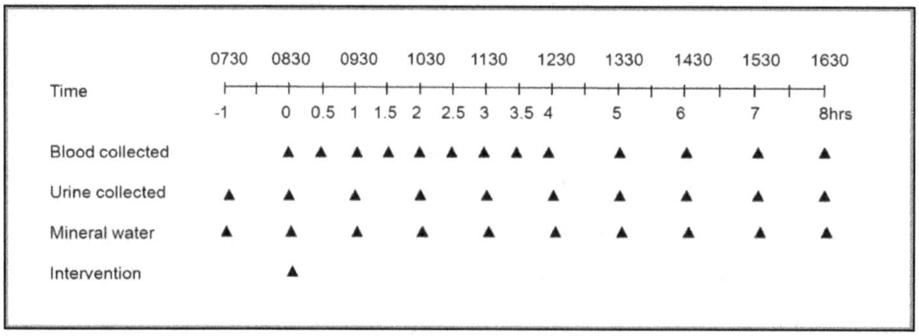

2.2. Study Design

The randomised cross-over pharmacokinetic study design comprised eight hours of sampling after a single dose of 1.5 *Sungold* kiwifruit (containing ~200 mg vitamin C) or chewable vitamin C tablets (total of 200 mg vitamin C) with a three-week washout period between the two clinic days (Figure 1) [20]. Following an overnight fast, the participants had a venous cannula inserted and blood samples were collected at baseline, and every 30 min post-intervention for the first four hours, then every hour for the next four hours. The cannulae were flushed with up to 10 mL sterile saline after each sampling. Urine was collected at baseline, after emptying the bladder an hour earlier, and then every hour post-intervention for the next eight hours. Mineral water (75 mL) was provided every hour and a cheese sandwich at four hours post-intervention. One of the nine participants did not carry out the vitamin C tablet supplementation arm of the study.

2.3. Interventions

Chewable orange-flavoured vitamin C tablets were provided by Tishcon Corp., Westbury, NY, USA. Analysis of the tablets indicated that they contained 49 mg of vitamin C per tablet. Participants received a single dose of four tablets, equivalent to ~196 mg vitamin C.

Gold kiwifruit (*Actinidia chinensis* var. *Sungold*) were provided by Zespri International Ltd., Mount Maunganui, New Zealand, and were stored at ≤4 °C. The vitamin C content of the kiwifruit was monitored by HPLC with electrochemical detection [21]. HPLC analysis indicated there was 162 ± 18 mg vitamin C per 100 g fruit ($n = 5$). Participants consumed 1.5 kiwifruit, without the skin (*i.e.*, ~78% of 103 ± 8.4 g fruit); therefore the actual amount of vitamin C consumed was estimated to be ~194 mg per 1.5 kiwifruit.

2.4. Sample Collection and Processing

Plasma. Peripheral blood was collected into 4 mL K_3-EDTA vacutainer tubes, which were kept on ice at all times. Samples were centrifuged at 4 °C to pellet cells and the plasma was collected and kept on ice for extraction of ascorbate. Plasma samples were treated with an equal volume of ice-cold 0.54 M perchloric acid containing the metal chelator DTPA (100 µmol/L) to precipitate protein [21]. The de-proteinated supernatants were stored at −80 °C until HPLC analysis.

Urine. Urine was collected into pre-weighed 50 mL sample containers and an aliquot was removed for urinary creatinine determinations. Urine samples were treated with an equal volume of ice-cold 0.54 M perchloric acid containing the metal chelator DTPA (100 µmol/L) to precipitate protein [21]. The de-proteinated supernatants were stored at −80 °C until HPLC analysis.

2.5. Plasma and Urine Analysis

Creatinine. Urinary creatinine was determined by the Jaffe reaction using an Abbot c8000 analyser (Canterbury Health Laboratories, Christchurch, New Zealand).

Ascorbate. The ascorbate content of the plasma and urine was analysed using reverse-phase HPLC, with a Synergi 4 µ Hydro-RP 80A column and an ESA Coulochem II electrochemical detector, as previously described in detail [13]. In order to measure total ascorbate (reduced and oxidised), duplicate samples were reduced with tris(2-carboxyethyl)phosphine hydrochloride as described previously [22].

2.6. Data and Statistical Analysis

Area under the plasma and urinary ascorbate time-concentration curve calculations were determined using the trapezoidal rule as described previously [23]. The increase in circulating ascorbate (by weight) was calculated using Nadler's formula for estimating total blood volume [24] and the increase in urinary ascorbate (by weight) was calculated from the total volume of urine collected. Data are represented as mean ± SD for group characteristics or mean ± SEM for comparisons between group means. Analysis of paired data was determined using two-tailed Students *t*-test with P <0.05 indicating statistical difference. Two way analysis of variance with Fisher pairwise multiple comparison procedure was carried out using SigmaStat software (version 11, Systat Software Inc., San Jose, CA, USA).

3. Results

3.1. Participant Characteristics

At screening, the participants' mean ± SD age was 24 ± 5 years, weight was 78 ± 10 kg, height was 180 ± 8 cm, and BMI was 24 ± 2 kg/m^2. The participants selected for this study had "healthy" (*i.e.*, >50 μmol/L) fasting plasma ascorbate concentrations, their mean ± SD at screening being 67 ± 17 μmol/L (n = 9). This was to avoid the potentially confounding effects of preferential tissue uptake in individuals with suboptimal ascorbate status at baseline, which could affect the comparative ascorbate levels observed in plasma and urine. Urinary ascorbate levels were detectible in the subjects at baseline, further indicating that plasma ascorbate levels were at or above the renal threshold.

Figure 2. Change in plasma ascorbate uptake following ingestion of 200 mg vitamin C (•) or 1.5 Sungold kiwifruit (○). Data represent mean ± SEM (n = 9). Baseline plasma ascorbate concentrations were 61 ± 6 μmol/L and 66 ± 6 μmol/L for the vitamin C and kiwifruit groups, respectively. Two way analysis of variance with Fisher pairwise multiple comparison procedure indicated a significant increase in plasma ascorbate from 0.5 h post intervention (P = 0.008), but no significant difference between the two interventions (P = 0.645).

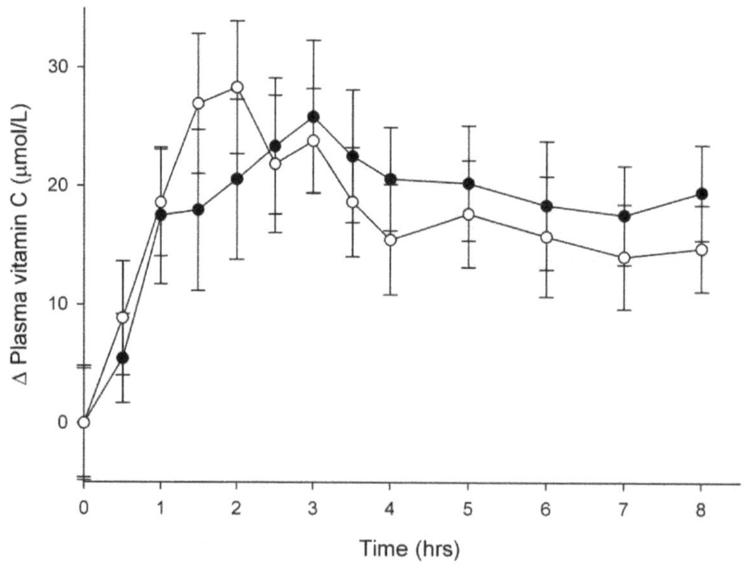

3.2. Vitamin C Uptake into Plasma

Plasma ascorbate levels, following ingestion of either 200 mg vitamin C tablets or 1.5 Sungold kiwifruit (providing an equivalent dose of ~200 mg vitamin C), are shown in Figure 2. A statistically significant increase in plasma ascorbate was observed as early as 0.5 h post intervention ($P = 0.008$). No significant differences in the plasma time-concentration curves were observed between the two interventions ($P = 0.645$). Area under the ascorbate time-concentration curves also indicated no difference between the two interventions (Table 1). An estimate of the total increase in plasma ascorbate indicated that all of the ingested vitamin C tablet and kiwifruit-derived vitamin C accumulated in plasma over the eight-hour time course (Table 1).

Table 1. Area under the plasma and urinary ascorbate time-concentration curves (AUC) and total increase in plasma and urinary ascorbate. Subjects were supplemented with 200 mg vitamin C or 1.5 Sungold kiwifruit and ascorbate concentrations in plasma and urine were determined over the eight hours post intervention.

	Vitamin C (200 mg) [a]	Kiwifruit (1.5 Sungold) [a]	*P* value [b]
Plasma AUC (h × μmol/L)	220 ± 23	237 ± 13	0.483
Plasma ascorbate (mg) [c]	211 ± 18	227 ± 16	0.496
Urinary AUC (h × μmol/mmol creatinine)	618 ± 133	856 ± 118	0.004
Urinary ascorbate (mg)	74 ± 14	101 ± 10	0.033

[a] Data represent mean ± SEM; [b] *P* values were determined using paired two-tailed Students *t*-test. [c] Total blood volumes were estimated using Nadler's formula [24].

Figure 3. Change in urinary ascorbate excretion following ingestion of 200 mg vitamin C (●) or 1.5 Sungold kiwifruit (○). Data represent mean ± SEM ($n = 9$). Baseline urinary ascorbate concentrations were 10 ± 4 μmol/mmol creatinine and 14 ± 3 μmol/mmol creatinine for the vitamin C and kiwifruit groups, respectively. Two way analysis of variance with Fisher pairwise multiple comparison procedure indicated a significant increase in plasma vitamin C from two hours post intervention ($P < 0.001$), as well as a significant difference between the two interventions ($P = 0.016$).

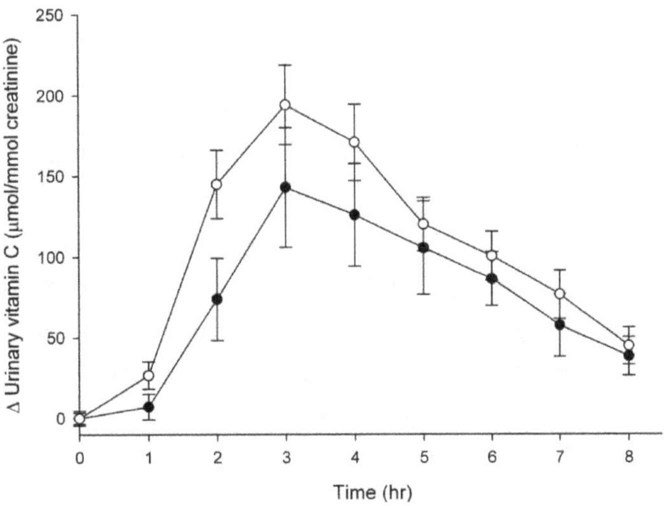

3.3. Vitamin C Excretion in Urine

Urinary ascorbate excretion was monitored over the eight hours following intervention with vitamin C tablets or Sungold kiwifruit and standardised to urinary creatinine concentrations (Figure 3). There was a significant increase in ascorbate excretion from two hours post intervention

($P < 0.001$) and also a significant difference between the two interventions, with enhanced ascorbate excretion observed in the kiwifruit group ($P = 0.016$, Figure 3). This difference was confirmed with ascorbate area under the time-concentration curves (Table 1). The total increase in ascorbate excretion over the eight hours indicated ~40% and ~50% excretion of the ingested dose from the supplement and kiwifruit arms, respectively (Table 1).

4. Discussion

Our pharmacokinetic study has shown comparable plasma uptake of synthetic and kiwifruit-derived vitamin C in subjects with "healthy" (*i.e.*, >50 μmol/L) baseline ascorbate status. Several other pharmacokinetic studies have shown comparable plasma uptake of vitamin C supplied in synthetic form *versus* that in fruit juices [15,23,25]. Nelson *et al.* [26] used an intestinal triple lumen tube perfusion model to investigate the absorption of synthetic vitamin C and that from an orange juice solution. This method allowed direct measurement of intraluminal events and showed no difference in the absorption of vitamin C from the two test solutions. Some pharmacokinetic studies have shown small or transient decreases in plasma ascorbate levels in the presence of fruit juices [16,18]. The physiological relevance of these small or transient differences is, however, likely minimal.

Vinson and Bose are the only investigators to have shown increased uptake of vitamin C, in the presence of citrus fruit extract, using a pharmacokinetic study design [27,28]. Their initial study, carried out in guinea pigs, indicated that vitamin C provided in a citrus fruit medium took longer to reach peak plasma concentrations compared with a synthetic vitamin C solution and also provided a larger area under the plasma ascorbate concentration-time curve [27]. These investigators also observed a comparable trend in human subjects supplemented with 500 mg vitamin C in the presence or absence of a citrus fruit extract [28]. The citrus extract delayed maximal plasma levels by one hour and provided a 35% increase in vitamin C levels.

The different outcomes observed in the pharmacokinetic studies discussed above could be explained by differences in study design and subjects. For example, the doses of vitamin C used varied by more than 10-fold, from 30 mg to 500 mg. Vitamin C bioavailability is non-linear [29] and although ~100% bioavailability is observed at a vitamin C dose of 200 mg, doses exceeding this exhibit decreased intestinal uptake [19]. Doses of 500 mg vitamin C are also significantly higher than would be obtained through a normal daily diet. Furthermore, the participants in these pharmacokinetic studies exhibited varying baseline plasma ascorbate levels, from 35 μmol/L to 75 μmol/L, the former being non-saturating and the latter being saturating levels of ascorbate [21]. These different baseline levels may affect vitamin C uptake and clearance kinetics as it is likely that there will be preferential uptake into cells and tissues in individuals with suboptimal vitamin C status [21,30]. Thus, it is possible that kiwifruit-derived vitamin C may exhibit different uptake kinetics in individuals with sub-optimal ascorbate status at baseline.

We observed a transient increase in urinary excretion when ascorbate was supplied as kiwifruit compared with tablets. Vinson and Bose [28] observed increased excretion of ascorbate when given in the presence of citrus fruit extract, but only in individuals who had been saturated with vitamin C prior to beginning the study. Similarly, others have shown small or transient increases in ascorbate excretion in the presence of fruit juice in pre-saturated subjects [17,18]. In contrast, Uchida *et al.* [15] recently reported decreased ascorbate excretion when given in the presence of acerola juice. Decreased excretion of fruit-derived vitamin C was observed in subjects with low baseline ascorbate status [15,28], supporting the premise that baseline ascorbate status may affect comparative vitamin C bioavailability.

The mechanism whereby kiwifruit enhances urinary excretion of ascorbate without affecting plasma levels is unkown. Certain dietary fibres, such as hemicellulose, which is present in kiwifruit [31], have been shown to increase the excretion of ascorbate [32]. The flavonoid quercetin, found in kiwifruit [33], is a reversible, non-competitive inhibitor of ascorbate transport by SVCT1 [34]. Due to the low intestinal bioavailabiltiy of flavonoids [6], this mechanism would be expected to occur primarily in the intestinal lumen. Although we did not observe an effect of kiwifruit on plasma uptake of ascorbate, alternative mechanisms for intestinal uptake have been implicated using SVCT1 knockout mice [35]. An alternative, hypothetical mechanism may involve a kiwifruit-derived metabolite, which is excreted into urine and thus selectively inhibits ascorbate reabsorption via SVCT1 in the kidney tubules. Urinary excretion of ascorbate may be advantageous with respect to diseases or infections of the urinary tract [36,37].

5. Conclusions

Our pharmacokinetic study has shown comparable plasma uptake of synthetic and kiwifruit-derived vitamin C and enhanced urinary excretion of kiwifruit-derived vitamin C, although the ~10% increase in total excretion is unlikely to be physiologically significant. Of interest, in our subjects with >50 μmol/L to saturating baseline plasma ascorbate, ~50%–60% of the ingested ascorbate was unaccounted for by urinary excretion, despite complete plasma uptake. This indicates possible tissue uptake even in individuals with supposedly "healthy" or "optimal" plasma ascorbate status.

Acknowledgments

We thank the young men who participated in this study, Jo Kepple and her staff at Primorus Clinical Trials Unit, Lynley Drummond for consultation on study design, Heather Webb for technical assistance, and Juliet Pullar for editing the manuscript. Sources of Support: Co-funding was provided by the New Zealand Ministry of Business, Innovation & Employment and Zespri International Ltd., Mount Maunganui, New Zealand.

References

1. Tsao, C.S. An Overview of Ascorbic Acid Chemistry and Biochemistry. In *Vitamin C in Health and Disease*; Packer, L., Fuchs, J., Eds.; Marcel Dekker: New York, NY, USA, 1997; pp. 25–58.
2. Sauberlich, H.E. A History of Scurvy and Vitamin C. In *Vitamin C in Health and Disease*; Packer, L., Fuchs, J., Eds.; Marcel Dekker: New York, NY, USA, 1997; pp. 1–24.

3. Ivanov, V.; Carr, A.C.; Frei, B. Red wine antioxidants bind to human lipoproteins and protect them from metal ion-dependent and -independent oxidation. *J. Agric. Food Chem.* **2001**, *49*, 4442–4449.
4. Beker, B.Y.; Sonmezoglu, I.; Imer, F.; Apak, R. Protection of ascorbic acid from copper(II)-catalyzed oxidative degradation in the presence of flavonoids: Quercetin, catechin and morin. *Int. J. Food Sci. Nutr.* **2011**, *62*, 504–512.
5. Clemetson, C.A.; Andersen, L. Plant polyphenols as antioxidants for ascorbic acid. *Ann. N. Y. Acad. Sci.* **1966**, *136*, 341–376.
6. Lotito, S.B.; Frei, B. Consumption of flavonoid-rich foods and increased plasma antioxidant capacity in humans: Cause, consequence, or epiphenomenon? *Free Radic. Biol. Med.* **2006**, *41*, 1727–1746.
7. Carr, A.; Frei, B. Does vitamin C act as a pro-oxidant under physiological conditions? *FASEB J.* **1999**, *13*, 1007–1024.
8. Tsukaguchi, H.; Tokui, T.; Mackenzie, B.; Berger, U.V.; Chen, X.Z.; Wang, Y.; Brubaker, R.F.; Hediger, M.A. A family of mammalian Na^+-dependent L-ascorbic acid transporters. *Nature* **1999**, *399*, 70–75.
9. Savini, I.; Rossi, A.; Pierro, C.; Avigliano, L.; Catani, M.V. SVCT1 and SVCT2: Key proteins for vitamin C uptake. *Amino Acids* **2008**, *34*, 347–355.
10. Parada, J.; Aguilera, J.M. Food microstructure affects the bioavailability of several nutrients. *J. Food Sci.* **2007**, *72*, R21–R32.
11. Kamp, F.; Jandel, D.; Hoenicke, I.; Pietrzk, K.; Gross, R.; Trugo, N.M.; Donangelo, C.M. Bioavailability of iron, zinc, folate, and vitamin C in the IRIS multi-micronutrient supplement: Effect of combination with a milk-based cornstarch porridge. *Food Nutr. Bull.* **2003**, *24* (3 Suppl.), 20–26.
12. Mangels, A.R.; Block, G.; Frey, C.M.; Patterson, B.H.; Taylor, P.R.; Norkus, E.P.; Levander, O.A. The bioavailability to humans of ascorbic acid from oranges, orange juice and cooked broccoli is similar to that of synthetic ascorbic acid. *J. Nutr.* **1993**, *123*, 1054–1061.
13. Carr, A.C.; Bozonet, S.M.; Pullar, J.M.; Simcock, J.W.; Vissers, M.C. A randomised steady-state bioavailability study of synthetic and natural (kiwifruit-derived) vitamin C. *Nutrients* **2013**, *5*, 3684–3695.
14. Vissers, M.C.M.; Bozonet, S.M.; Pearson, J.F.; Braithwaite, L.J. Dietary ascorbate affects steady state tissue levels in vitamin C-deficient mice: Tissue deficiency after sub-optimal intake and superior bioavailability from a food source (kiwifruit). *Am. J. Clin. Nutr.* **2011**, *93*, 292–301.
15. Uchida, E.; Kondo, Y.; Amano, A.; Aizawa, S.; Hanamura, T.; Aoki, H.; Nagamine, K; Koizumi, T.; Maruyama, N.; Ishigami, A. Absorption and excretion of ascorbic acid alone and in acerola (*Malpighia emarginata*) juice: Comparison in healthy Japanese subjects. *Biol. Pharm. Bull.* **2011**, *34*, 1744–1747.
16. Bates, C.J.; Jones, K.S.; Bluck, L.J. Stable isotope-labelled vitamin C as a probe for vitamin C absorption by human subjects. *Br. J. Nutr.* **2004**, *91*, 699–705.
17. Jones, E.; Hughes, R.E. The influence of bioflavonoids on the absorption of vitamin C. *IRCS Med. Sci.* **1984**, *12*, 320.

18. Pelletier, O.; Keith, M.O. Bioavailability of synthetic and natural ascorbic acid. *J. Am. Diet. Assoc.* **1974**, *64*, 271–275.
19. Levine, M.; Conry-Cantilena, C.; Wang, Y.; Welch, R.W.; Washko, P.W.; Dhariwal, K.R.; Park, J.B.; Lazarev, A.; Graumlich, J.K.; King, J.; *et al.* Vitamin C pharmacokinetics in healthy volunteers: Evidence for a recommended dietary allowance. *Proc. Natl. Acad. Sci. USA* **1996**, *93*, 3704–3709.
20. Kondo, Y.; Higashi, C.; Iwama, M.; Ishihara, K.; Handa, S.; Mugita, H.; Maruyama, N.; Koga, H.; Ishigami, A. Bioavailability of vitamin C from mashed potatoes and potato chips after oral administration in healthy Japanese men. *Br. J. Nutr.* **2012**, *107*, 885–892.
21. Carr, A.C.; Pullar, J.M.; Moran, S.; Vissers, M.C.M. Bioavailability of vitamin C from kiwifruit in non-smoking males: Determination of 'healthy' and 'optimal' intakes. *J. Nutr. Sci.* **2012**, *1*, e14. doi:10.1017/jns.2012.15.
22. Sato, Y.; Uchiki, T.; Iwama, M.; Kishimoto, Y.; Takahashi, R.; Ishigami, A. Determination of dehydroascorbic acid in mouse tissues and plasma by using tris(2-carboxyethyl)phosphine hydrochloride as reductant in metaphosphoric acid/ethylenediaminetetraacetic acid solution. *Biol. Pharm. Bull.* **2010**, *33*, 364–369.
23. Carter, B.; Monsivais, P.; Drewnowski, A. Absorption of folic acid and ascorbic acid from nutrient comparable beverages. *J. Food Sci.* **2010**, *75*, H289–H293.
24. Nadler, S.B.; Hidalgo, J.H.; Bloch, T. Prediction of blood volume in normal human adults. *Surgery* **1962**, *51*, 224–232.
25. Guarnieri, S.; Riso, P.; Porrini, M. Orange juice *vs.* vitamin C: Effect on hydrogen peroxide-induced DNA damage in mononuclear blood cells. *Br. J. Nutr.* **2007**, *97*, 639–643.
26. Nelson, E.W.; Streiff, R.R.; Cerda, J.J. Comparative bioavailability of folate and vitamin C from a synthetic and a natural source. *Am. J. Clin. Nutr.* **1975**, *28*, 1014–1019.
27. Vinson, J.A.; Bose, P. Comparative bioavailability of synthetic and natural vitamin C in guinea pigs. *Nutr. Rep. Int.* **1983**, *27*, 875–879.
28. Vinson, J.A.; Bose, P. Comparative bioavailability to humans of ascorbic acid alone or in a citrus extract. *Am. J. Clin. Nutr.* **1988**, *48*, 601–604.
29. Graumlich, J.F.; Ludden, T.M.; Conry-Cantilena, C.; Cantilena, L.R., Jr.; Wang, Y.; Levine, M. Pharmacokinetic model of ascorbic acid in healthy male volunteers during depletion and repletion. *Pharm. Res.* **1997**, *14*, 1133–1139.
30. Carr, A.C.; Bozonet, S.M.; Pullar, J.M.; Simcock, J.W.; Vissers, M.C. Human skeletal muscle ascorbate is highly responsive to changes in vitamin C intake and plasma concentrations. *Am. J. Clin. Nutr.* **2013**, *97*, 800–807.
31. Sims, I.M.; Monro, J.A. Fiber: Composition, structures, and functional properties. *Adv. Food Nutr. Res.* **2013**, *68*, 81–99.
32. Keltz, F.R.; Kies, C.; Fox, H.M. Urinary ascorbic acid excretion in the human as affected by dietary fiber and zinc. *Am. J. Clin. Nutr.* **1978**, *31*, 1167–1171.
33. Lee, D.E.; Shin, B.J.; Hur, H.J.; Kim, J.H.; Kim, J.; Kang, N.J.; Kim, D.O.; Lee, C.Y.; Lee, K.W.; Lee, H.J. Quercetin, the active phenolic component in kiwifruit, prevents hydrogen peroxide-induced inhibition of gap-junction intercellular communication. *Br. J. Nutr.* **2010**, *104*, 164–170.

34. Song, J.; Kwon, O.; Chen, S.; Daruwala, R.; Eck, P.; Park, J.B.; Levine, M. Flavonoid inhibition of sodium-dependent vitamin C transporter 1 (SVCT1) and glucose transporter isoform 2 (GLUT2), intestinal transporters for vitamin C and glucose. *J. Biol. Chem.* **2002**, *277*, 15252–15260.
35. Corpe, C.P.; Tu, H.; Eck, P.; Wang, J.; Faulhaber-Walter, R.; Schnermann, J.; Margolis, S.; Padayatty, S.; Sun, H.; Wang, Y.; Nussbaum, R.L.; Espey, M.G.; Leine, M. Vitamin C transporter Slc23a1 links renal reabsorption, vitamin C tissue accumulation, and perinatal survival in mice. *J. Clin. Investig.* **2010**, *120*, 1069–1083.
36. Yalcin, O.; Karatas, F.; Erulas, F.A.; Ozdemir, E. The levels of glutathione peroxidase, vitamin A, E, C and lipid peroxidation in patients with transitional cell carcinoma of the bladder. *BJU Int.* **2004**, *93*, 863–866.
37. Ochoa-Brust, G.J.; Fernandez, A.R.; Villanueva-Ruiz, G.J.; Velasco, R.; Trujillo-Hernandez, B.; Vasquez, C. Daily intake of 100 mg ascorbic acid as urinary tract infection prophylactic agent during pregnancy. *Acta Obstet. Gynecol. Scand.* **2007**, *86*, 783–787.

5

Ascorbic Acid and the Brain: Rationale for the Use against Cognitive Decline

Fiona E. Harrison [1], **Gene L. Bowman** [2] **and Maria Cristina Polidori** [3,*]

[1] Division of Diabetes, Endocrinology and Metabolism, Department of Medicine, Vanderbilt University Medical Center, Nashville, TN 37232, USA; E-Mail: fiona.harrison@vanderbilt.edu

[2] Brain Institute, Department of Neurology, NIA–Aging and Alzheimer's Disease Center Oregon Health and Science University, Portland, OR 97239, USA; E-Mail: bowmang@ohsu.edu

[3] Geriatrics Department, University of Cologne Medical Faculty, Cologne 50937, Germany

* Author to whom correspondence should be addressed; E-Mail: maria.polidori-nelles@uk-koeln.de

---

Abstract: This review is focused upon the role of ascorbic acid (AA, vitamin C) in the promotion of healthy brain aging. Particular attention is attributed to the biochemistry and neuronal metabolism interface, transport across tissues, animal models that are useful for this area of research, and the human studies that implicate AA in the continuum between normal cognitive aging and age-related cognitive decline up to Alzheimer's disease. Vascular risk factors and comorbidity relationships with cognitive decline and AA are discussed to facilitate strategies for advancing AA research in the area of brain health and neurodegeneration.

Keywords: ascorbic acid; vitamin C; brain; cognitive function; alzheimer's disease; dementia; aging; elderly; endothelial function; blood-brain barrier; SVCT (sodium-dependent vitamin C transporter)

---

1. Introduction

Ascorbic acid (AA; Vitamin C) is a remarkable water-soluble antioxidant concentrated predominately in citrus fruits, strawberries and vegetables (e.g., spinach and broccoli) and found in many supplement formulations (LPI Micronutrient Information Center). The adequate functioning of the human organism in general, and of the brain in particular, is highly dependent on AA, but humans are completely dependent on dietary sources due to the evolutionary process leaving us a gene incapable of producing the enzyme gulonolactone oxidase needed to yield AA from glucose [1]. Thus, humans require a constant stream of AA from the diet and rely on robust "carrier" transport and "barrier" integrity mechanisms to meet the brain's demand. AA is the most powerful water-soluble antioxidant of the organism, and key to preventing oxidative lipid damage in biological systems [2]. It forms the first line of antioxidant defence under many types of oxidizing conditions. It can rapidly intercept free radicals in the aqueous phase before they attack lipids [3]. As an antioxidant, AA also provides protection against oxidative stress-induced cellular damage by neutralization of lipid hydroperoxyl (LHP) radicals and by protecting proteins from alkylation by electrophilic lipid peroxidation activity [4].

Several pathological processes can involve the production of free radicals, antioxidant depletion, oxidative and nitrosative stress including vascular disease and cognitive impairments seen in aging older adults (Dementia of Alzheimer's type). Dementia, with its most prevalent form, Alzheimer's disease (AD), is characterized by an insidious progressive nature that usually begins with memory deficits followed by disturbances in other cognitive domains that eventually reach a level that impacts functions of daily life. Age–related dementias also disrupt the family unit, which must often scramble to meet day-to-day care requirements to compensate for loss of independence. The economic conditions associated with this phenomenon of disability and dependence is an enormous and pressing threat to public health. The major risk factor for dementia and AD remains to be advanced age; therefore the projected impact of AD can be estimated by frequency in strata of the population. For example, in the US about 14% of the older adult population age 65 and older carry a diagnosis of dementia and age 85 and older is about 47%. In either case, these cohort effects will stress the value of anti-AD strategies while general practitioners, geriatricians, neurologists and health care professionals all around the globe are projected to face over 115 million people with dementia from all causes by 2050 [5].

The pathological hallmarks of AD include a loss in synaptic function and accumulation of extracellular amyloid-β plaques and intraneuronal neurofibrillary tangles. Oxidative stress displays chronological primacy in the onset of AD, and in its prephase, mild cognitive impairment (MCI) [6–9]. Thus, preventive therapy that is safe and effective for reducing oxidative damage seen early in neurodegenerative disorders and applied before the onset of dementia is a public health priority.

This overview will focus on the biological rationale for the avoidance of AA deficiency in the promotion of healthy brain aging. We include discussion on the biochemistry and transport of AA, much of which has been clarified through basic research using genetically modified mouse models, and also the clinical studies designed to better understand the influence over cognitive health in our aging populations.

2. Ascorbic Acid Biochemistry and Transport

AA concentration is higher in the brain than almost all other organs, and in fact may only be equaled in concentration in the adrenal glands. Scurvy, the classical clinical syndrome of AA deficiency, is rare, although not unheard of, in developed populations, but sub-clinical deficiency is still widespread, particularly in at-risk populations such as the elderly, hospitalized and those with poor access to good nutrition. One or more symptoms of scurvy were observed in 18 out of 145 (12%) of elderly patients on admission to hospital, and all but one of this group were classed as being AA deficient as confirmed from plasma levels [10]. Interestingly, 7 of the 23 (30%) controls (no signs of clinical scurvy) also had AA deficiency according to plasma levels, and all of the patients included in the study were classed as having depleted serum AA. Animal studies have shown that brain preferentially retains AA at the expense of other organs with cerebellar, hippocampal and cortical areas appearing to retain AA the most effectively under conditions of depletion which may have a bearing on diseases that target specific areas of the brain [11]. However, the brain is unable to hold maximal or optimal or even sufficient levels in the face of chronic insufficiency, which may have important effects on pathological aging and neurodegenerative diseases. Some populations, such as the elderly and smokers likely require even higher intakes of AA [12]. Roles for AA are widespread and include its vital role as an antioxidant as well as action as a cofactor for a number of dioxygenase enzymes involved in the synthesis of carnitine, collagen, and neurotransmitters including dopamine, norepinephrine and serotonin (reviewed [13]). AA can inhibit LDL oxidation and increase resistance of LDL to oxidation (for review, see [4,14]). AA also plays a role in the function of endothelial nitric oxide synthase (eNOS) by recycling the eNOS cofactor, tetrahydrobiopterin, which is relevant for arterial elasticity and blood pressure regulation [4,15]. Each of these roles plus atherogenic factors may contribute to the preventative role of AA in the development of cognitive impairment.

Evidence of altered glutamate transport (e.g., changes in EAAT2 and EAAT3 transporters) is seen in human AD postmortem samples, particularly in patients with hippocampal sclerosis [16]. AA is released from astrocytes as glutamate is taken up, and this relationship is termed a hetero-exchange although this does not fully represent how the two processes are tethered [17,18]. It is presumed that AA moderates the oxidative stress induced by glutamate [19] and so is protective against overstimulation and cell death. This relationship has been more closely investigated in relation to Huntington's disease [20–22], which also involves cell death. GLT-1 is a high affinity transporter that relies on Na-dependent transport across an electrochemical gradient for rapid removal of glutamate from the synapse. It is sensitive to oxidative stress, and disruption of the transporter leads to glutamate accumulation and hyperstimulation of receptors. Memantine is the first of a new class of drugs for AD that blocks NMDA receptors and its efficacy suggests that further research into glutamatergic signaling and AD is warranted. Therefore, as the role of glutamate transport and NMDA receptors in AD becomes clearer, this may be revealed as another key area where high intracellular AA levels are critical for brain health.

Further excitement has recently been generated in the field of epigenetics with a potential new answer for why AA is concentrated so strongly in CSF and brain parenchyma (reviewed in [23]). Nutrition is perhaps the quintessential example of environmental modification of the genome, and recent work has highlighted a direct role for AA that cannot be replicated with other antioxidants. 5-mc (5-methylcytosine) is oxidized to 5-hmc (5-hydroxymethylcytosine) as part of dynamic DNA demethylation. This reaction, and further oxidation of 5-hmc, are both catalyzed by the activity of TET (ten-eleven translocation) dioxygenase enzymes, for which AA is a critical co-factor (needed for the reduction of iron Fe^{3+} to its active form Fe^{2+}) [24–26]. Thus AA is vital for neuronal repair as well as new cell generation and here may play a direct role in the transcription and expression of hundreds of different genes. 5-hmc and Tet proteins are abundant in brain and knockout of Tet1 in mice indicated that it may be involved in synaptic plasticity and memory extinction in addition to DNA methylation [27]. The specific relation to AD and other degenerative disorders is not yet clear, but this exciting field may provide new clues.

AA is a one-electron donor that readily reacts with a range of reactive oxygen species (ROS) to neutralize or decrease their reactivity. Loss of the electron leads to formation of the ascorbate free radical, which can be efficiently recycled to ascorbic acid through enzymatic means (summarized in Figure 1). Ascorbate radicals react preferentially with themselves forming ascorbic acid and dehydroascorbate. This oxidized form of AA can also be recycled back to ascorbic acid, although in some cases it undergoes irreversible ring opening and may be lost. AA also supports the regeneration of other antioxidants, such as vitamin E and glutathione (GSH), in biological tissues, thus combatting oxidative stress through various pathways. This close relationship between GSH and AA is such that AA has often been observed to "take the first hit" for GSH in response to oxidative stressors, and GSH is involved in reduction of dehydroascorbate to ascorbate [28].

Figure 1. Summary of ascorbic acid oxidation and recycling. Adapted from [13].

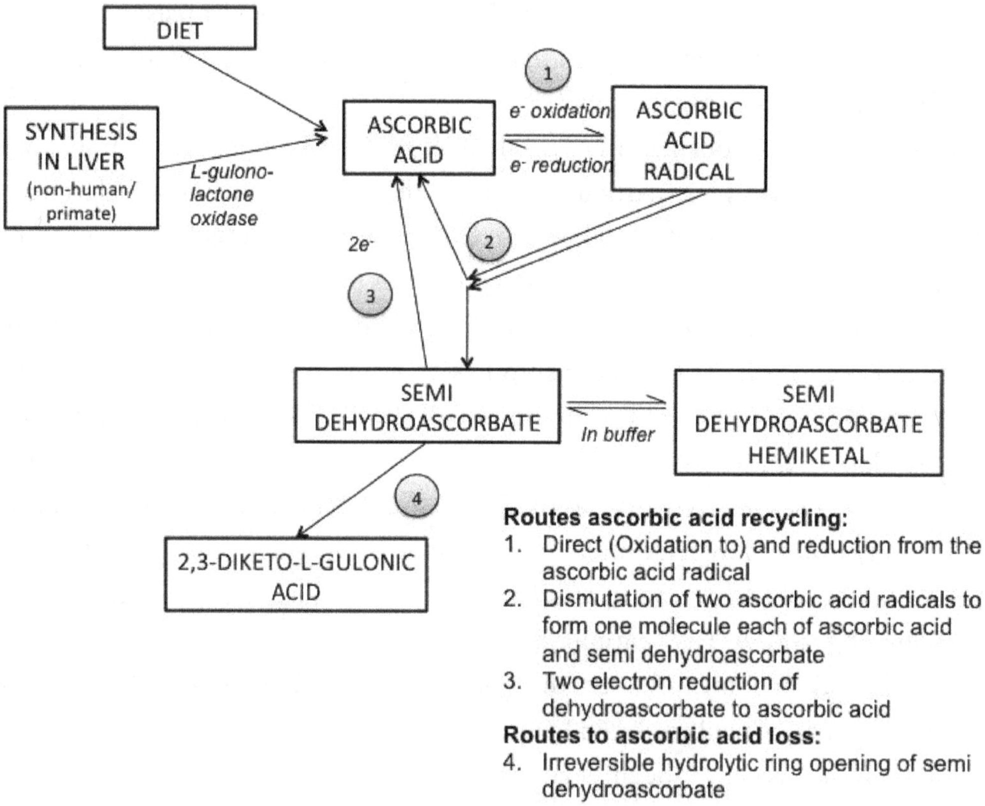

It should also be considered that AA and some of its degradation products may be involved in some potentially damaging functions [29]. For example, the Maillard reaction, most commonly studied in relation to food, is also a step in the formation of advanced glycation end products (AGEs). Evidence from a mouse model that selectively over-expressed the vitamin C transporter SVCT2 in the eye [30] implicated AA in age-related damage to crystalline proteins in the lens. There is also some debate as to the potential pro-oxidant role of AA via the Fenton reaction. AA reacts with metal ions in enzymes (e.g., hydroxylases, oxygenases) that require them to be in a reduced state for optimal enzyme function. *In vitro*, reactions with these ions can lead to the production of hydroxyl radicals and other reactive molecules. *In vivo*, catalytic metal ions are less available as their levels are typically kept in check in healthy individuals by metal binding proteins (e.g., ferritin, transferrin). Thus, *in vivo*, the evidence typically supports the antioxidant roles of AA (reviewed in detail [31,32]). One exception may be in the case of iron overload. A limited pro-oxidant effect of increased dietary AA, seen as elevated liver malondialdehyde in combination with decreased glutathione peroxidase, was found in mice fed supplemental dietary iron (although only in the lower and not the high iron diet group) [33]. It should be noted though that this study was performed under conditions of AA sufficiency, in wild-type mice that synthesize their own AA. Such an effect of pro-oxidation reactions was not found in plasma from adults or pre-term infants [3], or in AA- and iron-supplemented guinea pigs [34] and in general AA is not considered a risk factor even in patients with hereditary hemochromatosis [35]. High iron is thought to be a risk factor for AD [36] although the data are equivocal. In a study of 116 AD patients compared to 89 healthy controls, dysregulated iron homeostasis (lower serum iron, ferritin and transferrin, combined with several genetic markers for altered iron metabolism) was associated with AD [37]. The full relationship between AA, iron and AD may warrant further investigation. A further indication of the complexity of the relationships between AA, amyloid and oxidative damage is that in isolated rat brain mitochondria, and in the presence of AA and iron, amyloid-β_{1-42} was actually found to have an antioxidant effect and prevent formation of hydrogen peroxide, presumably through metal chelation [38]. Although aggregated amyloid-β_{1-42} cannot be argued to be healthy in brain tissue, this finding certainly raises interest for researchers in this field who have typically considered amyloid-β to be solely detrimental and an inducer of ROS.

Details of the complexity of the transport of AA within the central nervous system have been understood for almost half a century. Seminal work by Hammarström [39] using radio-labeled AA in guinea pigs first showed that peripherally-administered AA did indeed reach the brain, but that it appeared to travel via the choroid plexus and not traverse the blood brain barrier directly. Reports that AA levels in the CSF exceeded those found in blood, and were less affected by variations in plasma AA, suggested the existence of an active and saturable transporter for AA in the choroid plexus, which was then determined to be the case [40]. The sodium dependent vitamin C transporter 2 (SVCT2) itself was not described until much later but is responsible for transport both at the choroid plexus and in the neurons. There are two sodium-dependent vitamin C transporters, SVCT1 and SVCT2, which are responsible for transport of AA. Distribution of the two transporters varies across organs [41–43], but SVCT2 is the only transporter expressed in the brain. Regulation of the active transport of AA by these transporters may also vary across organs and in particular disease states (reviewed [44]). It allows for accumulation of AA in cells against the concentration gradient in SVCT2-dependent tissues. Following characterization of SVCT1 [43,45] single nucleotide polymorphisms (SNPs) were identified in both SVCT1 and SVCT2 and some studies are now being performed to ascertain how they alter AA status and whether they confer additional risk for diseases [46,47]. Several SNPs have been identified in the *SLC23A1* gene coding for SVCT1, and it is argued that this may be less constrained than the *SLC23A2* gene [45,48]. Altered function of the SVCT1 would have important effects on AA absorption and excretion and so would impact nutritional requirements. One synonymous and three nonsynonymous SNPs resulted in diminished vitamin C uptake in *Xenopus laevis* oocytes [49]. One of these SNPs led to an 80% decrease in uptake, and was found to have a relative occurrence of 6%–17% in African-Americans [49]. These studies are of interest to brain research because it is presumed that such SNPs could cause chronically lower circulating AA levels, which would also potentially affect brain levels. Although fewer SVCT2 SNPs have been identified, these could have an even greater effect on brain AA levels and impact disease progression.

Expression of SVCT2 mRNA and protein varies in brain and other organs during development, presumably directly linked to very high, and changing AA levels during this critical period Nevertheless developmental regulation appears to be particularly specialized and AA regulation of SVCT2 is not common to all cell types, nor to all ages. Thus, SVCT1 and SVCT2 expression, including in brain, is regulated by several disease states associated with oxidative stress (e.g., streptozotocin-induced diabetes and middle cerebral artery occlusion) [50,51] supporting the idea of potential for change in neurodegenerative disorders such as AD. Brain levels of AA in humans are dependent on the SVCT2 (see Figure 2) but also on dietary intake and intestinal absorption via SVCT1. Given that AA can also mediate the permeability of endothelial cell layers in culture [52,53], it can be seen that individual variability in either SVCT1 or SVCT2 transporter function could directly impact brain levels and vasculature in a similar manner to dietary deficiency. One particularly interesting question that may yet be answered with animal studies is the question of how SVCT2 transporter function may change with age and disease status and what impact this would have on AA levels. SVCT2 mRNA and protein both vary during development showing an inverse correlation with brain AA levels, whereas no such changes were seen in brain during AA deficiency in gulo-/- mice indicating that adult brain is unable to respond to long periods of deficiency by altering transport [54–56]. Changes in transporter function have not, to our knowledge, been studied in normally aging or AD mouse models, but if transporter function varied among groups, this could lower both CSF and intraneuronal AA levels independently of dietary intake and circulating AA levels.

There are several animals that, like humans, do not synthesize their own AA including guinea pigs, primates and some fish [57]. Nevertheless, transport is conserved across species and study of AA transporters *in situ* can be conducted in most animal models. Cell lines and primary culture techniques are available to study different organs and tissues, which have yielded useful information on expression, membrane location and transport kinetics of SVCT1 and SVCT2 in, for example, intestinal CaCo-2 cells, epithelial cells, endothelial cells, hepatocytes, muscle, intervertebral discs, Schwann cells and others [58–65]. An important consideration is that SVCT2 is regulated to some degree both by AA levels and by oxidative stress and can therefore develop in culture, as seen in astrocytes [66,67], which renders this approach potentially problematic. Other weaknesses of culture systems include the difficulties of maintaining a constant AA level in the media because it is so readily oxidized to dehydroascorbate. Dehydroascorbate can be lost reasonably quickly and can be transported into cells via glucose transporters and then recycled back to ascorbate within the cell. HPLC methods for measuring AA are very accurate if care is taken with sample preparation to minimize loss, and radiolabeled AA is available for assays for quantification in culture. Nevertheless to accurately model human *in vivo* situations, particularly in reference to specific diseases such as AD, animal models are also needed.

Different AA levels across brain regions have been reported in human and rodent brains [11,68,69]. Figure 2 shows a schematic representation of the distribution of SVCT2 (red, solid line) in the brain, and SVCT1 in intestines (green, dotted line). SVCT2 is highly, but not necessarily regularly, distributed throughout the brain. Figure components are not drawn to scale.

Figure 2. Location and distribution of SVCT1 and SVCT2 transporters and their importance in maintaining optimal brain ascorbic acid levels.

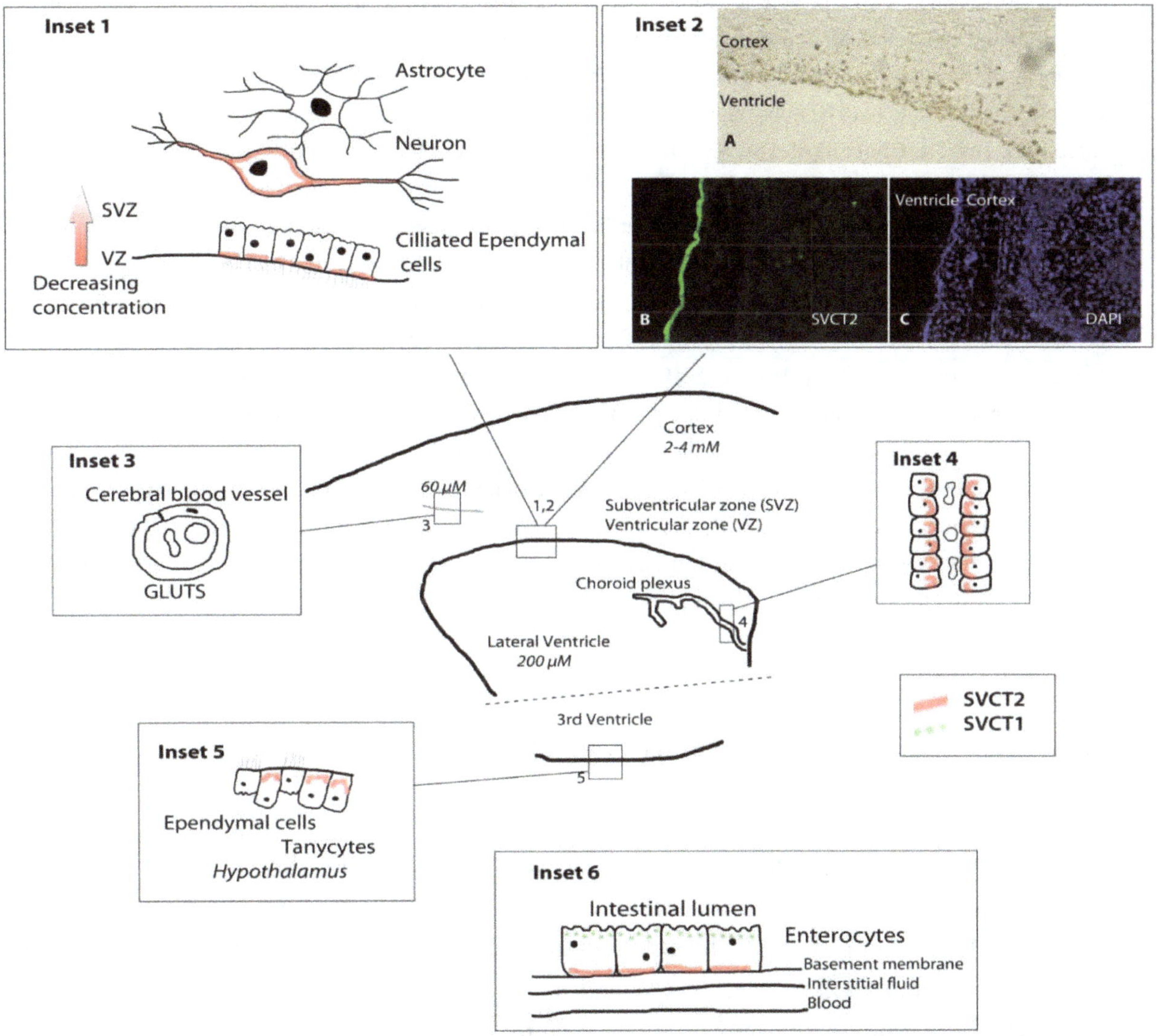

Inset 1. Cortex and lining of lateral ventricle. It was originally proposed that AA might follow a pattern of decreasing concentration with increasing distance from the ventricles following a pattern of diffusion [68]. It has since been shown that SVCT2 and AA distribution (indicated by red coloring) depend on cell type and correlate with neuronal density [70,71]. *In situ* hybridization in adult rat showed SVCT2 distribution throughout the brain, with highest expression in olfactory bulbs, hippocampus, cerebellum, cortex and choroid plexus [42]. High SVCT2 expression is seen in the ependymal cells lining the ventricular walls, with decreasing concentration in more external areas of the cortex by *in situ* hybridization and immunohistochemistry techniques [71]; **Neurons.** Primary culture of embryonic (E17) neurons shows SVCT2 in soma and cell processes [71]. Primary culture of mouse hippocampal cultures (E16–17) showed punctate staining of SVCT2 in axons [72]. Using immunohistochemical techniques in hippocampus, SVCT2 was observed in cell bodies but not processes by immunohistochemistry [73]; **Astrocytes** take up

dehydroascorbate via glucose transporters (GLUTS) and recycle it to ascorbic acid, which can be taken up by neurons. SVCT2 was not observed in astrocytes by *in situ* hybridization in adult rat brain, even following excitotoxic stimulation with quinolinic acid, although SVCT2 was observed through Northern blot technique in cultured astrocytes from rat embryo [66,74]; **Inset 2. Cortex and lining of lateral ventricle.** Panels A–C show cortex and ventricle. In panel A, AA is stained with silver stain [75] and can be seen at its most concentrated closest to the ventricle lining. In panel B, fluorescent stain for the S19 antibody staining for SVCT2 shows high expression in cells along the ventricle lining. Panel C shows DAPI stain for cell bodies. (Images courtesy of J.M. May); **Inset 3. Cross-section of Cerebral blood vessel.** There is no SVCT2 present in blood vessels in the brain. Glucose transporters (GLUTS) are found in endothelial cells and may transport dehydroascorbate. This contributes a negligible amount to brain AA stores under normal circumstances because there is typically competitive inhibition by glucose. An exception to this state may be after transient ischemia in which case SVCT2 has been shown to develop in mice [76]; **Inset 4. Choroid plexus.** SVCT2 is located throughout the choroid plexus for transfer of AA from blood to CSF. High expression of SVCT2 in choroid plexus cells has been shown by *in situ* hybridization in several studies [42,71,74]; **Inset 5. Tanycytes associated with the hypothalamus in the wall of the third ventricle.** Tanycytes are highly specialized hypothalamic glial cells that are capable of forming tight junctions and participate in the formation of the barrier between CSF and brain tissue. SVCT2 has been shown by *in situ* hybridization and immunohistochemistry in different subtypes of tanycytes in mouse brain [75]; **Inset 6. SVCT1 and SVCT2 expression in the intestine**. Expression of both transporters allows for uptake of AA from food and distribution around the body (and to brain). SVCT1 is located on the apical side of the enterocytes and is responsible for taking up AA as it passes through the intestinal lumen. SVCT2 is located on the basolateral side of cells. This is thought to be more important in animals that can synthesize their own AA, but do not consume an AA rich diet, and must still supply enterocytes with AA from blood [60]. Similar localization of SVCT1 on the apical membrane with SVCT2 found on the basolateral membrane is also seen in kidney cells. How AA passes out of the cells into the interstitial fluid and blood supply is still not confirmed, and is a conundrum given the typical direction of the SVCT2 for uptake into cells.

3. Ascorbic Acid Transport and Synthesis: Animal Models

Early work on AA and the effects of deficiency was accomplished using guinea pigs that are among the few non-primate mammals that naturally lack a functional *gulo* gene [77]. These studies on the course and effects of scurvy were conducted even before the identification of ascorbic acid as vitamin C [78,79] with inclusion of "the antiscorbutic factor" [80], (such as in fresh raw cabbage). Guinea pigs are particularly sensitive to AA (and other) deficiencies [81,82], and are still a highly utilized model for a number of human disease states, for example in relation to dyslipidemia (reviewed in [83]). The recent (since 2000) increased focus on mouse models results from the ability to use genetically altered mouse lines to impact both transport and synthesis in the same animals. Much more is known about the mouse genome than guinea pig and in many cases the models have been also bred to the same background strain making experiments directly comparable. Data can thus be interpreted, and experiments planned, with reference to the huge literature of biomedical and pharmaceutical research that has already taken place in mice making disease and treatment-relevant findings much more likely. Brief descriptions of the relevant mouse models, including gulo knockout mice, and SVCT1/2 knockout models and SVCT2 transgenic mice are reported hereafter.

Gulo knockout mice: Gulo knockout mice carry an inactivated form of the gene L-gulono-γ-lactone oxidase and are thus completely dependent on dietary AA [84]. These mice, when maintained on sub-optimal supplementation levels, are the closest to the human state of lifetime AA dietary deficiency. Knockout mice fed low levels of AA have decreased antioxidant capacity and also altered cholesterol metabolism and exhibit profound changes in vasculature. Oxidative stress has since been confirmed in these mice in adults and during development [11,85,86]. These mice also have an aberrant behavioral phenotype including poorer sensorimotor skills, and altered response to activity-inducing effects of cholinergic and dopaminergic compounds scopolamine and methamphetamine even when adequately supplemented as adults [86–88]. It is proposed that these changes result from low AA during some part of the developmental process. AA deficient gulo mice have been the subject of metabolomics profiling which has identified metabolic shifts as a response to oxidative stress of AA deficiency (e.g., upregulation of glutathione production, decreased carnitine production) [89]. Neutrophils from AA deficient gulo mice are more likely to undergo necrosis than normal apoptosis. They are not recognized by macrophages and thus clearance is also affected [90]. Such responses are important in any disease where inflammation is a factor, such as AD. Senescence marker protein 30 (SMP30) was first identified as a protein that decreased with age. Sequencing and creation of an SMP30 knockout mouse later identified this protein as the gulo enzyme [91,92]. These mice are likewise dependent on dietary AA and under conditions of deficiency their brains are susceptible to oxidative stress (generation of superoxide) [93,94]. A further mouse line exhibiting spontaneous bone fracture derived from in-bred balb/c mice [95] does not synthesize AA [96]. These mice die at an early age if not supplemented, and have been used for studies of AA level and gene transcription [97], however, this line is much less well-described. Disruption to catecholamine levels in brain and adrenal glands has been shown in each of these mouse lines [98,99]. Such data that follow a consistent pattern across the different mouse models are a strong support for the role of AA in any particular area and also of the validity of the models themselves.

SVCT1 knockout mice: SVCT1 knockout mice are viable and fertile [49]. They excrete significantly more AA in the urine than wild type and heterozygous littermates and have lower circulating blood levels. In addition to this loss of renal reabsorption of AA, uptake into liver was also dramatically decreased. Also of interest is the lower brain levels in these mice, presumably linked to lower circulating levels because SVCT1 is not expressed in brain and so should not have a direct effect (Figure 3).

SVCT2 knockout mice: The first report of the SVCT2 knockout mouse described homozygous mice that did not survive past birth (newborns never take a first breath) and had almost undetectable AA levels in all organs measured (brain, liver, adrenal glands, kidney, pituitary glands, pancreas and muscle) [100]. Subsequent studies found that AA levels were also decreased in placenta and lung as well as brain and other organs reported previously [101]. These low AA levels were associated with increased oxidative stress and cell death. Hemorrhaging, initially only reported in cortical areas [100] was also seen in the brain stem area which may contribute to the lack of breathing in the newborn mice, particularly because no obvious problems were identified in the lung in the earlier study. Primary cultured cells from hippocampi of embryonic SVCT2 knockout mice showed decreased neuronal activity, stunted neurite outgrowth and were much more sensitive to exogenously administered oxidative stress [72]. Investigation into catecholamine systems in these mice has yielded mixed data. One report showed large decreases (50%) of norepinephrine in the adrenal glands with no change in dopamine levels, whereas smaller changes in the brain (decrease of 20%–25%) were not significant for either dopamine or norepinephrine in SVCT2 knockout mice [102]. Additionally, morphological differences in the chromaffin cells of the adrenal glands were also noted in this study. Other reports have shown significant alteration to dopamine and norepinephrine systems, including metabolites, in embryonic SVCT2 knockout and SVCT2 transgenic (described below) brains [103].

Figure 3. Direct comparison of cortex levels of ascorbic acid in different mouse lines run concurrently. All mice used were male, aged 9–12 months (retired breeders).

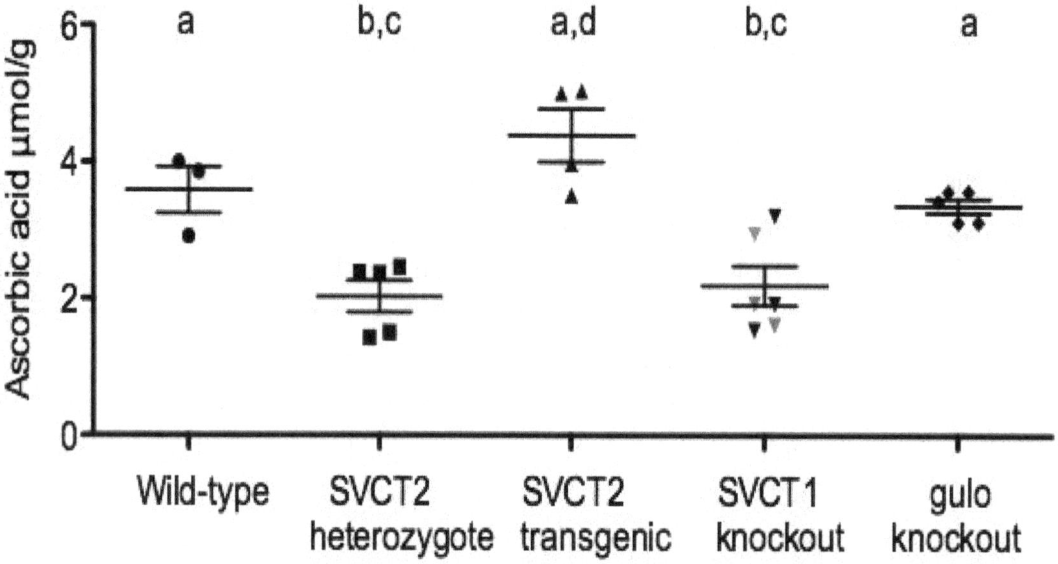

Increase in AA in SVCT2-Tg mice is dependent on level of over-expression, which varies among mice and in this small sample was only 1.3-2.0-fold compared to wild-type (not shown). Brain levels did not differ between supplemented (black triangles) and non-supplemented (grey triangles) SVCT1 knockout mice so combined average is shown. Normal brain levels can be achieved in gulo knockout mice with supplementation of at least 0.33 g/L, (shown here at supplementation with 1.0 g/L). Mean AA levels that share a superscript do not differ. Differing superscripts indicate significant difference [(a, b)] $p < 0.05$, [(c, d)] $p < 0.001$ by Univariate ANOVA with Tukey *post-hoc* comparisons (overall group effect $F(4,18) = 13.0$, $p < 0.001$).

SVCT2 transgenic mice: Recently, a new mouse line has been created that expresses additional copies of the SVCT2 [104]. This mouse has increased SVCT2 mRNA expression in all organs measured and a related increase in AA level in all organs except the liver, with up to two-fold increases in the brain, depending on mRNA expression. These mice were otherwise phenotypically indistinguishable from wild type but were more resistant to a severe oxidative stress in lung induced by paraquat. Although not designed to represent an attainable human situation, these mice may be able to inform on SVCT2 regulation and the role of vitamin C in high oxidative stress situations such as neurodegenerative disease.

4. Relation of Mice Models to Human Studies

A number of shortcomings exist to studies of AA in humans, such as accurate assessment of intake and determination of tissue levels of AA (discussed below). Thus, information from animal models can be critical to understanding changes in the brains of humans under AA deficiency. The gulo and SVCT2 knockout models have already been used to model long-term AA deficiency in disease states such as Alzheimer's disease, diabetes and atherosclerosis [88,105–107] by crossing them with other mouse models of disease (e.g., APP/PSEN1, ApoE). These models can even be crossed together to create *in vivo* models of extreme deficiency [108], although these may be less directly applicable to the human case. One key advantage to such models is the ability to investigate numerous biochemical correlates to disease and nutritional deficiency, including behavioral and cognition changes. Of course there are weaknesses to any animal model, particularly when genetic changes are artificially manufactured, and follow an all-or-none approach rather than the gradations of functional change from mutations seen in the general population. Nevertheless, the availability of models to study all aspects of transport and synthesis together provides a very strong future for pre-clinical AA research. It is important to note, however, that the changes reported in these models, particularly oxidative damage, or changes in neurotransmitter function, are not specific to Alzheimer's disease, and in fact are relevant to many types of neurodegenerative diseases, and to an extent in normal as well as pathological aging. For example, none of these mouse models exhibits robust cognitive deficits from AA deficiency alone. Future research must identify exact roles for AA in disease pathology, and how this can be applied specifically to Alzheimer's disease process as well as other disease states where applicable. This includes studying the impact of chronic deficiency resulting in sub-optimal brain levels, without clinical signs associated with scurvy. Knowledge of how AA transport and accumulation is regulated in specific brain areas, and how this may be affected by specific SNPs or disease states may permit better understanding of when and how best to intervene to correct levels, or how to identify populations that may be more at risk of deficiency.

5. Dietary Intake of Ascorbic Acid, Cognition and Alzheimer's Disease

Associations between risk for AD and AA intake have been investigated in several large population studies, both in the US and also in one large European sample. One early study appeared very promising when data was reported from the Chicago Healthy Aging Project (CHAP) showing that none of the 633 > 65 years old, dementia-free participants that supplemented with AA, developed AD over the follow up period (mean 4 years) [109]. Study of dietary intakes in the same cohort did not support the same protective effect of AA [110]. It may be that even the dietary levels ingested were insufficient for the protective effect and that supplements are necessary to maintain optimal levels. In the earlier study only supplementation was considered, as single nutrient, multi-vitamin or no supplement, without comment as to dose. In the latter study, while the median all-source intake was 124.7 mg/day, with 16.1% of population taking supplements of some kind, the intake ranges were very large. In the lowest quintile intake from food and supplements was estimated at below 93 mg/day and the highest quintile was between 310 and 2530 mg/day. In neither case are blood AA levels reported and thus it is difficult to accurately determine AA status in the different populations. The differences between dietary and synthetic AA intake, and their comparable bioavailability in humans, are discussed in this issue [111]. Self-reported AA intakes (alone or in combination with vitamin E) were not predictive of AD diagnosis in a cohort of nearly 5,000 participants aged 65 and older over the course of 5 years [112]. Nor were beneficial effects of AA intake observed in a study of 980 dementia-free men and women of the Washington Heights-Inwood Columbia Aging Project [113].

A more complex pattern of effects was reported in the Honolulu Asia Aging Study which comprised men aged 71 to 93 years [114]. In cognitively intact individuals, AA intake was associated with a higher likelihood for enhanced cognitive function. High AA and vitamin E intake were associated with lower likelihood for vascular dementia. In contrast, there was no relationship between AD diagnoses and AA intake. Findings from the Cache County Study [115] suggest that AA and vitamin E supplementation may have some synergistic effects in reducing risk for AD, but AA alone did not decrease risk for AD. Self reported intake questionnaires and telephone assessments of cognitive ability were used in the very large cohort of nearly 15,000 women in the Nurses health study. No consistent associations were found between AA and cognitive ability in this group [116,117].

Perhaps one of the most interesting results came from the Rotterdam Scan Study [118]. This large study of over 5000 participants reported an 18% reduced relative risk for AD with higher AA intake. Most revealing was that the most dramatic protective effects were seen in smokers. Smoking leads to rapid depletion of AA in plasma in addition to additional ROS generated following inhalation of smoke. It therefore seems likely that rescuing AA deficiency in this group may have been more useful than supplementing AA on top of dietary in healthier individuals.

If AA deficiency really is a key factor in the development of AD, then it might be expected that populations with poorer intake would be more prone to developing dementia, or follow a faster path of deterioration once diagnosed. For the most part these studies draw strength from the large sample sizes used, numbering in the thousands. On the other hand, reliance on dietary intake questionnaires may be problematic, particularly in a study of cognitive ability where reliability may be acutely affected by even mild changes in recall ability [119]. Current intake may not reflect lifetime dietary habits and given data that suggest that amyloid plaque burden begins to form well before middle age [120], intakes during younger adulthood may be equally as important as supplements taken by older adults, perhaps contributing to a biological buffer against disease pathogenesis. Overall, the two promising positive results are outweighed by the seven studies that did not confirm a link between AA and AD. Ideally, reliable biomarkers of diet should be employed instead, or preferably in addition to study of dietary intake [121]. Measurement of AA levels, preferably over several time points, permits determination of whether participants have deficient or depleted AA levels, and more importantly allow grouping according to AA level. In this way dietary *versus* supplemental intake is not as important as the resulting AA levels, and high level supplements, which, due to the limitations of the SVCT1 transporter in the intestines, may not functionally provide more AA than lower supplements or good diet, are not weighted more heavily and biasing results.

6. Blood Ascorbic Acid, Cognition and Alzheimer's Disease

For studies that have made measurements of biological AA levels in blood and/or CSF, the sample sizes are typically much lower than the population based studies described above (see Table 1). The logistics and cost of so many measurements may be prohibitive, and even in studies that have a prospective aspect, true control groups are not possible. It would be unethical to maintain one group of participants at low AA levels, and it is also not possible to control for lifetime dietary habits in these studies. Nevertheless, these cross sectional studies can certainly provide an accurate and useful picture of typical nutrition profiles in various populations, alongside cognitive analyses.

Table 1. Observational Studies of Ascorbic Acid Status in Dementia and Non-Impaired Elders (NIE) adapted from [122].

Authors	Sample	Design and Methods	Conclusion	Association y/n
Goodwin, 1983 [123]	260 dementia-free men/women Age $\geq$ 60 year Community-dwelling	Cross-sectional Plasma, 3 day diet recall Halstead-Reitan Categories Test, WMS-R delayed	Plasma AA associated with higher verbal memory; elders in the 90th percentile of plasma AA had better calculating ability and delayed recall	y
Gale, 1996 [124]	921 men/women Age $\geq$ 65 year English-Scottish-Welsh	Cross-sectional Plasma Hodkinson test	Plasma AA $\leq$ 11.91 µM was associated with 1.6 higher odds of cognitive impairment (95% CI: 1.1–2.3). Less than 27 mg of AA intake per day was associated with 1.7 higher odds for impairment	y
Riviere, 1998 [125]	19 ctls MMSE 24–30 20 severe AD MMSE 0–9 24 mod AD MMSE 10–23	Cross-sectional Plasma Mini-nutritional assessment	Plasma AA was incrementally lower by degree of cognitive impairment in AD, this observation was not explained by lower intake of AA	y
Charlton, 2004 [126]	93 men/women 50 ctls 43 dementia Age $\geq$ 65	Cross-sectional Plasma Mini-nutritional assessment	Plasma AA was lower in subjects with dementia compared to controls, this observation was not explained by lower intake of AA	y
Polidori, 2002 [127]	75 women 40 ctls (85.4 ± 4.4 year) 35 AD (85.9 ± 5.5 y) Age-matched Mean age 85 year	Cross-sectional Plasma NINCDS-ADRDA criteria	Plasma AA was lower in AD than controls (18 ± 6 µM *vs.* 36 ± 6, $p < 0.001$) AD subjects had increased plasma lipid peroxidation and less resistance to peroxyl-radical	y
Polidori, 2004 [128]	141 55 ctls 63 AD 23 VD	Cross-sectional Plasma	Plasma AA was lower in AD and VD *versus* NIE, no differences between AD and VD	y
Perrig, 1997 [129]	442 men/women (n = 312/132) Community-dwelling Age $\geq$ 65 (mean 75)	Prospective, cross-sectional Plasma Memory, WAIS-R vocabulary test	Plasma AA in 1971 associated with better cognitive performance in 1993; plasma AA associated with better free recall, recognition, and vocabulary, but not priming and working-memory in cross-sectional analysis	y

AD, Alzheimer's disease; VD, vascular dementia; Ctls, control subjects; NIE, non-impaired elders; AA, ascorbic acid; MMSE, mini-mental state exam (Folstein); NINCDS-ADRDA, National Institute of Neurological and Communicative Disorders and Stroke and the Alzheimer's Disease and Related Disorders Association; WAIS-R, Wechsler Adult Intelligence Scale—revised.

An early study by Goodwin *et al.* [123] used the revealing method of dividing participants into percentiles according to AA status. Using these methods verbal memory recall and calculations were indeed associated with higher plasma AA. In contrast, and in support of the idea that deficiency can impact development of AD and other dementias Gale *et al.* [124] report a significantly increased risk for cognitive impairment in those with depleted (<12 μM) plasma AA or very low intake (<28 mg/day). Higher plasma AA was associated with better free recall, recognition and vocabulary, but not working memory in a prospective sample of older men (>65 years) [129]. In general, plasma levels of AA in the above studies have been consistently observed to be around 20 μM in patients with AD, *i.e.*, about the half of those measured in controls [7,125,127]. In agreement with studies showing that plasma AA levels are depleted in AD independent of dietary intake, peripheral AA depletion in AD patients with respect to controls has been repeatedly confirmed after correction for age, gender, fruit and vegetable intake, and comorbidities [7,125,127]. Another element strongly suggestive of low AA levels as a co-causal factor for neurodegeneration and AD rather than epiphenomenon of AD is the observation of similarly depleted plasma AA levels in both MCI patients and AD patients compared to controls [7]. Comparison of all these studies where effects are on particular subtypes of memory of cognition, *versus* disease risk, may indicate that avoiding deficiency, and optimally supplementing with AA may benefit different facets of cognitive health. Nevertheless, the directions of effect seem to be in the same direction.

7. Cerebrospinal Fluid Ascorbic Acid, Cognition, and Alzheimer's Disease

Examination of the AA in the CSF reflects nutrient content with direct access to the brain parenchyma. This proximal representation should be considered the gold standard of brain nutrition in living subjects [130]. Presumably owing to the more intrusive nature of the testing far fewer studies have reported CSF AA (Table 2).

Paraskevas *et al.* [131] report high variation in plasma AA levels in hospitalized groups of 17 AD, 19 amyotrophic lateral sclerosis and 15 control patients, but reasonably stable CSF levels. They conclude that maintenance of the plasma:CSF ratio must be due to appropriate action of the SVCT2 at the choroid plexus. Lack of data on dietary intakes and case classifications limit the full utility of this study. Quinn *et al.* [132] examined the cross-sectional differences in CSF and plasma AA between 10 AD cases *versus* 10 healthy controls. Another cross-sectional study conducted by Glaso *et al.* [133] examined the mean differences between plasma and CSF AA in women with and without dementia of AD type. In both of these studies mean plasma and CSF AA were less (although not significantly in [132]) and the CSF-to-plasma AA ratio was higher in AD *versus* controls.

Table 2. Observational studies of CSF Ascorbic Acid, Cognitive Function, and Alzheimer's disease * adapted from [122].

Authors	Sample & Design	Plasma, μM		CSF, μM		CSF:Plasma Ratio		Conclusion
		Ctls	AD	Ctls	AD	Ctls	AD	
Paraskevas, 1997 [131]	32 15 ctls (58 ± 12 year) 17 AD (62 ± 7 year) Men/women Age-gender matched Cross-sectional	43 ± 13	45 ± 19	166 ± 45	156 ± 38	3.6 ± 0.5	4.1 ± 1.6	No differences between AD and controls
Quinn, 2003 [132]	20 10 Ctls (MMSE 29 ± 1), 10 AD (MMSE 19 ± 7) Age-gender matched Mean age 66 y Cross-sectional	86 ± 39	58 ± 42	238 ± 48	207 ± 64	3.1 ± 1.1	5.0 ± 2.6	CSF: plasma AA ratio higher in AD ($p = 0.048$). Mean plasma and CSF AA were lower in AD, but not significantly.
Glaso, 2004 [133]	38 18 Ctls (MMSE 27), 20 AD (MMSE 16) Women Age-matched (75–85 year) Cross- sectional	80 ± 28	44 ± 25	167 ± 23	140 ± 37	2.1 ± 0.7	3.3 ± 1.4	CSF: serum AA ratio higher in AD *versus* controls ($p = 0.001$) but both plasma ($p = 0.002$) and CSF ($p = 0.038$) AA were lower in AD. Subjects were well-nourished and without vascular disease
Bowman, 2009 [134]	32 AD (MMSE 19 ± 5) Men/women Mean age 71 year Prospective		41 ± 30		129 ± 52		4.0 ± 1.6	Neither plasma nor CSF AA was predictive, but CSF: plasma AA ratio associated with slower cognitive decline over 1 year (age, gender, education, apoEe4, and cognitive function at baseline adjusted $p = 0.025$). Interaction between CSF AA Ratio and BBB integrity suggesting AA leaking from brain to periphery

Table 2. *Cont.*

Arlt 2012 [135]	23 AD men/women, already taking cholinesterase inhibitors. Randomized to AA (2 × 500 mg/day) and vitamin E (400 IU/day) (Age 67.7 ± 7.2, baseline MMSE 20.0 ± 5.3)	Baseline 201.4 ± 25.9, 1 month 229.9 ± 36.7, 12 months 233.6 ± 44.8	Not measured	No direct effect of antioxidants on performance, however supplements did increase AA and vitamin E in CSF, with antioxidant effect. Greater oxidation of CSF lipids was associated with faster decline of cognitive ability
	No supplements (Age 73.7 ± 5.3, baseline MMSE 21.7 ± 5.5)	Not measured	Not measured	
Galasko 2012 [136]	16 weeks with 500 mg/day AA, plus 800 IU alpha-tocopherol and 900 mg/day alpha-lipoic acid in subjects with mild to moderate AD	Not measured	Not measured	Measures of CSF oxidative stress were decreased, but amyloid and tau markers were not. Nor were there any beneficial effects on cognitive decline.

* Total of 79 AD and 43 controls with CSF AA analysis; Ctls, control subjects; AD, Alzheimer's disease subjects; MMSE, mini-mental state exam.

Ideally, such studies would be prospective, with baseline and later AA levels taken of both plasma and CSF AA across at least one year, in addition to cognitive assessment. One such prospective analysis also included CSF Albumin Index to reflect blood-brain barrier integrity in living probable mild to moderate AD patients over a year [134]. However, a higher CSF-to-plasma AA ratio was associated with a slower rate of decline although neither plasma nor CSF AA alone was predictive. The relationship between CSF AA ratio and rate of decline was attenuated when CSF Albumin Index (a validated measure of BBB integrity) was added to the regression model. These findings suggest that maintenance of high CSF-to-plasma AA ratio may be important to preventing cognitive decline in AD and that BBB impairment unfavorably alters this ratio. This study was unable to distinguish whether transport mechanisms for AA (*i.e.*, SVCT2) were disturbed as well as the integrity of the BBB since the CSF albumin index reflects only barrier disturbances to our knowledge. How much of this "barrier" impairment is accompanied by "carrier" dysfunction is one area for future research interest.

A recent study on dietary supplements examined the antioxidant effect of 1000 mg AA per day (two × 500 mg) plus 400 IU vitamin E in mild to moderate AD patients who were also taking cholinesterase inhibitors [135]. In this relatively small, open label study, one year of supplements did not have a direct effect on cognition. Nevertheless, the authors were able to successfully demonstrate that supplements led to higher AA and vitamin E in the CSF and also decreased lipid peroxidation in the CSF. Greater levels of oxidation were also associated with faster cognitive decline. Unfortunately CSF was only measured in the supplement group, and dietary intake, or baseline group differences were not accounted for (although none of the subjects was taking supplements at the start of the study). In an additional study supplementation for 16 weeks with 500 mg/d AA with 800 IU/d vitamin E and 900 mg/day alpha-lipoic acid in 24 mild to moderately affected AD patients screened to exclude cases of vascular disease, were compared to 18 controls [136]. The antioxidant mix was also found to decrease oxidative stress in the CSF (F_2-isoprostanes), however, no effects were seen on CSF $A\beta_{1\text{-}42}$, tau or *p*-tau. No improvements were seen in cognition, in fact this group appeared to suffer faster cognitive decline. Critically, all subjects in the study were allowed to continue taking their own vitamin supplements up to 200 mg/day AA, this included 52% of the antioxidant group and 43% of controls. AA levels at baseline or following treatment are not reported, and thus it is not possible to assess whether groups truly differ; 200 mg/day in a supplement plus a reasonable diet could permit AA repletion in the placebo group and mitigate the chance of seeing differences in cognition although the oxidative stress data clearly indicates benefits of the antioxidant cocktail. A recent review of several studies above concluded that CSF levels within normal range for AA (and folate and additional CSF proteins), despite lower plasma levels indicated preservation of choroid plexus function and AA transport into CSF [137]. However, they also discuss the lack of definitive data on potential for change in CSF volume or turnover.

8. Ascorbic Acid and Vascular Cognitive Aging

The primary focus of this review is on AD, both with and without a vascular component. The main pathological hallmarks of AD (amyloid and tau deposits, neuronal death, neurotransmitter signaling, synaptic density) are shared across cases because the nature of AD is multifactorial.

However, in the same way that many of these symptoms are also found in other cases of dementia, e.g., pure vascular dementia, frontotemporal dementia, dementia with lewy bodies, it can easily be argued that many of the findings described are related to neurodegeneration in general and are thus applicable to many dementias and even normal aging. Previous schools of thought have considered vascular- *versus* AD-type dementia cases as separate entities, however accumulating evidence suggests that vascular pathology plays a central role in AD onset and development [138–140]. In a community sample of older adults (75+ years) almost 50% of the clinically diagnosed AD cases showed a possible vascular component [141]. Similarly, the next most prevalent dementia form, vascular dementia, presents overlapping traditional hallmarks of AD including amyloid-β accumulation. As a direct consequence of this complexity, a cure is difficult to find, and prevention becomes even more critical. The role of AA has recently been reviewed in relation to endothelial cell function, which may explain importance in its role in vascular health. In addition to the more well-known functions of AA such as synthesis and deposition of collagen in the basement membrane and antioxidant defense against ROS, other roles include stimulating endothelial proliferation, inhibiting apoptosis, and sparing endothelial cell-derived nitric oxide to help modulate blood flow [15].

The ability of AA to prevent age-associated cognitive decline and dementia risk may require a population with high vascular risk. AA has demonstrated some ability to reduce vascular risk factors and more recently vascular comorbidities are being acknowledged as important factors to reduce for prevention of age related dementias [138,139,142–147]. Some of the "vascular" mechanisms include: (1) reducing carotid intima-media-thickness [2,148]; (2) reducing lipid peroxidation [3,4,149–151]; and (3) reducing endothelial dysfunction [15].

We recently observed healthy elderly in the lowest plasma AA tertile at higher risk of carotid intima-media thickness >1.2 mm; a threshold established as pathologic by the European Society of Hypertension and the European Society of Cardiology 2007. It should be noted that this relationship was not appreciated with other antioxidants that include: uric acid, vitamins A and E, and enzymatic enzymes superoxide dismutase and glutathione oxidase activity. Another study of 8453 participants in NHANES II concluded that individuals with plasma AA ≥ 45.4 μM had a 21%–25% reduced risk for CVD-related death and a 25%–29% reduced risk of all-cause mortality compared to the participants with plasma AA < 23 μM [152]. In the European Prospective Investigation into Cancer and Nutrition (EPIC)-Norfolk study [153] a 33% lower risk of developing coronary heart disease was shown in subjects with the highest plasma AA compared to the lowest (mean, 27.6 μM) over six years of follow up. Long in advance to these results, the EPIC-Norfolk study had found that plasma AA concentrations in 8860 men and 10,636 women were inversely correlated to mortality from all causes and CVD. In this study, each 20 μmol/liter increase in plasma AA was associated with a 20%–30% reduction in risk for all-cause and CVD mortality [154]. When 563 elderly men were randomly allocated to one of four treatment groups in a clinical trial that included dietary intervention, omega-3 supplementation, both or neither, carotid intima-media thickness progression over a three-year term was reduced in those undergoing dietary intervention that included daily AA intake [155]. Vitamin E [156] or combined antioxidants [157] in the dietary intervention groups were not successful.

These data suggest that AA has a role in modifying vascular risk factors and vascular disease, which could represent mechanisms by which AA might reduce dementia risk in people carrying this vascular risk profile [158].

Recent research has demonstrated that it is now possible to non-invasively measure AA (and GSH) levels in the human brain using MEGA-PRESS MRI (a type of spectroscopic MRI imaging) [159]. These techniques were used to compare AA, GSH and lactate in brain in 22 young (20 years) *versus* 22 normally aging (76.6 years) subjects [160]. The study reported decreased GSH and increased lactate with age, indicating oxidative damage, but no change in AA between the groups. The authors recruited candidates that ate less than five fruits and vegetables per day and did not take supplements, then provided food calculated to contain 30 mg/1000 kcal in an attempt to provide all subjects with the recommended daily intake. Thus, potential group differences were already minimized, and at ~60 mg/day circulating and brain AA levels may still have been sub-optimal in all subjects, reflected by the estimated brain levels of 0.4–1.2 μmol/g (their Figure 3 [160]) tissue wet weight. It is reported that brain AA content was not associated with AA in blood, however these data are not recorded. So although this study does not provide a definitive statement of AA in brain in the elderly, development of this fascinating and ingenious technique to measure AA in brain may add a critical factor to future studies of the role of AA in the brain.

9. Conclusion

This review highlights several key points relating to the role of AA in healthy brain aging: (1) both human and animal studies demonstrate AA deficiency in association with oxidative stress markers, and oxidative stress is a consistent observation in AD; (2) there is inconsistency among the large observational studies relating dietary intake of AA to cognition. However, it remains unclear whether this inconsistency is methodological in nature (e.g., the subjective dietary surveys used to capture AA intake) since biomarkers of both AA (and oxidative stress) present more consistent results favouring an important role for AA in cognitive health; (3) there are genetic (SVCT1 and SVCT2 SNPs) and non-genetic (e.g., age) factors that modulate AA absorption and assimilation, which could indicate an increased demand for AA in subsets of the population such as the elderly and those with an AD diagnosis. Thus, we do not suggest that AA deficiency in isolation can explain AD neuro- and psycho-pathology, however, we do propose more research focused on investigating the specific role of AA in AD pathogenesis with meticulous attention to the study design (e.g., people with low AA and high vascular risk may be best suited for intervention). This activity should provide more conclusive data on this remarkable micronutrient highly concentrated in the brain.

Acknowledgments

FEH is supported by grant AG038739 from the NIA. GLB is supported by grant NIH/NCCAM AT004777 and NIH/NIA AG043398. The authors would like to thank Jack Petros for technical assistance in tissue collection and measurement of ascorbic acid levels.

References

1. Nishikimi, M.; Fukuyama, R.; Minoshima, S.; Yagi, K. Cloning and chromosomal mapping of the human nonfunctional gene for L-gulono-gamma-lactone oxidase, the enzyme for L-ascorbic acid biosynthesis missing in man. *J. Biol. Chem.* **1994**, *269*, 13685–13688.
2. Frei, B.; England, L.; Ames, B.N. Ascorbate is an outstanding antioxidant in human blood plasma. *Proc. Natl. Acad. Sci. USA* **1989**, *86*, 6377–6381.
3. Berger, T.M.; Polidori, M.C.; Dabbagh, A.; Evans, P.J.; Halliwell, B.; Morrow, J.D.; Roberts, L.J., II; Frei, B. Antioxidant activity of vitamin C in iron-overloaded human plasma. *J. Biol. Chem.* **1997**, *272*, 15656–15660.
4. Traber, M.G.; Stevens, J.F. Vitamins C and E: Beneficial effects from a mechanistic perspective. *Free Radic. Biol. Med.* **1997**, *51*, 1000–1013.
5. Prince, M.; Bryce, R.; Albanese, E.; Wimo, A.; Ribeiro, W.; Ferri, C.P. The global prevalence of dementia: A systematic review and metaanalysis. *Alzheimer's Dement.* **2013**, *9*, 63–75 e62.
6. Pratico, D.; Clark, C.M.; Liun, F.; Rokach, J.; Lee, V.Y.; Trojanowski, J.Q. Increase of brain oxidative stress in mild cognitive impairment: A possible predictor of Alzheimer disease. *Arch. Neurol.* **2002**, *59*, 972–976.
7. Rinaldi, P.; Polidori, M.C.; Metastasio, A.; Mariani, E.; Mattioli, P.; Cherubini, A.; Catani, M.; Cecchetti, R.; Senin, U.; Mecocci, P. Plasma antioxidants are similarly depleted in mild cognitive impairment and in Alzheimer's disease. *Neurobiol. Aging* **2003**, *24*, 915–919.
8. Mecocci, P.; Polidori, M.C. Antioxidant clinical trials in mild cognitive impairment and Alzheimer's disease. *Biochim. Biophys. Acta* **2012**, *1822*, 631–638.
9. Mangialasche, F.; Kivipelto, M.; Mecocci, P.; Rizzuto, D.; Palmer, K.; Winblad, B.; Fratiglioni, L. High plasma levels of vitamin E forms and reduced Alzheimer's disease risk in advanced age. *J. Alzheimer's Dis. (JAD)* **2010**, *20*, 1029–1037.
10. Raynaud-Simon, A.; Cohen-Bittan, J.; Gouronnec, A.; Pautas, E.; Senet, P.; Verny, M.; Boddaert, J. Scurvy in hospitalized elderly patients. *J. Nutr. Health Aging* **2010**, *14*, 407–410.
11. Harrison, F.E.; Green, R.J.; Dawes, S.M.; May, J.M. Vitamin C distribution and retention in the mouse brain. *Brain Res.* **2010**, *1348*, 181–186.
12. Brubacher, D.; Moser, U.; Jordan, P. Vitamin C concentrations in plasma as a function of intake: A meta-analysis. *Int. J. Vitam Nutr. Res.* **2000**, *70*, 226–237.
13. Harrison, F.E.; May, J.M. Vitamin C function in the brain: vital role of the ascorbate transporter SVCT2. *Free Radic Biol. Med.* **2009**, *46*, 719–730.
14. Kaliora, A.C.; Dedoussis, G.V.; Schmidt, H. Dietary antioxidants in preventing atherogenesis. *Atherosclerosis* **2006**, *187*, 1–17.
15. May, J.M.; Harrison, F.E. Role of Vitamin C in the Function of the Vascular Endothelium. *Antioxid. Redox Signal.* **2013**, *19*, 2068–2083.
16. Proper, E.A.; Hoogland, G.; Kappen, S.M.; Jansen, G.H.; Rensen, M.G.; Schrama, L.H.; van Veelen, C.W.; van Rijen, P.C.; van Nieuwenhuizen, O.; Gispen, W.H.; *et al.* Distribution of glutamate transporters in the hippocampus of patients with pharmaco-resistant temporal lobe epilepsy. *Brain* **2002**, *125*, 32–43.

17. Wilson, J.X.; Peters, C.E.; Sitar, S.M.; Daoust, P.; Gelb, A.W. Glutamate stimulates ascorbate transport by astrocytes. *Brain Res.* **2000**, *858*, 61–66.
18. Estrada-Sanchez, A.M.; Rebec, G.V. Corticostriatal dysfunction and glutamate transporter 1 (GLT1) in Huntington's disease: Interactions between neurons and astrocytes. *Basal Ganglia* **2012**, *2*, 57–66.
19. Ballaz, S.; Morales, I.; Rodriguez, M.; Obeso, J.A. Ascorbate prevents cell death from prolonged exposure to glutamate in an *in vitro* model of human dopaminergic neurons. *J. Neurosci. Res.* **2013**, *91*, 1609–1617.
20. Dorner, J.L.; Miller, B.R.; Klein, E.L.; Murphy-Nakhnikian, A.; Andrews, R.L.; Barton, S.J.; Rebec, G.V. Corticostriatal dysfunction underlies diminished striatal ascorbate release in the R6/2 mouse model of Huntington's disease. *Brain Res.* **2009**, *1290*, 111–120.
21. Rebec, G.V.; Pierce, R.C. A vitamin as neuromodulator: Ascorbate release into the extracellular fluid of the brain regulates dopaminergic and glutamatergic transmission. *Prog. Neurobiol.* **1994**, *43*, 537–565.
22. Rebec, G.V.; Barton, S.J.; Marseilles, A.M.; Collins, K. Ascorbate treatment attenuates the Huntington behavioral phenotype in mice. *Neuroreport* **2003**, *14*, 1263–1265.
23. Spector, R.; Johanson, C.E. The nexus of vitamin homeostasis and DNA synthesis and modification in mammalian brain. *Mol. Brain* **2014**, *7*, 3.
24. Blaschke, K.; Ebata, K.T.; Karimi, M.M.; Zepeda-Martinez, J.A.; Goyal, P.; Mahapatra, S.; Tam, A.; Laird, D.J.; Hirst, M.; Rao, A.; *et al.* Vitamin C induces Tet-dependent DNA demethylation and a blastocyst-like state in ES cells. *Nature* **2013**, *500*, 222–226.
25. Yin, R.; Mao, S.Q.; Zhao, B.; Chong, Z.; Yang, Y.; Zhao, C.; Zhang, D.; Huang, H.; Gao, J.; Li, Z.; *et al.* Ascorbic acid enhances Tet-mediated 5-methylcytosine oxidation and promotes DNA demethylation in mammals. *J. Am. Chem. Soc.* **2013**, *135*, 10396–10403.
26. Minor, E.A.; Court, B.L.; Young, J.I.; Wang, G. Ascorbate induces ten-eleven translocation (Tet) methylcytosine dioxygenase-mediated generation of 5-hydroxymethylcytosine. *J. Biol. Chem.* **2013**, *288*, 13669–13674.
27. Rudenko, A.; Dawlaty, M.M.; Seo, J.; Cheng, A.W.; Meng, J.; Le, T.; Faull, K.F.; Jaenisch, R.; Tsai, L.H. Tet1 is critical for neuronal activity-regulated gene expression and memory extinction. *Neuron* **2013**, *79*, 1109–1122.
28. Meister, A. Glutathione, ascorbate, and cellular protection. *Cancer Res.* **1994**, *54*, 1969s–1975s.
29. Smuda, D.G.M. Maillard degradation pathways of vitamin C. *Angew. Chem. Int. Ed.* **2013**, *52*, 4887–4891.
30. Fan, X.; Reneker, L.W.; Obrenovich, M.E.; Strauch, C.; Cheng, R.; Jarvis, S.M.; Ortwerth, B.J.; Monnier, V.M. Vitamin C mediates chemical aging of lens crystallins by the Maillard reaction in a humanized mouse model. *Proc. Natl. Acad. Sci. USA* **2006**, *103*, 16912–16917.
31. Carr, A.; Frei, B. Does vitamin C act as a pro-oxidant under physiological conditions? *FASEB J.* **1999**, *13*, 1007–1024.
32. Halliwell, B. Vitamin C: Antioxidant or pro-oxidant *in vivo*? *Free Radic. Res.* **1996**, *25*, 439–454.
33. Premkumar, K.; Bowlus, C.L. Ascorbic acid does not increase the oxidative stress induced by dietary iron in C3H mice. *J. Nutr.* **2004**, *134*, 435–438.

34. Collis, C.S.; Yang, M.; Diplock, A.T.; Hallinan T.; Rice-Evans, C.A. Effects of co-supplementation of iron with ascorbic acid on antioxidant—Pro-oxidant balance in the guinea pig. *Free Radic. Res.* **1997**, *27*, 113–121.

35. Gerster, H. High-dose vitamin C: A risk for persons with high iron stores? *Int. J. Vitam Nutr. Res.* **1999**, *69*, 67–82.

36. Loef, M.; Walach, H. Copper and iron in Alzheimer's disease: A systematic review and its dietary implications. *Br. J. Nutr.* **2012**, *107*, 7–19.

37. Crespo, A.C.; Silva, B.; Marques, L.; Marcelino, E.; Maruta, C.; Costa, S.;Timoteo, A.; Vilares, A.; Couto, F.S.; Faustino, P.; *et al.* Genetic and biochemical markers in patients with Alzheimer's disease support a concerted systemic iron homeostasis dysregulation. *Neurobiol. Aging* **2014**, *35*, 777–785.

38. Sinha, M.; Bhowmick, P.; Banerjee, A.; Chakrabarti, S. Antioxidant role of amyloid beta protein in cell-free and biological systems: Implication for the pathogenesis of Alzheimer disease. *Free Radic. Biol. Med.* **2013**, *56*, 184–192.

39. Hammarstrom, L. Autoradiographic studies on the distribution of C14-labelled ascorbic acid and dehydroascorbic acid. *Acta Physiol. Scand.* **1966**, *70*, 3–83.

40. Spector, R.; Lorenzo, A.V. Ascorbic acid homeostasis in the central nervous system. *Am. J. Physiol.* **1973**, *225*, 757–763.

41. Savini, I.; Rossi, A.; Pierro, C.; Avigliano, L.; Catani, M.V. SVCT1 and SVCT2: Key proteins for vitamin C uptake. *Amino Acids* **2008**, *34*, 347–355.

42. Tsukaguchi, H.; Tokui, T.; Mackenzie, B.; Berger, U.V.; Chen, X.Z.; Wang, Y.; Brubaker, R.F.; Hediger, M.A. A family of mammalian Na+-dependent L-ascorbic acid transporters. *Nature* **1999**, *399*, 70–75.

43. Wang, Y.; Mackenzie, B.; Tsukaguchi, H.; Weremowicz, S.; Morton, C.C.; Hediger, M.A. Human vitamin C (L-ascorbic acid) transporter SVCT1. *Biochem. Biophys. Res. Commun.* **2000**, *267*, 488–494.

44. Lindblad, M.; Tveden-Nyborg, P.; Lykkesfeldt, J. Regulation of Vitamin C Homeostasis during Deficiency. *Nutrients* **2013**, *5*, 2860–2879.

45. Erichsen, H.C.; Eck, P.; Levine, M.; Chanock, S. Characterization of the genomic structure of the human vitamin C transporter SVCT1 (SLC23A2). *J. Nutr.* **2001**, *131*, 2623–2627.

46. Erichsen, H.C.; Peters, U.; Eck, P.; Welch, R.; Schoen, R.E.; Yeager, M.; Levine, M.; Hayes, R.B.; Chanock, S. Genetic variation in sodium-dependent vitamin C transporters SLC23A1 and SLC23A2 and risk of advanced colorectal adenoma. *Nutr. Cancer* **2008**, *60*, 652–659.

47. Michels, A.J.; Hagen, T.M.; Frei, B. Human genetic variation influences vitamin C homeostasis by altering vitamin C transport and antioxidant enzyme function. *Annu. Rev. Nutr.* **2013**, *33*, 45–70.

48. Eck, P.; Erichsen, H.C.; Taylor, J.G.; Corpe, C.; Chanock, S.J.; Levine, M. Genomic and functional analysis of the sodium-dependent vitamin C transporter SLC23A1-SVCT1. *Genes Nutr.* **2007**, *2*, 143–145.

49. Corpe, C.P.; Tu, H.; Eck, P.; Wang, J.; Faulhaber-Walter, R.; Schnermann, J.; Margolis, S.; Padayatty, S.; Sun, H.; Wang, Y.; *et al.* Vitamin C transporter Slc23a1 links renal reabsorption, vitamin C tissue accumulation, and perinatal survival in mice. *J. Clin. Investig.* **2010**, *120*, 1069–1083.
50. Hierro, C.; Monte, M.J.; Lozano, E.; Gonzalez-Sanchez, E.; Marin, J.J.; Macias, R.I. Liver metabolic/oxidative stress induces hepatic and extrahepatic changes in the expression of the vitamin C transporters SVCT1 and SVCT2. *Eur. J. Nutr.* **2014**, *53*, 401–412.
51. Gess, B.; Sevimli, S.; Strecker, J.K.; Young, P.; Schabitz, W.R. Sodium-dependent vitamin C transporter 2 (SVCT2) expression and activity in brain capillary endothelial cells after transient ischemia in mice. *PLoS One* **2011**, *6*, e17139.
52. May, J.M.; Qu, Z.C. Ascorbic acid prevents increased endothelial permeability caused by oxidized low density lipoprotein. *Free Radic. Res.* **2010**, *44*, 1359–1368.
53. May, J.M.; Qu, Z.C. Ascorbic acid prevents oxidant-induced increases in endothelial permeability. *Biofactors* **2011**, *37*, 46–50.
54. Amano, A.; Aigaki, T.; Maruyama, N.; Ishigami, A. Ascorbic acid depletion enhances expression of the sodium-dependent vitamin C transporters, SVCT1 and SVCT2, and uptake of ascorbic acid in livers of SMP30/GNL knockout mice. *Arch. Biochem. Biophys.* **2010**, *496*, 38–44.
55. Meredith, M.E.; Harrison, F.E.; May, J.M. Differential regulation of the ascorbic acid transporter SVCT2 during development and in response to ascorbic acid depletion. *Biochem. Biophys. Res. Commun.* **2011**, *414*, 737–742.
56. Nualart, F.; Castro, T.; Low, M.; Henriquez, J.P.; Oyarce, K.; Cisternas, P.; Garcia, A.; Yanez, A.J.; Bertinat, R.; Montecinos, V.P.; *et al.* Dynamic expression of the sodium-vitamin C co-transporters, SVCT1 and SVCT2, during perinatal kidney development. *Histochem. Cell Biol.* **2013**, *139*, 233–247.
57. Jimenez-Fernandez, E.; Ponce, M.; Zuasti, E.; Fernandez-Diaz, C.; Manchado, M.; Infante, C. Molecular characterization and transcriptional regulation of the sodium-dependent vitamin C transporter genes (slc23a1 and slc23a2) in a teleost fish, the Senegalese sole (Solea senegalensis). *Comp. Biochem. Physiol. Part B Biochem. Mol. Biol.* **2012**, *161*, 208–218.
58. Gess, B.; Lohmann, C.; Halfter, H.; Young, P. Sodium-dependent vitamin C transporter 2 (SVCT2) is necessary for the uptake of L-ascorbic acid into Schwann cells. *Glia* **2010**, *58*, 287–299.
59. Maulen, N.P.; Henriquez, E.A.; Kempe, S.; Carcamo, J.G.; Schmid-Kotsas, A.; Bachem, M.; Grunert, A.; Bustamante, M.E.; Nualart, F.; Vera, J.C. Up-regulation and polarized expression of the sodium-ascorbic acid transporter SVCT1 in post-confluent differentiated CaCo-2 cells. *J. Biol. Chem.* **2003**, *278*, 9035–9041.
60. Boyer, J.C.; Campbell, C.E.; Sigurdson, W.J.; Kuo, S.M. Polarized localization of vitamin C transporters, SVCT1 and SVCT2, in epithelial cells. *Biochem. Biophys. Res. Commun.* **2005**, *334*, 150–156.
61. MacDonald, L.; Thumser, A.E.; Sharp, P. Decreased expression of the vitamin C transporter SVCT1 by ascorbic acid in a human intestinal epithelial cell line. *Br. J. Nutr.* **2002**, *87*, 97–100.

62. Varma, S.; Sobey, K.; Campbell, C.E.; Kuo, S.M. Hierarchal contribution of N- and C-terminal sequences to the differential localization of homologous sodium-dependent vitamin C transporters, SVCT1 and SVCT2, in epithelial cells. *Biochemistry* **2009**, *48*, 2969–2980.
63. May, J.M.; Li, L.; Qu, Z.C. Oxidized LDL up-regulates the ascorbic acid transporter SVCT2 in endothelial cells. *Mol. Cell. Biochem.* **2010**, *343*, 217–222.
64. Qiao, H.; May, J.M. Development of ascorbate transporters in brain cortical capillary endothelial cells in culture. *Brain Res.* **2008**, *1208*, 79–86.
65. Chothe, P.P.; Chutkan, N.; Sangani, R.; Wenger, K.H.; Prasad, P.D.; Thangaraju, M.; Hamrick, M.W.; Isales, C.M.; Ganapathy, V.; Fulzele, S. Sodium-coupled vitamin C transporter (SVCT2): expression, function, and regulation in intervertebral disc cells. *Spine J.* **2013**, *13*, 549–557.
66. Berger, U.V.; Hediger, M.A. The vitamin C transporter SVCT2 is expressed by astrocytes in culture but not *in situ*. *Neuroreport* **2000**, *11*, 1395–1399.
67. Korcok, J.; Yan, R.; Siushansian, R.; Dixon, S.J.; Wilson, J.X. Sodium-ascorbate cotransport controls intracellular ascorbate concentration in primary astrocyte cultures expressing the SVCT2 transporter. *Brain Res.* **2000**, *881*, 144–151.
68. Oke, A.F.; May, L.; Adams, R.N. Ascorbic acid distribution patterns in human brain. A comparison with nonhuman mammalian species. *Ann. N. Y. Acad. Sci.* **1987**, *498*, 1–12.
69. Mefford, I.N.; Oke, A.F.; Adams, R.N. Regional distribution of ascorbate in human brain. *Brain Res.* **1981**, *212*, 223–226.
70. Rice, M.E.; Russo-Menna, I. Differential compartmentalization of brain ascorbate and glutathione between neurons and glia. *Neuroscience* **1998**, *82*, 1213–1223.
71. Caprile, T.; Salazar, K.; Astuya, A.; Cisternas, P.; Silva-Alvarez, C.; Montecinos, H.; Millan, C.; de Los Angeles Garcia, M.; Nualart, F. The Na+-dependent L-ascorbic acid transporter SVCT2 expressed in brainstem cells, neurons, and neuroblastoma cells is inhibited by flavonoids. *J. Neurochem.* **2009**, *108*, 563–577.
72. Qiu, S.; Li, L.; Weeber, E.J.; May, J.M. Ascorbate transport by primary cultured neurons and its role in neuronal function and protection against excitotoxicity. *J. Neurosci. Res.* **2007**, *85*, 1046–1056.
73. Mun, G.H.; Kim, M.J.; Lee, J.H.; Kim, H.J.; Chung, Y.H.; Chung, Y.B.; Kang, J.S.; Hwang, Y.I.; Oh, S.H.; Kim, J.G.; *et al.* Immunohistochemical study of the distribution of sodium-dependent vitamin C transporters in adult rat brain. *J. Neurosci. Res.* **2006**, *83*, 919–928.
74. Garcia Mde, L.; Salazar, K.; Millan, C.; Rodriguez, F.; Montecinos, H.; Caprile, T.; Silva, C.; Cortes, C.; Reinicke, K.; Vera, J.C.; *et al.* Sodium vitamin C cotransporter SVCT2 is expressed in hypothalamic glial cells. *Glia* **2005**, *50*, 32–47.
75. Chinoy, N.J.; Sanjeevan, A.G. On the specificity of alcoholic acidic silver nitrate reagent for the histochemical localization of ascorbic acid. A reappraisal. *Histochemistry* **1978**, *56*, 275–282.
76. Berger, U.V.; Lu, X.C.; Liu, W.; Tang, Z.; Slusher, B.S.; Hediger, M.A. Effect of middle cerebral artery occlusion on mRNA expression for the sodium-coupled vitamin C transporter SVCT2 in rat brain. *J. Neurochem.* **2003**, *86*, 896–906.

77. McHenry, E.W.; Reedman, E.J.; Sheppard, M. The physiological properties of ascorbic acid: An effect upon the weights of guinea-pigs. *Biochem. J.* **1938**, *32*, 1302–1304.

78. Svirbely, J.L.; Szent-Gyorgyi, A. The chemical nature of vitamin C. *Biochem. J.* **1932**, *26*, 865–870.

79. Szent-Gyorgyi, A.H.W.N. "Hexuronic Acid" (Ascorbic Acid) as the Antiscorbutic Factor. *Nature* **1933**, *131*, 24.

80. Anderson WES, A.H. The effect of acute scurvy on the subsequent nutrition and growth of guinea pigs. *J. Biol. Chem.* 1924, *61*, 181–191.

81. Burk, R.F.; Christensen, J.M.; Maguire, M.J.; Austin, L.M.; Whetsell, W.O., Jr.; May, J.M.; Hill, K.E.; Ebner, F.F. A combined deficiency of vitamins E and C causes severe central nervous system damage in guinea pigs. *J. Nutr.* **2006**, *136*, 1576–1581.

82. Hill, K.E.; Motley, A.K.; May, J.M.; Burk, R.F. Combined selenium and vitamin C deficiency causes cell death in guinea pig skeletal muscle. *Nutr. Res.* **2009**, *29*, 213–219.

83. Frikke-Schmidt, H.; Lykkesfeldt, J. Role of marginal vitamin C deficiency in atherogenesis: *In vivo* models and clinical studies. *Basic Clin. Pharmacol. Toxicol.* **2009**, *104*, 419–433.

84. Maeda, N.; Hagihara, H.; Nakata, Y.; Hiller, S.; Wilder, J.; Reddick, R. Aortic wall damage in mice unable to synthesize ascorbic acid. *Proc. Natl. Acad. Sci. USA* **2000**, *97*, 841–846.

85. Harrison, F.E.; Meredith, M.E.; Dawes, S.M.; Saskowski, J.L.; May, J.M. Low ascorbic acid and increased oxidative stress in gulo(−/−) mice during development. *Brain Res.* **2010**, *1349*, 143–152.

86. Harrison, F.E.; Yu, S.S.; Van Den Bossche, K.L.; Li, L.; May, J.M.; McDonald, M.P. Elevated oxidative stress and sensorimotor deficits but normal cognition in mice that cannot synthesize ascorbic acid. *J. Neurochem.* **2008**, *106*, 1198–1208.

87. Chen, Y.; Curran, C.P.; Nebert, D.W.; Patel, K.V.; Williams, M.T.; Vorhees, C.V. Effect of vitamin C deficiency during postnatal development on adult behavior: functional phenotype of Gulo(−/−) knockout mice. *Genes Brain Behav.* **2012**, *11*, 269–277.

88. Harrison, F.E.; May, J.M.; McDonald, M.P. Vitamin C deficiency increases basal exploratory activity but decreases scopolamine-induced activity in APP/PSEN1 transgenic mice. *Pharmacol. Biochem. Behav.* **2010**, *94*, 543–552.

89. Duggan, G.E.; Joan Miller, B.; Jirik, F.R.; Vogel, H.J. Metabolic profiling of vitamin C deficiency in Gulo−/− mice using proton NMR spectroscopy. *J. Biomol. NMR* **2011**, *49*, 165–173.

90. Vissers, M.C.; Wilkie, R.P. Ascorbate deficiency results in impaired neutrophil apoptosis and clearance and is associated with up-regulation of hypoxia-inducible factor 1alpha. *J. Leukoc. Biol.* **2007**, *81*, 1236–1244.

91. Ishigami, A.; Fujita, T.; Handa, S.; Shirasawa, T.; Koseki, H.; Kitamura, T.; Enomoto, N.; Sato, N.; Shimosawa, T.; Maruyama, N. Senescence marker protein-30 knockout mouse liver is highly susceptible to tumor necrosis factor-alpha- and Fas-mediated apoptosis. *Am. J. Pathol.* **2002**, *161*, 1273–1281.

92. Kondo, Y.; Inai, Y.; Sato, Y.; Handa, S.; Kubo, S.; Shimokado, K.; Goto, S.; Nishikimi, M.; Maruyama, N.; Ishigami, A. Senescence marker protein 30 functions as gluconolactonase in L-ascorbic acid biosynthesis, and its knockout mice are prone to scurvy. *Proc. Natl. Acad. Sci. USA* **2006**, *103*, 5723–5728.

93. Kondo, Y.; Sasaki, T.; Sato, Y.; Amano, A.; Aizawa, S.; Iwama, M.; Handa, S.; Shimada, N.; Fukuda, M.; Akita, M.; *et al.* Vitamin C depletion increases superoxide generation in brains of SMP30/GNL knockout mice. *Biochem. Biophys. Res. Commun.* **2008**, *377*, 291–296.

94. Son, T.G.; Zou, Y.; Jung, K.J.; Yu, B.P.; Ishigami, A.; Maruyama, N.; Lee, J. SMP30 deficiency causes increased oxidative stress in brain. *Mech. Ageing Dev.* **2006**, *127*, 451–457.

95. Beamer, W.G.; Rosen, C.J.; Bronson, R.T.; Gu, W.; Donahue, L.R.; Baylink, D.J.; Richardson, C.C.; Crawford, G.C.; Barker, J.E. Spontaneous fracture (sfx): A mouse genetic model of defective peripubertal bone formation. *Bone* **2000**, *27*, 619–626.

96. Mohan, S.; Kapoor, A.; Singgih, A.; Zhang, Z.; Taylor, T.; Yu, H.; Chadwick, R.B.; Chung, Y.S.; Donahue, L.R.; Rosen, C.; *et al.* Spontaneous fractures in the mouse mutant sfx are caused by deletion of the gulonolactone oxidase gene, causing vitamin C deficiency. *J. Bone Miner. Res.* **2005**, *20*, 1597–1610.

97. Jiao, Y.; Zhang, J.; Yan, J.; Stuart, J.; Gibson, G.; Lu, L.; Willaims, R.; Wang, Y.J.; Gu, W. Differential gene expression between wild-type and Gulo-deficient mice supplied with vitamin C. *Genet. Mol. Biol.* **2011**, *34*, 386–395.

98. Ward, M.S.; Lamb, J.; May, J.M.; Harrison, F.E. Behavioral and monoamine changes following severe vitamin C deficiency. *J. Neurochem.* **2013**, *124*, 363–375.

99. Amano, A.; Tsunoda, M.; Aigaki, T.; Maruyama, N.; Ishigami, A. Effect of ascorbic acid deficiency on catecholamine synthesis in adrenal glands of SMP30/GNL knockout mice. *Eur. J. Nutr.* **2014**, *53*, 177–185.

100. Sotiriou, S.; Gispert, S.; Cheng, J.; Wang, Y.; Chen, A.; Hoogstraten-Miller, S.; Miller, G.F.; Kwon, O.; Levine, M.; Guttentag, S.H.; *et al.* Ascorbic-acid transporter Slc23a1 is essential for vitamin C transport into the brain and for perinatal survival. *Nat. Med.* **2002**, *8*, 514–517.

101. Harrison, F.E.; Dawes, S.M.; Meredith, M.E.; Babaev, V.R.; Li, L.; May, J.M. Low vitamin C and increased oxidative stress and cell death in mice that lack the sodium-dependent vitamin C transporter SVCT2. *Free Radic. Biol. Med.* **2010**, *49*, 821–829.

102. Bornstein, S.R.; Yoshida-Hiroi, M.; Sotiriou, S.; Levine, M.; Hartwig, H.G.; Nussbaum, R.L.; Eisenhofer, G. Impaired adrenal catecholamine system function in mice with deficiency of the ascorbic acid transporter (SVCT2). *FASEB J.* **2003**, *17*, 1928–1930.

103. Meredith, M.E.; May, J.M. Regulation of embryonic neurotransmitter and tyrosine hydroxylase protein levels by ascorbic acid. *Brain Res.* **2013**, *1539*, 7–14.

104. Harrison, F.E.; Best, J.L.; Meredith, M.E.; Gamlin, C.R.; Borza, D.B.; May, J.M. Increased expression of SVCT2 in a new mouse model raises ascorbic acid in tissues and protects against paraquat-induced oxidative damage in lung. *PLoS One* **2012**, *7*, e35623.

105. Babaev, V.R.; Whitesell, R.R.; Li, L.; Linton, M.F.; Fazio, S.; May, J.M. Selective macrophage ascorbate deficiency suppresses early atherosclerosis. *Free Radic. Biol. Med.* **2011**, *50*, 27–36.

106. Babaev, V.R.; Li, L.; Shah, S.; Fazio, S.; Linton, M.F.; May, J.M. Combined vitamin C and vitamin E deficiency worsens early atherosclerosis in apolipoprotein E-deficient mice. *Arterioscler. Thromb. Vasc. Biol.* **2010**, *30*, 1751–1757.
107. Kook, S.Y.; Lee, K.M.; Kim, Y.; Cha, M.Y.; Kang, S.; Baik, S.H.; Lee, H.; Park, R.; Mook-Jung, I. High-dose of vitamin C supplementation reduces amyloid plaque burden and ameliorates pathological changes in the brain of 5XFAD mice. *Cell. Death Dis.* **2014**, *5*, e1083.
108. Pierce, M.R.; Diasio, D.L.; Rodrigues, L.M.; Harrison, F.E.; May, J.M. Combined vitamin C and E deficiency induces motor defects in gulo(−/−)/SVCT2(+/−) mice. *Nutr. Neurosci.* **2013**, *16*, 160–173.
109. Morris, M.C.; Beckett, L.A.; Scherr, P.A.; Hebert, L.E.; Bennett, D.A.; Field, T.S.; Evans, D.A. Vitamin E and vitamin C supplement use and risk of incident Alzheimer disease. *Alzheimer Dis. Assoc. Disord.* **1998**, *12*, 121–126.
110. Morris, M.C.; Evans, D.A.; Bienias, J.L.; Tangney, C.C.; Bennett, D.A.; Aggarwal, N.; Wilson, R.S.; Scherr, P.A. Dietary intake of antioxidant nutrients and the risk of incident Alzheimer disease in a biracial community study. *JAMA* **2002**, *287*, 3230–3237.
111. Carr, A.C.; Bozonet, S.M.; Pullar, J.M.; Simcock, J.W.; Vissers, M.C. A Randomized Steady-State Bioavailability Study of Synthetic *versus* Natural (Kiwifruit-Derived) Vitamin C. *Nutrients* **2013**, *5*, 3684–3695.
112. Gray, S.L.; Anderson, M.L.; Crane, P.K.; Breitner, J.C.; McCormick, W.; Bowen, J.D.; Teri, L.; Larson, E. Antioxidant vitamin supplement use and risk of dementia or Alzheimer's disease in older adults. *J. Am. Geriatr. Soc.* **2008**, *56*, 291–295.
113. Luchsinger, J.A.; Tang, M.X.; Shea, S.; Mayeux, R. Antioxidant vitamin intake and risk of Alzheimer disease. *Arch. Neurol.* **2003**, *60*, 203–208.
114. Masaki, K.H.; Losonczy, K.G.; Izmirlian, G.; Foley, D.J.; Ross, G.W.; Petrovitch, H.; Havlik, R.; White, L.R. Association of vitamin E and C supplement use with cognitive function and dementia in elderly men. *Neurology* **2000**, *54*, 1265–1272.
115. Zandi, P.P.; Anthony, J.C.; Khachaturian, A.S.; Stone, S.V.; Gustafson, D.; Tschanz, J.T.; Norton, M.C.; Welsh-Bohmer, K.A.; Breitner, J.C. Reduced risk of Alzheimer disease in users of antioxidant vitamin supplements: the Cache County Study. *Arch. Neurol.* **2004**, *61*, 82–88.
116. Grodstein, F.; Chen, J.; Willett, W.C. High-dose antioxidant supplements and cognitive function in community-dwelling elderly women. *Am. J. Clin. Nutr.* **2003**, *77*, 975–984.
117. Devore, E.E.; Kang, J.H.; Stampfer, M.J.; Grodstein, F. The association of antioxidants and cognition in the Nurses' Health Study. *Am. J. Epidemiol.* **2013**, *177*, 33–41.
118. Engelhart, M.J.; Geerlings, M.I.; Ruitenberg, A.; van Swieten, J.C.; Hofman, A.; Witteman, J.C.; Breteler, M.M. Dietary intake of antioxidants and risk of Alzheimer disease. *JAMA* **2002**, *287*, 3223–3229.
119. Bowman, G.L.; Shannon, J.; Ho, E.; Traber, M.G.; Frei, B.; Oken, B.S.; Kaye, J.A.; Quinn, J.F. Reliability and validity of food frequency questionnaire and nutrient biomarkers in elders with and without mild cognitive impairment. *Alzheimer Dis. Assoc. Disord.* **2011**, *25*, 49–57.
120. Rodrigue, K.M.; Kennedy, K.M.; Devous, M.D., Sr.; Rieck, J.R.; Hebrank, A.C.; Diaz-Arrastia, R.; Mathews, D.; Park, D.C. beta-Amyloid burden in healthy aging: Regional distribution and cognitive consequences. *Neurology* **2012**, *78*, 387–395.

121. Bowman, G.L.; Silbert, L.C.; Howieson, D.; Dodge, H.H.; Traber, M.G.; Frei, B.; Kaye, J.A.; Shannon, J.; Quinn, J.F. Nutrient biomarker patterns, cognitive function, and MRI measures of brain aging. *Neurology* **2012**, *78*, 241–249.
122. Bowman, G.L. Ascorbic acid, cognitive function, and Alzheimer's disease: A current review and future direction. *Biofactors* **2012**, *38*, 114–122.
123. Goodwin, J.S.; Goodwin, J.M.; Garry, P.J. Association between nutritional status and cognitive functioning in a healthy elderly population. *JAMA* **1983**, *249*, 2917–2921.
124. Gale, C.R.; Martyn, C.N.; Cooper, C. Cognitive impairment and mortality in a cohort of elderly people. *BMJ* **1996**, *312*, 608–611.
125. Riviere, S.; Birlouez-Aragon, I.; Nourhashemi, F.; Vellas, B. Low plasma vitamin C in Alzheimer patients despite an adequate diet. *Int. J. Geriatr. Psychiatry* **1998**, *13*, 749–754.
126. Charlton, K.E.; Rabinowitz, T.L.; Geffen, L.N.; Dhansay, M.A. Lowered plasma vitamin C, but not vitamin E, concentrations in dementia patients. *J. Nutr. Health Aging* **2004**, *8*, 99–107.
127. Polidori, M.C.; Mecocci, P. Plasma susceptibility to free radical-induced antioxidant consumption and lipid peroxidation is increased in very old subjects with Alzheimer disease. *J. Alzheimer's Dis. (JAD)* **2002**, *4*, 517–522.
128. Polidori, M.C.; Mattioli, P.; Aldred, S.; Cecchetti, R.; Stahl, W.; Griffiths, H.; Senin, U.; Sies, H.; Mecocci, P. Plasma antioxidant status, immunoglobulin g oxidation and lipid peroxidation in demented patients: relevance to Alzheimer disease and vascular dementia. *Dement. Geriatr. Cogn. Disord.* **2004**, *18*, 265–270.
129. Perrig, W.J.; Perrig, P.; Stahelin, H.B. The relation between antioxidants and memory performance in the old and very old. *J. Am. Geriatr. Soc.* **1997**, *45*, 718–724.
130. Spector, R. Nutrient transport systems in brain: 40 years of progress. *J. Neurochem.* **2009**, *111*, 315–320.
131. Paraskevas, G.P.; Kapaki, E.; Libitaki, G.; Zournas, C.; Segditsa, I.; Papageorgiou, C. Ascorbate in healthy subjects, amyotrophic lateral sclerosis and Alzheimer's disease. *Acta Neurol. Scand.* **1997**, *96*, 88–90.
132. Quinn, J.; Suh, J.; Moore, M.M.; Kaye, J.; Frei, B. Antioxidants in Alzheimer's disease-vitamin C delivery to a demanding brain. *J. Alzheimers Dis.* **2003**, *5*, 309–313.
133. Glaso, M.; Nordbo, G.; Diep, L.; Bohmer, T. Reduced concentrations of several vitamins in normal weight patients with late-onset dementia of the Alzheimer type without vascular disease. *J. Nutr. Health Aging* **20**04, *8*, 407–413.
134. Bowman, G.L.; Dodge, H.; Frei, B.; Calabrese, C.; Oken, B.S.; Kaye, J.A.; Quinn, J.F. Ascorbic acid and rates of cognitive decline in Alzheimer's disease. *J. Alzheimers Dis.* **2009**, *16*, 93–98.
135. Arlt, S.; Muller-Thomsen, T.; Beisiegel, U.K.; Ontush, A. Effect of One-Year Vitamin C- and E-Supplementation on Cerebrospinal Fluid Oxidation Parameters and Clinical Course in Alzheimer's Disease. *Neurochem. Res*. **2012**, *37*, 2706–2714.
136. Galasko, D.R.; Peskind, E.; Clark, C.M.; Quinn, J.F.; Ringman, J.M.; Jicha, G.A.; Cotman, C.; Cottrell, B.; Montine, T.J.; Thomas, R.G.; Aisen, P. Antioxidants for Alzheimer disease: A randomized clinical trial with cerebrospinal fluid biomarker measures. *Arch. Neurol.* **2012**, *69*, 836–841.

137. Spector, R.; Johanson, C.E. Sustained choroid plexus function in human elderly and Alzheimer's disease patients. *Fluids Barriers CNS* **2013**, *10*, 28.
138. Polidori, M.C.; Pientka, L. Bridging the pathophysiology of Alzheimer's disease with vascular pathology: The feed-back, the feed-forward, and oxidative stress. *J. Alzheimer's Dis. (JAD)* **2012**, *28*, 1–9.
139. Polidori, M.C.; Pientka, L.; Mecocci, P. A review of the major vascular risk factors related to Alzheimer's disease. *J. Alzheimer's Dis. (JAD)* **2012**, *32*, 521–530.
140. de la Torre, J.C. Cerebral hemodynamics and vascular risk factors: setting the stage for Alzheimer's disease. *J. Alzheimer's Dis. (JAD)* **2012**, *32*, 553–567.
141. Aguero-Torres, H.; Kivipelto, M.; von Strauss, E. Rethinking the dementia diagnoses in a population-based study: What is Alzheimer's disease and what is vascular dementia? A study from the kungsholmen project. *Dement. Geriatr. Cogn. Disord.* **2006**, *22*, 244–249.
142. de la Torre, J.C.; Stefano, G.B. Evidence that Alzheimer's disease is a microvascular disorder: The role of constitutive nitric oxide. *Brain Res. Brain Res. Rev.* **2000**, *34*, 119–136.
143. Polidori, M.C.; Mecocci, P.; Frei, B. Plasma vitamin C levels are decreased and correlated with brain damage in patients with intracranial hemorrhage or head trauma. *Stroke* **2001**, *32*, 898–902.
144. Knopman, D.; Boland, L.L.; Mosley, T.; Howard, G.; Liao, D.; Szklo, M.; McGovern, P.; Folsom, A.R. Cardiovascular risk factors and cognitive decline in middle-aged adults. *Neurology* **2001**, *56*, 42–48.
145. Polidori, M.C.; Pratico, D.; Savino, K.; Rokach, J.; Stahl, W.; Mecocci, P. Increased F2 isoprostane plasma levels in patients with congestive heart failure are correlated with antioxidant status and disease severity. *J. Card. Fail.* **2004**, *10*, 334–338.
146. Polidori, M.C.; Pratico, D.; Ingegni, T.; Mariani, E.; Spazzafumo, L.; Del Sindaco, P.; Cecchetti, R.; Yao, Y.; Ricci, S.; Cherubini, A.; *et al.* Effects of vitamin C and aspirin in ischemic stroke-related lipid peroxidation: Results of the AVASAS (Aspirin Versus Ascorbic acid plus Aspirin in Stroke) Study. *Biofactors* **2005**, *24*, 265–274.
147. Wendell, C.R.; Zonderman, A.B.; Metter, E.J.; Najjar, S.S.; Waldstein, S.R. Carotid intimal medial thickness predicts cognitive decline among adults without clinical vascular disease. *Stroke* **2009**, *40*, 3180–3185.
148. Frei, B. To C or not to C, that is the question! *J. Am. Coll. Cardiol.* **2003**, *42*, 253–255.
149. Polidori, M.C.; Mecocci, P.; Reimann, A.; Cherubini, A.; Cecchetti, R.; Briviba, K.; Stahl, W.; Sies, H.; Senin, U. Plasma lipid peroxidation and vitamin C status in healthy centenarians. *J. Am. Geriatr. Soc.* **1999**, *47*, 1038–1039.
150. Hunter, D.C.; Skinner, M.A.; Wolber, F.M.; Booth, C.L.; Loh, J.M.; Wohlers, M.; Stevenson, L.M.; Kruger, M.C. Consumption of gold kiwifruit reduces severity and duration of selected upper respiratory tract infection symptoms and increases plasma vitamin C concentration in healthy older adults. *Br. J. Nutr.* **2012**, *108*, 1235–1245.
151. Moretti, M.; Colla, A.; de Oliveira Balen, G.; dos Santos, D.B.; Budni, J.; de Freitas, A.E.; Farina, M.; Severo Rodrigues, A.L. Ascorbic acid treatment, similarly to fluoxetine, reverses depressive-like behavior and brain oxidative damage induced by chronic unpredictable stress. *J. Psychiatr. Res.* **2012**, *46*, 331–340.

152. Simon, J.A.; Hudes, E.S.; Tice, J.A. Relation of serum ascorbic acid to mortality among US adults. *J. Am. Coll. Nutr.* **2001**, *20*, 255–263.
153. Boekholdt, S.M.; Meuwese, M.C.; Day, N.E.; Luben, R.; Welch, A.; Wareham, N.J.; Khaw, K.T. Plasma concentrations of ascorbic acid and C-reactive protein, and risk of future coronary artery disease, in apparently healthy men and women: the EPIC-Norfolk prospective population study. *Br. J. Nutr.* **2006**, *96*, 516–522.
154. Khaw, K.T.; Bingham, S.; Welch, A.; Luben, R.; Wareham, N.; Oakes, S.; Day, N. Relation between plasma ascorbic acid and mortality in men and women in EPIC-Norfolk prospective study: A prospective population study. European Prospective Investigation into Cancer and Nutrition. *Lancet* **2001**, *357*, 657–663.
155. Ellingsen, I.; Seljeflot, I.; Arnesen, H.; Tonstad, S. Vitamin C consumption is associated with less progression in carotid intima media thickness in elderly men: A 3-year intervention study. *Nutr. Metab. Cardiovasc. Dis. (NMCD)* **2009**, *19*, 8–14.
156. Hodis, H.N.; Mack, W.J.; LaBree, L.; Mahrer, P.R.; Sevanian, A.; Liu, C.R.; Liu, C.H.; Hwang, J.; Selzer, R.H.; Azen, S.P. Alpha-tocopherol supplementation in healthy individuals reduces low-density lipoprotein oxidation but not atherosclerosis: The Vitamin E Atherosclerosis Prevention Study (VEAPS). *Circulation* **2002**, *106*, 1453–1459.
157. Zureik, M.; Galan, P.; Bertrais, S.; Mennen, L.; Czernichow, S.; Blacher, J.; Ducimetiere, P.; Hercberg, S. Effects of long-term daily low-dose supplementation with antioxidant vitamins and minerals on structure and function of large arteries. *Arterioscler. Thromb. Vasc. Biol.* **2004**, *24*, 1485–1491.
158. Luzzi, S.; Vella, L.; Bartolini, M.; Provinciali, L.; Silvestrini, M. Atherosclerosis in the evolution of Alzheimer's disease: Can treatment reduce cognitive decline? *J. Alzheimer's Dis. (JAD)* **2010**, *20*, 893–901.
159. Terpstra, M.; Marjanska, M.; Henry, P.G.; Tkac, I.; Gruetter, R. Detection of an antioxidant profile in the human brain *in vivo* via double editing with MEGA-PRESS. *Magn. Reson. Med.* **2006**, *56*, 1192–1199.
160. Emir, U.E.; Raatz, S.; McPherson, S.; Hodges, J.S.; Torkelson, C.; Tawfik, P.; White, T.; Terpstra, M. Noninvasive quantification of ascorbate and glutathione concentration in the elderly human brain. *NMR Biomed.* **2011**, *24*, 888–894.

6

Synthetic or Food-Derived Vitamin C—Are they Equally Bioavailable?

Anitra C. Carr * and Margreet C. M. Vissers

Centre for Free Radical Research, Department of Pathology and Biomedical Science, University of Otago, Christchurch, P.O. Box 4345, Christchurch 8140, New Zealand; E-Mail: margreet.vissers@otago.ac.nz

* Author to whom correspondence should be addressed; E-Mail: anitra.carr@otago.ac.nz;

Abstract: Vitamin C (ascorbate) is an essential water-soluble micronutrient in humans and is obtained through the diet, primarily from fruits and vegetables. *In vivo*, vitamin C acts as a cofactor for numerous biosynthetic enzymes required for the synthesis of amino acid-derived macromolecules, neurotransmitters, and neuropeptide hormones, and is also a cofactor for various hydroxylases involved in the regulation of gene transcription and epigenetics. Vitamin C was first chemically synthesized in the early 1930s and since then researchers have been investigating the comparative bioavailability of synthetic *versus* natural, food-derived vitamin C. Although synthetic and food-derived vitamin C is chemically identical, fruit and vegetables are rich in numerous nutrients and phytochemicals which may influence its bioavailability. The physiological interactions of vitamin C with various bioflavonoids have been the most intensively studied to date. Here, we review animal and human studies, comprising both pharmacokinetic and steady-state designs, which have been carried out to investigate the comparative bioavailability of synthetic and food-derived vitamin C, or vitamin C in the presence of isolated bioflavonoids. Overall, a majority of animal studies have shown differences in the comparative bioavailability of synthetic *versus* natural vitamin C, although the results varied depending on the animal model, study design and body compartments measured. In contrast, all steady state comparative bioavailability studies in humans have shown no differences between synthetic and natural vitamin C, regardless of the subject population, study design or intervention used. Some pharmacokinetic studies in humans have shown transient and small comparative differences between synthetic and natural vitamin C, although these differences are likely to have minimal physiological impact. Study design issues and future research directions are discussed.

Keywords: ascorbate; dietary vitamin C; bioavailability; animal studies; human studies; bioflavonoids

---

1. Introduction

Vitamin C (ascorbate) is an essential water-soluble micronutrient in humans and is obtained through the diet primarily from fruits and vegetables [1]. *In vivo*, it acts as a cofactor for numerous biosynthetic enzymes required for the synthesis of amino acid-derived macromolecules, neurotransmitters and neuropeptide hormones [2], and for various hydroxylases involved in the regulation of gene transcription and epigenetics [3,4]. Vitamin C is concentrated from the plasma into the body's organs and is found in particularly high concentrations in the pituitary and adrenal glands and in the corpus luteum [5], although skeletal muscle, brain, and liver comprise the largest body pools [6]. Most animals can synthesize vitamin C from glucose in the liver [7]; however, humans and a small selection of animal species have lost the ability to synthesize vitamin C due to mutations in the gene encoding L-gulono-γ-lactone oxidase, the terminal enzyme in the vitamin C biosynthetic pathway [8]. Therefore, an adequate and regular dietary intake is essential to prevent hypovitaminosis C and the potentially fatal deficiency disease, scurvy [9].

In the mid 1700s the Royal Navy surgeon James Lind carried out controlled dietary trials and determined that citrus fruit could cure individuals with scurvy (reviewed in [10]). However, it wasn't until the early 1900s that experimental scurvy was first produced in guinea pigs through dietary restriction and shown to be prevented by feeding the animals fresh fruits and vegetables. In the early 1930s vitamin C was isolated from fruit and vegetables and adrenal cortex and was named "hexuronic acid", which was shown to cure scurvy in guinea pigs and was subsequently renamed ascorbic acid to reflect its anti-scorbutic properties. Vitamin C was first chemically synthesized in 1933 [10] and, since the mid 1930s, the question of the comparative bioavailability of synthetic *versus* natural, food-derived vitamin C in animal models and human subjects has been a point of consideration.

The bioavailability of dietary vitamin C represents the proportion of the micronutrient that is absorbed by the intestines and is available for metabolic processes within the body. *In vivo* vitamin C levels are a function of uptake, metabolism, and excretion (see [11] for an excellent review of these processes). Vitamin C is actively transported into the body via two sodium-dependent vitamin C transporters, SVCT1 and SVCT2 [12,13]. These transporters exhibit different tissue distributions and uptake kinetics. SVCT1 is expressed in epithelial tissues and is primarily responsible for intestinal uptake and renal reabsorption of vitamin C, the latter helping to maintain whole body homeostasis [13]. SVCT2 is expressed in specialized and metabolically active tissues and is required for delivery of vitamin C to tissues with a high demand for the vitamin either for enzymatic reactions [2] and/or to help protect these tissues from oxidative stress [13]. Both of these transporters show significantly more affinity for the L- *versus* D-isoform of vitamin C (Figure 1) [12,14], and this selectivity likely explains earlier observations of significantly lower tissue accumulation and anti-scorbutic activity of D-ascorbic acid in guinea pigs [15,16]. Although D-ascorbic acid is a commonly added food preservative [17], administration of D- and L-ascorbic acid together does not affect the bioavailability of the latter in humans [18].

Through its action as a reducing agent and antioxidant, ascorbate undergoes one and two electron oxidations to produce the ascorbyl radical and dehydroascorbic acid (DHA) (Figure 1). Recent research has shown that DHA can be taken up by the facilitative glucose transporters GLUT2 and GLUT8 in the small intestine [19]. Cells are also able to transport DHA via GLUT1 and GLUT3 [20,21], followed by intracellular reduction to ascorbate [22,23]. However, transport via the GLUTs is in competition with glucose which is at relatively high concentrations throughout the body and although different fruits and vegetables have been shown to contain relatively high amounts of DHA [24], the *in vivo* contribution of DHA is uncertain due to its minimal circulating and organ levels [25,26] (although white blood cells may be an exception to this) [27,28].

Figure 1. Vitamin C in its reduced form (ascorbic acid), shown as both its L- and D-isomers, and its two electron oxidation form (dehydroascorbic acid, DHA). DHA can be readily reduced back to ascorbic acid *in vivo* via both chemical and enzymatic pathways [23].

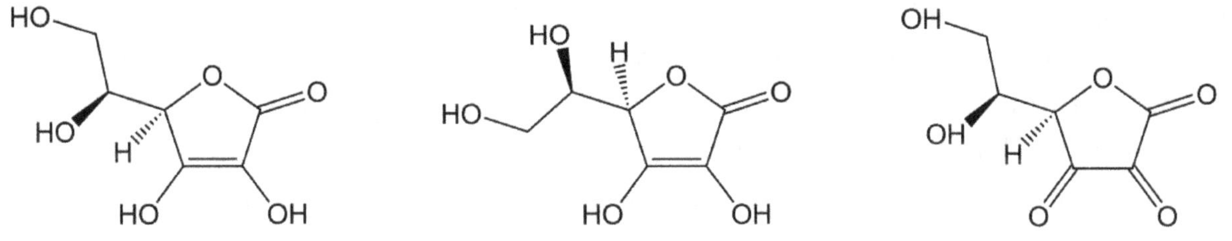

L-Ascorbic Acid **D-Ascorbic acid** **Dehydroascorbic acid**

Synthetic and food-derived vitamin C is chemically identical. However, fruit and vegetables are rich in numerous micronutrients (vitamins and minerals), dietary fiber, and phytochemicals (e.g., bioflavonoids), and the presence of some of these may affect the bioavailability of vitamin C. Vitamin C has long been known to interact with vitamin E by reducing the tocopheroxyl radical and regenerating native tocopherol [29]. Some fruit, such as kiwifruit, contain relatively high amounts of vitamin E and one animal study has indicated that vitamin E is able to preserve vitamin C *in vivo* [30]. Food-derived (and synthetic) vitamin C is well known to increase non-heme iron uptake and body status, likely via its ability to reduce iron from its ferric to ferrous state [31,32]. However, whether iron can affect vitamin C bioavailability is less clear [33–35]. Although iron has been shown to increase the uptake of vitamin C in cultured intestinal cells [33], human intervention studies have shown no effect of iron intake on vitamin C bioavailability [34,35]. One study has indicated that specific dietary fibers, such as hemicellulose and pectin, may affect the excretion of vitamin C [36], however, their influence on vitamin C uptake was not determined.

Plant-derived flavonoids have been of interest since the mid 1930s, when they were initially referred to as "vitamin P", primarily due to their effect on vascular permeability [37]. At the time, there was much debate in the literature regarding the role of "vitamin P" in experimental [38–42] and human scurvy [37,43–45]. Flavonoids can act as antioxidants via direct scavenging of free radicals [46,47] and/or chelation of redox-active metal ions [48,49]. As a result, it has been suggested that flavonoids may "spare" vitamin C and, thus, increase its bioavailability. Flavonoids have been shown to inhibit the *in vitro* oxidation of vitamin C [48–51], however, the *in vivo* relevance of metal-ion mediated oxidation of vitamin C is likely to be minimal as free metal ions are largely sequestered in the body [52]. Whether flavonoids can affect vitamin C uptake *in vivo* is uncertain due to the low plasma bioavailability of these compounds [53]. Thus, any interaction of flavonoids with vitamin C would be expected to occur primarily in the intestinal lumen prior to active uptake.

Of note, several *in vitro* studies have shown that various flavonoids can inhibit vitamin C and DHA uptake by their respective transporters. The flavonoid quercetin can reversibly inhibit SVCT1 expressed in *Xenopus* oocytes [54] and limited data from an animal model indicates that this may occur *in vivo* [54]. Quercetin and myricetin can inhibit the uptake of vitamin C and DHA into cultured monocytic (HL-60 and U937) and lymphocytic (Jurkat) cells via inhibition of GLUT1 and GLUT3 [55] and possibly also SVCT2, which is expressed in leukocytes [56]. Quercetin and phloretin can also inhibit the intestinal GLUT2 and GLUT8 transporters [19]. Thus, based on the above *in vitro* studies, it is unclear whether flavonoids will enhance *in vivo* vitamin C bioavailability through a sparing action, or decrease its bioavailability through inhibiting vitamin C transporters.

The effect of various purified flavonoids or flavonoid-rich fruits and vegetables on vitamin C bioavailability in different animal models and human subjects is discussed below. To test comparative vitamin C bioavailability, both steady-state and pharmacokinetic models have been used. The former monitors ascorbate levels in blood and/or urine following a number of weeks of supplementation, while the latter monitors transient changes in plasma levels and/or urinary excretion over the hours following ingestion of the vitamin C-containing test substance. The gold standard for analysis of vitamin C is HPLC with coulometric electrochemical detection due to its sensitivity and specificity [57]. Early studies, however, were limited primarily to colourimetric methods based on reduction of ferric iron compounds and are prone to interference by numerous other substances [57].

2. Vitamin C Bioavailability Studies Using Animal Models

There are a number of benefits to the use of animal models to investigate vitamin C bioavailability, particularly the ease of diet control and the ability to obtain tissues not normally accessible in human studies. However, results can vary widely depending on the animal model used and the different treatment and analytical methodologies employed. It should also be noted that not all of the animal models that have been used are naturally vitamin C deficient. The animal models of choice are the naturally vitamin C deficient guinea pig, and genetically scorbutic animal models, such as the Osteogenic Disorder Shionogi (ODS) rat [58], the L-gulono-γ-lactone oxidase (*Gulo*$^{-/-}$) knockout mouse [59], and the spontaneous bone fracture (*sfx*) mouse [60]. Although animal studies can provide useful information, translation of the findings to humans should always proceed with caution.

Studies investigating the comparative bioavailability of synthetic *versus* natural vitamin C in animal models are shown in Table 1. Studies carried out in guinea pigs showed enhanced uptake of vitamin C into specific organs (e.g., adrenals and spleen) in the presence of flavonoid-rich juices/extracts or purified plant flavonoids (e.g., hesperidin, rutin, and catechin) [42,61–64]. Vinson and Bose [65] carried out a pharmacokinetic study in guinea pigs and found a 148% increase in the area under the plasma ascorbate concentration-time curve when administered as citrus fruit media. They also noted that the citrus fruit group demonstrated delayed plasma vitamin C uptake compared with the synthetic vitamin C group [65]. Cotereau *et al.* [42] reported that animals given both vitmain C and catechin not only had four to eight-fold more vitamin C in the organs measured, but they were also the only group without scorbutic-type lesions. The latter finding was supported by a similar study showing fewer fresh hemorrhages in scorbutic guinea pigs receiving vitamin C with rutin or querceitin compared with vitamin C alone [66].

Several of the studies in Table 1, however, showed no differences in vitamin C accumulation in some organs (e.g., liver) [61–63,67]. Hughes *et al.* noted that the acerola cherry preparation they used was virtually flavonoid free due to dilution of the high vitamin C fruit extract, which they suggested may have accounted for its reduced efficacy compared with blackcurrant juice, which is flavonoid rich [64]. To account for the flavonoid-dependent differences in vitamin C uptake observed between the adrenals and livers of guinea pigs [62,63], Douglass and Kamp [62] noted that flavonols such as rutin are rapidly destroyed in liver tissue, but are relatively stable in adrenal homogenates. Papageorge *et al.* [63] also noted that when epinephrine oxidizes it can contribute to the destruction of vitamin C and thus the antioxidant effects of rutin may result in "sparing" of vitamin C in adrenals. A study by Levine's group [54] showed that the flavonoid quercetin can reversibly inhibit vitamin C intestinal transport and decrease plasma levels of the vitamin in the CD (Sprague-Dawley) rat, although it should be noted that this is not a vitamin C deficient animal model. Some of the variability observed in these different animal studies (Table 1) may be due to the varying ratios of flavonoid to vitamin C employed.

We recently carried out a comparative bioavailability study, using the *Gulo* mouse model, investigating the uptake of vitamin C from kiwifruit gel compared with synthetic vitamin C [68]. We found that the kiwifruit extract, which is rich in flavonoids [69,70], provided significantly higher serum, leukocyte, heart, liver, and kidney levels of vitamin C than the purified vitamin, suggesting some type of synergistic activity of the whole fruit in this model. As with Wilson *et al.* [61], we did not observe any difference between the two interventions with respect to vitamin C uptake into the brain. Indeed, there is significant retention of vitamin C in the brain during dietary depletion [64,68], suggesting a vital role for vitamin C in the brain. Thus, a significant proportion of animal studies show enhanced circulating and organ levels of vitamin C in the presence of food-derived or purified flavonoids.

Table 1. Vitamin C comparative bioavailability studies in animal models.

Animal Model	Intervention	Study Design	Vitamin C Analysis	Bioavailability Findings: Natural *vs.* Synthetic Vitamin C	Bioavailability Summary: Natural *vs.* Synthetic Vitamin C	Reference
Gulo$^{-/-}$ mice	0.5–5 mg/day vitamin C solution Kiwifruit gel	4 weeks intervention	HPLC-ECD	Kiwifruit ↑ serum, leukocyte, heart, liver, and kidney, but not brain vitamin C	Enhanced uptake in 5/6 pools	[68]
CD rats	60 mg/kg vitamin C gavage 15 mg/kg quercetin	Single dose; 4 h sampling	HPLC-ECD	Quercetin ↓ plasma vitamin C (at 4 h)	Decreased uptake in 1/1 pool	[54]
Guinea pigs	50 mg vitamin C solution Citrus fruit media	Single dose; 4 h sampling	Fluorometric (NQSA)	Citrus fruit media ↑ plasma AUC	Enhanced uptake in 1/1 pool	[65]
	1 mg/kg vitamin C (low vitamin C diet) 50 mg/kg orange peel extract 50 mg/kg hesperidin	26 days intervention	Colorimetric (DCPIP)	Orange peel extract ↑ adrenal, spleen and leukocyte, but not brain vitamin C; hesperidin ↑ adrenal and leukocyte, but not spleen vitamin C	Enhanced uptake in 3/4 pools	[61]
	5 mg/kg vitamin C solution Black current juice Acerola cherry juice	23 days intervention	Colorimetric (DCPIP)	Black current juice ↑ adrenal and spleen vitamin C; acerola cherry juice comparable adrenal and spleen vitamin C	Enhanced uptake in 2/2 organs	[64]
	0, 5 and 10 mg/kg vitamin C 50 mg rutin	3 weeks intervention	Colorimetric (DNPH)	Rutin ↑ adrenal, but not liver vitamin C	Enhanced uptake in 1/2 pools	[62]
	4 mg/kg vitamin C (low vitamin C diet) 10 mg rutin tablet 18 mg/kg vitamin C (adequate vitamin C diet) 10 mg rutin tablet	22 days intervention	Colorimetric (DNPH)	Rutin ↑ adrenal, but not liver or whole blood vitamin C of adequate animals	Enhanced uptake in 1/3 pools	[63]
	Basic diet 1 mg/animal catechin 10 mg/animal vitamin C Vitamin C + catechin	23 days intervention	Colorimetric (DCPIP)	Vitamin C + catechin ↑ liver, spleen, kidney, and adrenal vitamin C	Enhanced uptake in 4/4 organs	[42]
	0.5 mg/day vitamin C solution 1 mL lemon juice	20 days intervention	Colorimetric (DCPIP)	Lemon juice comparable plasma and adrenal vitamin C	Comparable uptake in 2/2 pools	[67]

NQSA: 1,2-naphthoquinone-4-sulfonic acid; AUC: area under the concentration-time curve; DNPH: 2,4-dinitrophenylhydrazine; DCPIP: 2,6-dichlorophenolindophenol.

3. Steady State Bioavailability Studies in Humans

An early report of several patients with scurvy whose plasma vitamin C levels did not increase with synthetic vitamin C alone, but only in the form of lemon juice [45], initially leant support to the "vitamin P"/flavonoid theory. However, in contrast to the animal studies, all steady state human studies (summarized in Table 2) have shown little difference in plasma and/or urine bioavailability between synthetic vitamin C and that from different fruits, fruit juices, and vegetables [35,71–76]. Mangels *et al.* [35] did observe a 20% lower plasma bioavailability of vitamin C from raw broccoli compared with cooked broccoli, however, this may have been due to differences in mechanical homogenization (chewing), a similar effect to that observed for carotenoid absorption from raw *versus* cooked carrots.

We recently carried out a steady state bioavailability study in young non-smoking men supplemented for six weeks with 50 mg/day vitamin C, in the form of a chewable vitamin C tablet or half a gold kiwifruit [77]. This dose was chosen as it lies on the steep part of the sigmoidal plasma uptake curve [78], thus enhancing the likelihood of detecting a difference between the two interventions. Although most steady state studies have used sequential or crossover study designs, we chose a randomized parallel arms design for a number of reasons. Block *et al.* [79] have previously observed a lower plasma vitamin C response to supplemental vitamin C in the second phase of a multiple depletion/repletion study. Furthermore, although washout of vitamin C could be monitored between the two phases of a cross-over study, it would not be possible to monitor washout of other kiwifruit-derived components, e.g., vitamin E, which may affect the second phase of a cross-over study due to potential *in vivo* interactions with the supplemental vitamin C [30].

Only one previous study has investigated the comparative bioavailability of synthetic *versus* natural vitamin C in leukocytes [71]. These investigators found no difference in leukocyte vitamin C uptake between synthetic vitamin C (in the presence or absence of rutin) and that in orange juice two hours after a single 75 mg dose [71]. Therefore, in addition to plasma, urine, and semen samples, we also isolated peripheral blood mononuclear cells and neutrophils before and after intervention. Due to ease of accessibility and isolation, peripheral blood leukocytes are often used as a marker for tissue vitamin C status, however, whether they are a good model for all organs and tissues is uncertain. In support of this premise our animal study indicated that different organs exhibited maximal vitamin C uptake at varying doses of the vitamin [68] and we have recently shown that human skeletal muscle exhibits greater relative uptake of vitamin C than leukocytes [80]. Therefore, we also carried out needle biopsies of skeletal muscle tissue (*vastus lateralis*), before and after intervention. In contrast to our earlier animal study [68], our human study clearly showed no differences in the steady-state bioavailability of kiwifruit-derived *versus* synthetic vitamin C to plasma, semen, peripheral blood leukocytes, and skeletal muscle tissue [77]. Thus, other nutrients and phytochemicals present in kiwifruit are neither enhancing nor inhibiting the uptake of vitamin C from the whole fruit in humans.

Table 2. Steady state comparative bioavailability studies in humans.

Subjects	Intervention	Study Design	Vitamin C Analysis	Bioavailability Findings: Natural *vs.* Synthetic Vitamin C	Bioavailability Summary: Natural *vs.* Synthetic Vitamin C	Reference
36 non-smoking males 18–35 years	50 mg/day vitamin C tablet Gold kiwifruit (50 mg vitamin C)	6 weeks of supplementation; Parallel design	HPLC-ECD	Kiwifruit comparable plasma, urine, semen, mononuclear cell, neutrophil and muscle tissue vitamin C	Comparable uptake in 6/6 pools	[77]
11 non-smoking women 21–39 years	69 mg/day vitamin C capsule Orange juice (66 mg vitamin C)	2 weeks of supplementation; Crossover design (2 week washout)	Colorimetric (DNPH)	Orange juice comparable plasma vitamin C	Comparable uptake in 1/1 pool	[76]
68 non-smoking males 30–59 years	108 mg/day vitamin C tablet Orange—pieces or juice Broccoli—cooked or raw	4 weeks of supplementation; Crossover design (4 week washout)	Colorimetric (DNPH)	Orange pieces/juice or cooked broccoli comparable plasma vitamin C; raw broccoli ↓ plasma vitamin C	Comparable uptake in 1/1 pool	[35]
14 men and women	75 mg/day vitamin C Papayas (75 mg/day vitamin C) Guava juice (75 mg/day vitamin C)	Sequential design	Colorimetric	Papayas and guava juice comparable plasma and urinary vitamin C	Comparable uptake in 2/2 pools	[72]
4 healthy young subjects	75 mg/day vitamin C tablets Raw cabbage (75 mg/day vitamin C) Tomato juice (75 mg/day vitamin C)	Pre-study saturation; Sequential design	Colorimetric	Raw cabbage and tomato juice comparable plasma and urinary vitamin C	Comparable uptake in 2/2 pools	[73]
7 college women	40 mg/day vitamin C solution Red raspberries (40 mg/day vitamin C)	Pre-study saturation; Sequential design	Colorimetric (DCPIP)	Raspberries comparable blood and urinary vitamin C	Comparable uptake in 2/2 pools	[74]
12 young adults	100 mg/day vitamin C Orange juice (100 mg/day vitamin C)	Sequential design	Colorimetric (DCPIP)	Orange juice comparable urinary vitamin C	Comparable uptake in 1/1 pool	[75]

DNPH: 2,4-dinitrophenylhydrazine; DCPIP: 2,6-dichlorophenolindophenol.

4. Pharmacokinetic Bioavailability Studies in Humans

Pharmacokinetic studies show transient changes in plasma vitamin C levels and urinary excretion over the hours following ingestion of the vitamin C-containing test substance (relevant studies are shown in Table 3). Supplemental vitamin C typically takes about two hours to reach maximal plasma levels following ingestion. An early animal study found that vitamin C provided in citrus fruit media took longer to reach peak plasma concentrations compared with a synthetic vitamin C solution and also provided a larger area under the plasma vitamin C concentration-time curve [65]. These same investigators observed a comparable trend in human subjects supplemented with 500 mg vitamin C in the presence or absence of a citrus fruit extract [81]. The citrus fruit extract delayed maximal plasma levels by one hour and provided a 35% increase in vitamin C bioavailability. Interestingly, the citrus fruit extract increased 24 h urinary vitamin C excretion in participants pre-saturated with vitamin C, but decreased excretion in non-saturated participants compared with synthetic vitamin C alone. This suggests that the baseline vitamin C status of the individual may affect the comparative bioavailability of vitamin C. Although two other studies showed increased urinary excretion in vitamin C pre-saturated subjects in the presence of fruit juice [71,82], another pre-saturation study showed comparable plasma levels and 24 h urinary excretion in the presence of mixed bioflavonoids [83]. It should be noted that doses of 500 mg vitamin C have reduced intestinal bioavailability [78] and are significantly higher than would be obtained through a normal daily diet.

A number of pharmacokinetic studies have shown comparable bioavailability of vitamin C supplied in synthetic form or in the presence of foods or fruit juices [84–88]. Nelson *et al.* [88] used an intestinal triple lumen tube perfusion model to investigate the absorption of synthetic vitamin C and that from an orange juice solution. This method allows direct measurement of intraluminal events and showed no difference in the absorption of vitamin C from the two test solutions. A few pharmacokinetic studies have shown transient decreases in plasma vitamin C levels and/or urinary excretion at specific time points in the presence of food and fruit juices [34,71,84,85]. The physiological relevance of these transient differences is, however, likely minimal.

We recently carried out a pharmacokinetic bioavailability study of synthetic *versus* kiwifruit-derived vitamin C in nine non-smoking males (aged 18–35 years) who had "healthy" or "optimal" (*i.e.*, >50 μmol/L) baseline levels of plasma vitamin C [89]. The participants received either a chewable tablet (200 mg vitamin C) or the equivalent dose from gold kiwifruit. Fasting blood and urine were collected half hourly to hourly over the eight hours following intervention. Plasma ascorbate levels increased from 0.5 h post intervention, although no significant differences in the plasma time-concentration curves were observed between the two interventions. An estimate of the total increase in plasma ascorbate indicated complete uptake of the ingested vitamin C tablet and kiwifruit-derived vitamin C. There was an increase in urinary ascorbate excretion, relative to urinary creatinine, from two hours post intervention. There was also a significant difference between the two interventions, with enhanced ascorbate excretion observed in the kiwifruit group. Urinary excretion was calculated as ~40% and ~50% of the ingested dose from the vitamin C tablet and kiwifruit arms, respectively. Overall, our pharmacokinetic study showed comparable relative bioavailability of kiwifruit-derived vitamin C and synthetic vitamin C [89].

Table 3. Pharmacokinetic comparative bioavailability studies in humans.

Subjects	Intervention	Study Design	Vitamin C Analysis	Plasma Uptake	Urinary Excretion	Reference
9 non-smoking males 18–35 years	200 mg vitamin C tablet Gold kiwifruit (200 mg vitamin C)	8 h sampling; Crossover design (3 week washout)	HPLC-ECD	Kiwifruit comparable plasma vitamin C and AUC	Kiwifruit ↑ urinary vitamin C and AUC (relative to creatinine)	[89]
5 non-smoking males 22–27 years	50 mg vitamin C solution; 282 g mashed potato (50 mg vitamin C) 87 g potato chips (50 mg vitamin C) Placebo	8 h sampling; Crossover design (4 week washout)	HPLC-ECD	Mashed potatoes ↓ plasma vitamin C (at 1 to 2.5 h); potato chips ↓ AUC	Mashed potatoes ↓ urinary vitamin C (at 3 h)	[84]
5 non-smoking males 22–26 years	50–500 mg vitamin C solution 100 mL acerola juice (50 mg vitamin C)	6 h sampling; Crossover design	HPLC-ECD	Acerola juice comparable plasma vitamin C and AUC	Acerola juice ↓ urinary vitamin C (at 1, 2 and 5 h)	[85]
12 males 20–35 years	284 mg vitamin C drink 590 mL orange juice (68 mg vitamin C) Placebo (milk)	4.5 h sampling; Crossover design (1 week washout)	Colorimetric (TPTZ)	Orange juice comparable bioavailability (AUC/concentration)	ND	[86]
7 non-smoking females	150 mg vitamin C solution 300 mL orange juice (150 mg vitamin C) Placebo	8 h sampling; Crossover design (2 week washout)	HPLC-UV	Orange juice comparable plasma vitamin C	ND	[87]
7 non-smokers 26–59 years	30 mg vitamin C solution 200 mL red grape juice (30 mg vitamin C)	4 h sampling; Crossover design (3–4 week washout)	Fluorometric (phenylene diamine)	Grape juice ↓ plasma vitamin C (at 16 to 28 min)	ND	[34]
9 healthy subjects 19–41 years	500 mg vitamin C tablet Mixed bioflavonoids Placebo	1 g/day vitamin C for 2 weeks pre-study; 8 h sampling; Crossover design (1 week washout)	Colorimetric (DNPH)	Bioflavonoids comparable AUC	Bioflavonoids comparable 24 h vitamin C excretion	[83]
12 non-smoking subjects 18–41 years	500 mg vitamin C solution 2 g citrus extract Placebo	Subgroup had 1 g/day vitamin C for 2 weeks pre-study; 8 h sampling; Crossover design (1 week washout)	Fluorometric	Citrus extract ↑ AUC	Citrus extract ↓ 24 h vitamin C excretion in non-saturated subjects and ↑ 24 h vitamin C excretion in saturated subjects	[81]

Table 3. *Cont.*

5 men 21–25 years	500 mg vitamin C solution 500 mg vitamin C in blackcurrant juice	100 mg/day vitamin C for 1 month pre-study; 8 h sampling; Crossover design (1 week washout)	Colorimetric (Indophenol dye)	ND	Blackcurrant juice slight ↑ 8 h vitamin C excretion in saturated subjects	[82]
15 normal subjects (4 smokers) 20–42 years	70 mg/h vitamin C solution Orange juice	Intestinal perfusion; Tandem design	Colorimetric (DNPH)	Orange juice comparable intestinal absorption	ND	[88]
12 men (6 smokers) 23–44 years	75 mg vitamin C solution 400 mg rutin Orange juice (75 mg vitamin C)	Pre- and post-saturation with 1 mg/day vitamin C; 2–24 h sampling; Crossover design (1 day washout)	Colorimetric	Orange juice and rutin ↓ plasma vitamin C (at 2 h)	Orange juice slight ↑ 24 h vitamin C excretion	[71]

AUC: area under the concentration-time curve; ND: not determined; DNPH: 2,4-dinitrophenylhydrazine; TPTZ: 2,4,6-tris(2-pyridyl)-*s*-triazine.

5. Vitamin C Bioavailability from Different Tablet Formulations

Doses of vitamin C up to 2000 mg/day are considered safe for general consumption [90]. However, pharmacokinetic studies indicate that ingestion of single doses of vitamin C greater than 200 mg have lower relative bioavailability [78], indicating that ingestion of several smaller doses each day is preferable to a single large dose. A number of studies have investigated the relative bioavailability of vitamin C from different tablet formulations and have shown that slow-release formulations provide superior vitamin bioavailability [91–94]. Salts of vitamin C, such as sodium and calcium ascorbate (Ester-C), have also been tested. Animal studies indicated that Ester-C (which contains calcium ascorbate, as well as DHA and calcium threonate) was absorbed more readily and excreted less rapidly than ascorbic acid [95] and had superior anti-scorbutic activity in ODS rats [96]. Johnston and Luo [83], however, found no significant differences between Ester-C and ascorbic acid bioavailability in humans. Nevertheless, Ester-C has been shown to be better tolerated in individuals sensitive to acidic foods [97].

6. Conclusions

Overall, a majority of animal studies have shown differences in the comparative bioavailability of synthetic *versus* food-derived vitamin C, or vitamin C in the presence of isolated bioflavonoids, although the results varied depending on the animal model, study design and body compartments measured. In contrast, all steady state comparative bioavailability studies in humans have shown no differences between synthetic and natural vitamin C, regardless of the subject population, study design or intervention used. Some pharmacokinetic studies in humans have shown transient and small comparative differences between synthetic and natural vitamin C, although these differences are likely to have minimal physiological impact. Thus, not only do the reviewed studies reiterate the injunction that the findings of animal studies should not be directly translated to humans [98,99], but it is also apparent that additional comparative bioavailability studies in humans are unwarranted.

Although synthetic and food-derived vitamin C appear to be equally bioavailable in humans, ingesting vitamin C as part of a whole food is considered preferable because of the concomitant consumption of numerous other macro- and micronutrients and phytochemicals, which will confer additional health benefits. Numerous epidemiological studies have indicated that higher intakes of fruit and vegetables are associated with decreased incidence of stroke [100], coronary heart disease [101], and cancers at various sites [102,103]. Vitamin C status is one of the best markers for fruit and vegetable intake [104], and food-derived vitamin C is associated with decreased incidence of numerous chronic diseases [1], however, whether the observed health effects of fruit and vegetable ingestion are due to vitamin C and/or other plant-derived components is currently unknown. With respect to coronary heart disease, strong evidence exists for a protective effect of vegetables, moderate evidence for fruit and dietary vitamin C and insufficient evidence for supplemental vitamin C [105]. Some meta-analyses support the premise that dietary vitamin C is more protective than supplements [106], while others show reduced disease incidence with supplemental but not dietary vitamin C [107].

A major limitation with epidemiological studies is that they show only an association between dietary vitamin C intake and disease risk and cannot ascertain whether different sources of vitamin C (*i.e.*, food-derived *versus* supplement) are a cause, consequence, or simply a correlate of the particular end-point measured. Interpretations can also vary significantly depending on the input of different confounders [108]. Furthermore, epidemiological studies rely predominantly on food frequency questionnaires [109,110] and 24 h dietary recalls [111] to ascertain vitamin C intakes from foods and/or supplements [112]. This methodology has numerous limitations [113] and correlations with vitamin C status can vary depending on the methods employed as well as numerous other external factors [114]. Pooled or meta-analyses of epidemiological studies are particularly problematic due to the combining of variable study designs, cohorts and endpoints, often resulting in dilution or misinterpretation of study findings.

The gold standard for determining causality is the double-blind randomized placebo controlled clinical trial. Although this type of study design works well for comparing the effects of drugs against a placebo, it does not work for nutrients, such as vitamin C, which are already in the food chain and are required for life, *i.e.*, there is no true placebo. Numerous other methodological issues have been identified with the design of many clinical trials investigating the health effects of vitamin C [115]. For example, a major flaw with many vitamin C intervention studies is the use of study populations with already adequate or even saturating vitamin C levels, which significantly decreases the likelihood of observing any effects of the intervention. Thus, it is recommended that study populations are comprised of individuals with sub-optimal vitamin C status (*i.e.*, <50 µmol/L plasma vitamin C) or that sub-group analysis is carried out on the low vitamin C sub-populations [116]. With pharmacokinetic studies, both unsaturated and saturated individuals can be used, but comparative bioavailability studies have shown that results may vary depending on the baseline vitamin C status of the study subjects. Furthermore, the vitamin C doses chosen for intervention are critical since doses above 200 mg have decreased intestinal uptake [78], indicating that if higher doses are warranted then these should be provided as multiple doses of ~200 mg each to ensure complete bioavailability.

The comparative health effects of supplemental *versus* food-derived vitamin C will only be determined through the use of appropriate and well-designed studies. Determination of the physiological effects or health outcomes of intervention with synthetic *versus* natural vitamin C will depend largely on the endpoints measured. Only a handful of comparative intervention studies have been carried out to assess specific physiological or health endpoints. Guarnieri *et al.* [89] investigated potential protection of mononuclear leukocytes from supplemented individuals against *ex vivo* oxidative DNA damage. Although they found comparable vitamin C bioavailability between a single portion of orange juice (containing 150 mg vitamin C) and a synthetic vitamin C drink of the same dosage, they showed that only the orange juice protected the leukocytes from *ex vivo* oxidative DNA damage [89]. However, how closely *ex vivo* oxidation of DNA resembles events occurring *in vivo* is debatable and results could also vary significantly depending on the type of oxidative stress. Johnston *et al.* [76] compared plasma lipid peroxidation in individuals who had been supplemented with either orange juice or synthetic vitamin C (~70 mg/day) for two weeks. They found comparable vitamin C bioavailability and a similar reduction in lipid peroxidation with both interventions [76]. Several studies have assessed the effects of synthetic and natural vitamin C, or vitamin C in the presence of bioflavonoids, on the common cold. Two earlier studies showed a lack of an effect of vitamin C (~200 mg/day), with and without purified bioflavonoids, on the prevention and cure of the common cold [117,118]. Another study indicated that synthetic vitamin C (80 mg/day) and orange juice both decreased the symptoms of the common cold compared with placebo, but there were no differences between the two interventions [119].

As alluded to in the introduction, vitamin C is known to enhance the bioavailability of other nutrients, such as vitamin E [30] and non-heme iron [31,32], which may enhance the health effects of vitamin C-containing foods. Bioflavonoids are also known to have numerous biological activities [120]. Recently vitamin C has been shown to modulate specific biological activities of quercetin and tea polyphenols [121,122]. Thus, future studies may elucidate the physiological relevance of these interactions.

Acknowledgments

Co-funding was provided by the New Zealand Ministry of Business, Innovation & Employment and Zespri International Ltd., Mount Maunganui, New Zealand.

References

1. Carr, A.C.; Frei, B. Toward a new recommended dietary allowance for vitamin C based on antioxidant and health effects in humans. *Am. J. Clin. Nutr.* **1999**, *69*, 1086–1107.
2. Englard, S.; Seifter, S. The biochemical functions of ascorbic acid. *Annu. Rev. Nutr.* **1986**, *6*, 365–406.
3. Ozer, A.; Bruick, R.K. Non-heme dioxygenases: Cellular sensors and regulators jelly rolled into one? *Nat. Chem. Biol.* **2007**, *3*, 144–153.
4. Monfort, A.; Wutz, A. Breathing-in epigenetic change with vitamin C. *EMBO Rep.* **2013**, *14*, 337–346.
5. Hornig, D. Distribution of ascorbic acid, metabolites and analogues in man and animals. *Ann. N. Y. Acad. Sci.* **1975**, *258*, 103–118.
6. Omaye, S.T.; Schaus, E.E.; Kutnink, M.A.; Hawkes, W.C. Measurement of vitamin C in blood components by high-performance liquid chromatography. Implication in assessing vitamin C status. *Ann. N. Y. Acad. Sci.* **1987**, *498*, 389–401.
7. Tsao, C.S. An Overview of Ascorbic Acid Chemistry and Biochemistry. In *Vitamin C in Health and Disease*; Packer, L., Fuchs, J., Eds.; Marcel Dekker: New York, NY, USA, 1997; pp. 25–58.
8. Nishikimi, M.; Fukuyama, R.; Minoshima, S.; Shimizu, N.; Yagi, K. Cloning and chromosomal mapping of the human nonfunctional gene for L-gulono-γ-lactone oxidase, the enzyme for L-ascorbic acid biosynthesis missing in man. *J. Biol. Chem.* **1994**, *269*, 13685–13688.
9. Krebs, H.A. The Sheffield Experiment on the vitamin C requirement of human adults. *Proc. Nutr. Soc.* **1953**, *12*, 237–246.

10. Sauberlich, H.E. A History of Scurvy and Vitamin C. In: *Vitamin C in Health and Disease*; Packer, L., Fuchs, J., Eds.; Marcel Dekker: New York, NY, USA, 1997; pp. 1–24.
11. Michels, A.J.; Hagen, T.M.; Frei, B. Human genetic variation influences vitamin C homeostasis by altering vitamin C transport and antioxidant enzyme function. *Annu. Rev. Nutr.* **2013**, *33*, 45–70.
12. Tsukaguchi, H.; Tokui, T.; Mackenzie, B.; Berger, U.V.; Chen, X.Z.; Wang, Y.; Brubaker, R.F.; Hediger, M.A. A family of mammalian Na^+-dependent L-ascorbic acid transporters. *Nature* **1999**, *399*, 70–75.
13. Savini, I.; Rossi, A.; Pierro, C.; Avigliano, L.; Catani, M.V. SVCT1 and SVCT2: Key proteins for vitamin C uptake. *Amino Acids* **2008**, *34*, 347–355.
14. Rumsey, S.C.; Welch, R.W.; Garraffo, H.M.; Ge, P.; Lu, S.F.; Crossman, A.T.; Kirk, K.L.; Levine, M. Specificity of ascorbate analogs for ascorbate transport. Synthesis and detection of [(125)I]6-deoxy-6-iodo-L-ascorbic acid and characterization of its ascorbate-specific transport properties. *J. Biol. Chem.* **1999**, *274*, 23215–23222.
15. Goldman, H.M.; Gould, B.S.; Munro, H.N. The antiscorbutic action of L-ascorbic acid and D-isoascorbic acid (erythorbic acid) in the guinea pig. *Am. J. Clin. Nutr.* **1981**, *34*, 24–33.
16. Hughes, R.E.; Hurley, R.J. The uptake of D-araboascorbic acid (D-isoascorbic acid) by guinea-pig tissues. *Br. J. Nutr.* **1969**, *23*, 211–216.
17. Levine, M. Fruits and vegetables: There is no substitute. *Am. J. Clin. Nutr.* **1996**, *64*, 381–382.
18. Sauberlich, H.E.; Tamura, T.; Craig, C.B.; Freeberg, L.E.; Liu, T. Effects of erythorbic acid on vitamin C metabolism in young women. *Am. J. Clin. Nutr.* **1996**, *64*, 336–346.
19. Corpe, C.P.; Eck, P.; Wang, J.; Al-Hasani, H.; Levine, M. Intestinal dehydroascorbic acid (DHA) transport mediated by the facilitative sugar transporters, GLUT2 and GLUT8. *J. Biol. Chem.* **2013**, *288*, 9092–9101.
20. Rumsey, S.C.; Kwon, O.; Xu, G.W.; Burant, C.F.; Simpson, I.; Levine, M. Glucose transporter isoforms GLUT1 and GLUT3 transport dehydroascorbic acid. *J. Biol. Chem.* **1997**, *272*, 18982–18989.
21. Vera, J.C.; Rivas, C.I.; Fischbarg, J.; Golde, D.W. Mammalian facilitative hexose transporters mediate the transport of dehydroascorbic acid. *Nature* **1993**, *364*, 79–82.
22. Washko, P.W.; Wang, Y.; Levine, M. Ascorbic acid recycling in human neutrophils. *J. Biol. Chem.* **1993**, *268*, 15531–15535.
23. Corti, A.; Casini, A.F.; Pompella, A. Cellular pathways for transport and efflux of ascorbate and dehydroascorbate. *Arch. Biochem. Biophys.* **2010**, *500*, 107–115.
24. Nishiyama, I.; Yamashita, Y.; Yamanaka, M.; Shimohashi, A.; Fukuda, T.; Oota, T. Varietal difference in vitamin C content in the fruit of kiwifruit and other actinidia species. *J. Agric. Food Chem.* **2004**, *52*, 5472–5475.
25. Dhariwal, K.R.; Hartzell, W.O.; Levine, M. Ascorbic acid and dehydroascorbic acid measurements in human plasma and serum. *Am. J. Clin. Nutr.* **1991**, *54*, 712–716.
26. Ogiri, Y.; Sun, F.; Hayami, S.; Fujimura, A.; Yamamoto, K.; Yaita, M.; Kojo, S. Very low vitamin C activity of orally administered L-dehydroascorbic acid. *J. Agric. Food Chem.* **2002**, *50*, 227–229.

27. Welch, R.W.; Wang, Y.; Crossman, A., Jr.; Park, J.B.; Kirk, K.L.; Levine, M. Accumulation of vitamin C (ascorbate) and its oxidized metabolite dehydroascorbic acid occurs by separate mechanisms. *J. Biol. Chem.* **1995**, *270*, 12584–12592.
28. Wang, Y.; Russo, T.A.; Kwon, O.; Chanock, S.; Rumsey, S.C.; Levine, M. Ascorbate recycling in human neutrophils: Induction by bacteria. *Proc. Natl. Acad. Sci. USA* **1997**, *94*, 13816–13819.
29. Packer, J.E.; Slater, T.F.; Willson, R.L. Direct observation of a free radical interaction between vitamin E and vitamin C. *Nature* **1979**, *278*, 737–738.
30. Tanaka, K.; Hashimoto, T.; Tokumaru, S.; Iguchi, H.; Kojo, S. Interactions between vitamin C and vitamin E are observed in tissues of inherently scorbutic rats. *J. Nutr.* **1997**, *127*, 2060–2064.
31. Beck, K.; Conlon, C.A.; Kruger, R.; Coad, J.; Stonehouse, W. Gold kiwifruit consumed with an iron-fortified breakfast cereal meal improves iron status in women with low iron stores: A 16-week randomised controlled trial. *Br. J. Nutr.* **2011**, *105*, 101–109.
32. Hallberg, L.; Brune, M.; Rossander, L. Effect of ascorbic acid on iron absorption from different types of meals. Studies with ascorbic-acid-rich foods and synthetic ascorbic acid given in different amounts with different meals. *Hum. Nutr. Appl. Nutr.* **1986**, *40*, 97–113.
33. Scheers, N.M.; Sandberg, A.S. Iron regulates the uptake of ascorbic acid and the expression of sodium-dependent vitamin C transporter 1 (SVCT1) in human intestinal Caco-2 cells. *Br. J. Nutr.* **2011**, *105*, 1734–1740.
34. Bates, C.J.; Jones, K.S.; Bluck, L.J. Stable isotope-labelled vitamin C as a probe for vitamin C absorption by human subjects. *Br. J. Nutr.* **2004**, *91*, 699–705.
35. Mangels, A.R.; Block, G.; Frey, C.M.; Patterson, B.H.; Taylor, P.R.; Norkus, E.P.; Levander, O.A. The bioavailability to humans of ascorbic acid from oranges, orange juice and cooked broccoli is similar to that of synthetic ascorbic acid. *J. Nutr.* **1993**, *123*, 1054–1061.
36. Keltz, F.R.; Kies, C.; Fox, H.M. Urinary ascorbic acid excretion in the human as affected by dietary fiber and zinc. *Am. J. Clin. Nutr.* **1978**, *31*, 1167–1171.
37. Rusznyak, S.; Szent-Gyorgyi, A. Vitamin P: Flavonols as vitamins. *Nature* **1936**, *138*, 27.
38. Bentsath, A.; Rusznyak, S.; Szent-Gyorgyi, A. Vitamin nature of flavones. *Nature* **1936**, *138*, 798.
39. Bentsath, A.; Rusznyak, S.; Szent-Gyorgyi, A. Vitamin P. *Nature* **1937**, *139*, 326–327.
40. Rusznyak, S.; Benko, A. Experimental vitamin P deficiency. *Science* **1941**, *94*, 25.
41. Zilva, S.S. Vitamin P. *Biochem. J.* **1937**, *31*, 915–919.
42. Cotereau, H.; Gabe, M.; Géro, E.; Parrot, J.-L. Influence of vitamin P (vitamin C_2) upon the amount of ascorbic acid in the organs of the guinea pig. *Nature* **1948**, *161*, 557.
43. Scarborough, H. Deficiency of vitamin C and vitamin P in man. *Lancet* **1940**, *236*, 644–647.
44. Scarborough, H. Vitamin P. *Biochem. J.* **1939**, *33*, 1400–1407.
45. Elmby, A.; Warburg, E. The inadequacy of synthetic ascorbic acid as an antiscorbutic agent. *Lancet* **1937**, *230*, 1363–1365.
46. Ivanov, V.; Carr, A.C.; Frei, B. Red wine antioxidants bind to human lipoproteins and protect them from metal ion-dependent and -independent oxidation. *J. Agric. Food Chem.* **2001**, *49*, 4442–4449.

47. Bors, W.; Michel, C.; Saran, M. Flavonoid antioxidants: Rate constants for reactions with oxygen radicals. *Methods Enzymol.* **1994**, *234*, 420–429.
48. Beker, B.Y.; Sonmezoglu, I.; Imer, F.; Apak, R. Protection of ascorbic acid from copper(II)-catalyzed oxidative degradation in the presence of flavonoids: Quercetin, catechin and morin. *Int. J. Food Sci. Nutr.* **2011**, *62*, 504–512.
49. Clemetson, C.A.; Andersen, L. Plant polyphenols as antioxidants for ascorbic acid. *Ann. N. Y. Acad Sci.* **1966**, *136*, 341–376.
50. Harper, K.A.; Morton, A.D.; Rolfe, E.J. The phenolic compounds of blackcurrant juice and their protective effect on ascorbic acid III. The mechansim of ascorbic acid oxidation and its inhibition by flavonoids. *Int. J. Food Sci. Technol.* **1969**, *4*, 255–267.
51. Clegg, K.M.; Morton, A.D. The phenolic compounds of blackcurrant juice and their protective effect on ascorbic acid II. The stability of ascorbic acid in model systems containing some of the phenolic compounds associated with blackcurrant juice. *Int. J. Food Sci. Technol.* **1968**, *3*, 277–284.
52. Carr, A.; Frei, B. Does vitamin C act as a pro-oxidant under physiological conditions? *FASEB J.* **1999**, *13*, 1007–1024.
53. Lotito, S.B.; Frei, B. Consumption of flavonoid-rich foods and increased plasma antioxidant capacity in humans: Cause, consequence, or epiphenomenon? *Free Radic. Biol. Med.* **2006**, *41*, 1727–1746.
54. Song, J.; Kwon, O.; Chen, S.; Daruwala, R.; Eck, P.; Park, J.B.; Levine, M. Flavonoid inhibition of sodium-dependent vitamin C transporter 1 (SVCT1) and glucose transporter isoform 2 (GLUT2), intestinal transporters for vitamin C and Glucose. *J. Biol. Chem.* **2002**, *277*, 15252–15260.
55. Park, J.B.; Levine, M. Intracellular accumulation of ascorbic acid is inhibited by flavonoids via blocking of dehydroascorbic acid and ascorbic acid uptakes in HL-60, U937 and Jurkat cells. *J. Nutr.* **2000**, *130*, 1297–1302.
56. Corpe, C.P.; Lee, J.H.; Kwon, O.; Eck, P.; Narayanan, J.; Kirk, K.L.; Levine, M. 6-Bromo-6-deoxy-L-ascorbic acid: An ascorbate analog specific for Na^+-dependent vitamin C transporter but not glucose transporter pathways. *J. Biol. Chem.* **2005**, *280*, 5211–5220.
57. Washko, P.W.; Welch, R.W.; Dhariwal, K.R.; Wang, Y.; Levine, M. Ascorbic acid and dehydroascorbic acid analyses in biological samples. *Anal. Biochem.* **1992**, *204*, 1–14.
58. Mizushima, Y.; Harauchi, T.; Yoshizaki, T.; Makino, S. A rat mutant unable to synthesize vitamin C. *Experientia* **1984**, *40*, 359–361.
59. Maeda, N.; Hagihara, H.; Nakata, Y.; Hiller, S.; Wilder, J.; Reddick, R. Aortic wall damage in mice unable to synthesize ascorbic acid. *Proc. Natl. Acad. Sci. USA* **2000**, *97*, 841–846.
60. Mohan, S.; Kapoor, A.; Singgih, A.; Zhang, Z.; Taylor, T.; Yu, H.; Chadwick, R.B.; Chung, Y.S.; Donahue, L.R.; Rosen, C.; *et al.* Spontaneous fractures in the mouse mutant *sfx* are caused by deletion of the gulonolactone oxidase gene, causing vitamin C deficiency. *J. Bone Miner. Res.* **2005**, *20*, 1597–1610.
61. Wilson, H.K.; Price-Jones, C.; Hughes, R.E. The influence of an extract of orange peel on the growth and ascorbic acid metabolism of young guinea-pigs. *J. Sci. Food Agric.* **1976**, *27*, 661–666.

62. Douglass, C.D.; Kamp, G.H. The effect of orally administered rutin on the adrenal ascorbic acid level in guinea pigs. *J. Nutr.* **1959**, *67*, 531–536.
63. Papageorge, E.; Mitchell, G.L., Jr. The effect of oral administration of rutin on blood, liver and adrenal ascorbic acid and on liver and adrenal cholesterol in guinea pigs. *J. Nutr.* **1949**, *37*, 531–540.
64. Hughes, R.E.; Hurley, R.J.; Jones, P.R. The retention of ascorbic acid by guinea-pig tissues. *Br. J. Nutr.* **1971**, *26*, 433–438.
65. Vinson, J.A.; Bose, P. Comparative bioavailability of synthetic and natural vitamin C in guinea pigs. *Nutr. Rep. Int.* **1983**, *27*, 875–879.
66. Ambrose, A.M.; De, E.F. The value of rutin and quercetin in scurvy. *J. Nutr.* **1949**, *38*, 305–317.
67. Todhunter, E.N.; Robbins, R.C.; Ivey, G.; Brewer, W. A comparison of the utilization by guinea pigs of equivalent amounts of ascorbic acid (vitamin C) in lemon juice and in crystalline form. *J. Nutr.* **1940**, *19*, 113–120.
68. Vissers, M.C.M.; Bozonet, S.M.; Pearson, J.F.; Braithwaite, L.J. Dietary ascorbate affects steady state tissue levels in vitamin C-deficient mice: Tissue deficiency after sub-optimal intake and superior bioavailability from a food source (kiwifruit). *Am. J. Clin. Nutr.* **2011**, *93*, 292–301.
69. Latocha, P.; Krupa, T.; Wolosiak, R.; Worobiej, E.; Wilczak, J. Antioxidant activity and chemical difference in fruit of different *Actinidia* sp. *Int J. Food Sci. Nutr.* **2010**, *61*, 381–394.
70. Fiorentino, A.; D'Abrosca, B.; Pacifico, S.; Mastellone, C.; Scognamiglio, M.; Monaco, P. Identification and assessment of antioxidant capacity of phytochemicals from kiwi fruits. *J. Agric. Food Chem.* **2009**, *57*, 4148–4155.
71. Pelletier, O.; Keith, M.O. Bioavailability of synthetic and natural ascorbic acid. *J. Am. Diet. Assoc.* **1974**, *64*, 271–275.
72. Hartzler, E.R. The availability of ascorbic acid in papayas and guavas. *J. Nutr.* **1945**, *30*, 355–365.
73. Clayton, M.M.; Borden, R.A. The availability for human nutrition of the vitamin C in raw cabbage and home-canned tomato juice. *J. Nutr.* **1943**, *25*, 349–369.
74. Todhunter, E.N.; Fatzer, A.S. A comparison of the utilization by college women of equivalent amounts of ascorbic acid (vitamin C) in red raspberries and in crystalline form. *J. Nutr.* **1940**, *19*, 121–130.
75. Hawley, E.E.; Stephens, D.J.; Anderson, G. The excretion of vitamin C in normal individuals following a comparable quantitative administration in the form of orange juice, cevitamic acid by mouth and cevitamic acid intravenously. *J. Nutr.* **1936**, *11*, 135–145.
76. Johnston, C.S.; Dancho, C.L.; Strong, G.M. Orange juice ingestion and supplemental vitamin C are equally effective at reducing plasma lipid peroxidation in healthy adult women. *J. Am. Coll. Nutr.* **2003**, *22*, 519–523.
77. Carr, A.C.; Bozonet, S.M.; Pullar, J.M.; Simcock, J.W.; Vissers, M.C. A randomised steady-state bioavailability study of synthetic and natural (kiwifruit-derived) vitamin C. *Nutrients* **2013**, *5*, 3684–3695.

78. Levine, M.; Conry-Cantilena, C.; Wang, Y.; Welch, R.W.; Washko, P.W.; Dhariwal, K.R.; Park, J.B.; Lazarev, A.; Graumlich, J.F.; King, J.; *et al.* Vitamin C pharmacokinetics in healthy volunteers: Evidence for a recommended dietary allowance. *Proc. Natl. Acad. Sci. USA* **1996**, *93*, 3704–3709.
79. Block, G.; Mangels, A.R.; Patterson, B.H.; Levander, O.A.; Norkus, E.P.; Taylor, P.R. Body weight and prior depletion affect plasma ascorbate levels attained on identical vitamin C intake: A controlled-diet study. *J. Am. Coll. Nutr.* **1999**, *18*, 628–637.
80. Carr, A.C.; Bozonet, S.M.; Pullar, J.M.; Simcock, J.W.; Vissers, M.C. Human skeletal muscle ascorbate is highly responsive to changes in vitamin C intake and plasma concentrations. *Am. J. Clin. Nutr.* **2013**, *97*, 800–807.
81. Vinson, J.A.; Bose, P. Comparative bioavailability to humans of ascorbic acid alone or in a citrus extract. *Am. J. Clin. Nutr.* **1988**, *48*, 601–604.
82. Jones, E.; Hughes, R.E. The influence of bioflavonoids on the absorption of vitamin C. *IRCS J. Med. Sci.* **1984**, *12*, 320.
83. Johnston, C.S.; Luo, B. Comparison of the absorption and excretion of three commercially available sources of vitamin C. *J. Am. Diet. Assoc.* **1994**, *94*, 779–781.
84. Kondo, Y.; Higashi, C.; Iwama, M.; Ishihara, K.; Handa, S.; Mugita, H.; Maruyama, N.; Koga, H.; Ishigami, A. Bioavailability of vitamin C from mashed potatoes and potato chips after oral administration in healthy Japanese men. *Br. J. Nutr.* **2012**, *107*, 885–892.
85. Uchida, E.; Kondo, Y.; Amano, A.; Aizawa, S.; Hanamura, T.; Aoki, H.; Nagamine, K.; Koizumi, T.; Maruyama, N.; Ishigami, A. Absorption and excretion of ascorbic acid alone and in acerola (*Malpighia emarginata*) juice: Comparison in healthy japanese subjects. *Biol. Pharm. Bull.* **2011**, *34*, 1744–1747.
86. Carter, B.; Monsivais, P.; Drewnowski, A. Absorption of folic acid and ascorbic acid from nutrient comparable beverages. *J. Food Sci.* **2010**, *75*, H289–H293.
87. Guarnieri, S.; Riso, P.; Porrini, M. Orange juice *vs* vitamin C: Effect on hydrogen peroxide-induced DNA damage in mononuclear blood cells. *Br. J. Nutr.* **2007**, *97*, 639–643.
88. Nelson, E.W.; Streiff, R.R.; Cerda, J.J. Comparative bioavailability of folate and vitamin C from a synthetic and a natural source. *Am. J. Clin. Nutr.* **1975**, *28*, 1014–1019.
89. Carr, A.C.; Bozonet, S.M.; Vissers, M.C.M. A randomised cross-over pharmacokinetic bioavailabiltiy study of synthetic *versus* kiwifruit-derived vitamin C. *Nutrients* **2013**, *5*, 3684–3695.
90. Hathcock, J.N.; Azzi, A.; Blumberg, J.; Bray, T.; Dickinson, A.; Frei, B.; Jialal, I.; Johnston, C.S.; Kelly, F.J.; Kraemer, K.; *et al.* Vitamins E and C are safe across a broad range of intakes. *Am. J. Clin. Nutr.* **2005**, *81*, 736–745.
91. Yung, S.; Mayersohn, M.; Robinson, J.B. Ascorbic acid absorption in humans: A comparison among several dosage forms. *J. Pharm. Sci.* **1982**, *71*, 282–285.
92. Bhagavan, H.N.; Wolkoff, B.I. Correlation between the disintegration time and the bioavailability of vitamin C tablets. *Pharm. Res.* **1993**, *10*, 239–242.
93. Sacharin, R.; Taylor, T.; Chasseaud, L.F. Blood levels and bioavailability of ascorbic acid after administration of a sustained-release formulation to humans. *Int. J. Vitam. Nutr. Res.* **1977**, *47*, 68–74.

94. Nyyssonen, K.; Poulsen, H.E.; Hayn, M.; Agerbo, P.; Porkkala-Sarataho, E.; Kaikkonen, J.; Salonen, R.; Salonen, J.T. Effect of supplementation of smoking men with plain or slow release ascorbic acid on lipoprotein oxidation. *Eur. J. Clin. Nutr.* **1997**, *51*, 154–163.
95. Bush, M.J.; Verlangieri, A.J. An acute study on the relative gastro-intestinal absorption of a novel form of calcium ascorbate. *Res. Commun. Chem. Pathol. Pharmacol.* **1987**, *57*, 137–140.
96. Verlangieri, A.J.; Fay, M.J.; Bannon, A.W. Comparison of the *anti*-scorbutic activity of L-ascorbic acid and Ester C in the non-ascorbate synthesizing Osteogenic Disorder Shionogi (ODS) rat. *Life Sci.* **1991**, *48*, 2275–2281.
97. Gruenwald, J.; Graubaum, H.J.; Busch, R.; Bentley, C. Safety and tolerance of ester-C compared with regular ascorbic acid. *Adv. Ther.* **2006**, *23*, 171–178.
98. Knight, A. Systematic reviews of animal experiments demonstrate poor human clinical and toxicological utility. *Altern. Lab. Anim.* **2007**, *35*, 641–659.
99. Seok, J.; Warren, H.S.; Cuenca, A.G.; Mindrinos, M.N.; Baker, H.V.; Xu, W.; Richards, D.R.; McDonald-Smith, G.P.; Gao, H.; Hennessy, L.; *et al.* Genomic responses in mouse models poorly mimic human inflammatory diseases. *Proc. Natl. Acad. Sci. USA* **2013**, *110*, 3507–3512.
100. He, F.J.; Nowson, C.A.; MacGregor, G.A. Fruit and vegetable consumption and stroke: Meta-analysis of cohort studies. *Lancet* **2006**, *367*, 320–326.
101. Dauchet, L.; Amouyel, P.; Hercberg, S.; Dallongeville, J. Fruit and vegetable consumption and risk of coronary heart disease: A meta-analysis of cohort studies. *J. Nutr.* **2006**, *136*, 2588–2593.
102. Steinmetz, K.A.; Potter, J.D. Vegetables, fruit, and cancer prevention: A review. *J. Am. Diet. Assoc.* **1996**, *96*, 1027–1039.
103. Riboli, E.; Norat, T. Epidemiologic evidence of the protective effect of fruit and vegetables on cancer risk. *Am. J. Clin. Nutr.* **2003**, *78*, 559S–569S.
104. Block, G.; Norkus, E.; Hudes, M.; Mandel, S.; Helzlsouer, K. Which plasma antioxidants are most related to fruit and vegetable consumption? *Am. J. Epidemiol.* **2001**, *154*, 1113–1118.
105. Mente, A.; de Koning, L.; Shannon, H.S.; Anand, S.S. A systematic review of the evidence supporting a causal link between dietary factors and coronary heart disease. *Arch. Intern. Med.* **2009**, *169*, 659–669.
106. Ye, Z.; Song, H. Antioxidant vitamins intake and the risk of coronary heart disease: Meta-analysis of cohort studies. *Eur. J. Cardiovasc. Prev. Rehabil.* **2008**, *15*, 26–34.
107. Knekt, P.; Ritz, J.; Pereira, M.A.; O'Reilly, E.J.; Augustsson, K.; Fraser, G.E.; Goldbourt, U.; Heitmann, B.L.; Hallmans, G.; Liu, S.; *et al.* Antioxidant vitamins and coronary heart disease risk: A pooled analysis of 9 cohorts. *Am. J. Clin. Nutr.* **2004**, *80*, 1508–1520.
108. Lawlor, D.A.; Davey Smith, G.; Kundu, D.; Bruckdorfer, K.R.; Ebrahim, S. Those confounded vitamins: What can we learn from the differences between observational *versus* randomised trial evidence? *Lancet* **2004**, *363*, 1724–1727.
109. Maserejian, N.N.; Giovannucci, E.L.; McVary, K.T.; McKinlay, J.B. Dietary, but not supplemental, intakes of carotenoids and vitamin C are associated with decreased odds of lower urinary tract symptoms in men. *J. Nutr.* **2011**, *141*, 267–273.

110. Osganian, S.K.; Stampfer, M.J.; Rimm, E.; Spiegelman, D.; Hu, F.B.; Manson, J.E.; Willett, W.C. Vitamin C and risk of coronary heart disease in women. *J. Am. Coll. Cardiol.* **2003**, *42*, 246–252.
111. Agarwal, M.; Mehta, P.K.; Dwyer, J.H.; Dwyer, K.M.; Shircore, A.M.; Nordstrom, C.K.; Sun, P.; Paul-Labrador, M.; Yang, Y.; Merz, C.N. Differing relations to early atherosclerosis between vitamin C from supplements *vs.* food in the Los Angeles atherosclerosis Study: A prospective cohort study. *Open Cardiovasc. Med. J.* **2012**, *6*, 113–121.
112. Henriquez-Sanchez, P.; Sanchez-Villegas, A.; Doreste-Alonso, J.; Ortiz-Andrellucchi, A.; Pfrimer, K.; Serra-Majem, L. Dietary assessment methods for micronutrient intake: A systematic review on vitamins. *Br. J. Nutr.* **2009**, *102*, S10–S37.
113. Thompson, F.E.; Byers, T. Dietary assessment resource manual. *J. Nutr.* **1994**, *124*, 2245S–2317S.
114. Dehghan, M.; Akhtar-Danesh, N.; McMillan, C.R.; Thabane, L. Is plasma vitamin C an appropriate biomarker of vitamin C intake? A systematic review and meta-analysis. *Nutr. J.* **2007**, *6*, 41.
115. Lykkesfeldt, J.; Poulsen, H.E. Is vitamin C supplementation beneficial? Lessons learned from randomised controlled trials. *Br. J. Nutr.* **2010**, *103*, 1251–1259.
116. Carr, A.C.; Pullar, J.M.; Moran, S.; Vissers, M.C.M. Bioavailability of vitamin C from kiwifruit in non-smoking males: Determination of 'healthy' and 'optimal' intakes. *J. Nutr. Sci.* **2012**, *1*, e14.
117. Franz, W.L.; Heyl, H.L.; Sands, G.W. Blood ascorbic acid level in bioflavonoid and ascorbic acid therapy of common cold. *J. Am. Med. Assoc.* **1956**, *162*, 1224–1226.
118. Arminio, J.J.; Johnston, J.H.; Tebrock, H.E. Usefulness of bioflavonoids and ascorbic acid in treatment of common cold. *J. Am. Med. Assoc.* **1956**, *162*, 1227–1233.
119. Baird, I.M.; Hughes, R.E.; Wilson, H.K.; Davies, J.E.; Howard, A.N. The effects of ascorbic acid and flavonoids on the occurrence of symptoms normally associated with the common cold. *Am. J. Clin. Nutr.* **1979**, *32*, 1686–1690.
120. Stevenson, D.E.; Hurst, R.D. Polyphenolic phytochemicals—Just antioxidants or much more? *Cell. Mol. Life Sci.* **2007**, *64*, 2900–2916.
121. Gao, Y.; Li, W.; Jia, L.; Li, B.; Chen, Y.C.; Tu, Y. Enhancement of (−)-epigallocatechin-3-gallate and theaflavin-3-3′-digallate induced apoptosis by ascorbic acid in human lung adenocarcinoma SPC-A-1 cells and esophageal carcinoma Eca-109 cells via MAPK pathways. *Biochem. Biophys. Res. Commun.* **2013**, *438*, 370–374.
122. Calero, C.I.; Beltran Gonzalez, A.N.; Gasulla, J.; Alvarez, S.; Evelson, P.; Calvo, D.J. Quercetin antagonism of GAB receptors is prevented by ascorbic acid through a redox-independent mechanism. *Eur. J. Pharmacol.* **2013**, doi:10.1016/j.ejphar.2013.07.044.

7

Myths, Artifacts and Fatal Flaws: Identifying Limitations and Opportunities in Vitamin C Research

Alexander J. Michels * and Balz Frei

Linus Pauling Institute, 307 Linus Pauling Science Center, Oregon State University, Corvallis, OR 97331, USA; E-Mail: balz.frei@oregonstate.edu

* Author to whom correspondence should be addressed; E-Mail: michelsa@onid.orst.edu;

Abstract: Research progress to understand the role of vitamin C (ascorbic acid) in human health has been slow in coming. This is predominantly the result of several flawed approaches to study design, often lacking a full appreciation of the redox chemistry and biology of ascorbic acid. In this review, we summarize our knowledge surrounding the limitations of common approaches used in vitamin C research. In human cell culture, the primary issues are the high oxygen environment, presence of redox-active transition metal ions in culture media, and the use of immortalized cell lines grown in the absence of supplemental ascorbic acid. Studies in animal models are also limited due to the presence of endogenous ascorbic acid synthesis. Despite the use of genetically altered rodent strains lacking synthesis capacity, there are additional concerns that these models do not adequately recapitulate the effects of vitamin C deprivation and supplementation observed in humans. Lastly, several flaws in study design endemic to randomized controlled trials and other human studies greatly limit their conclusions and impact. There also is anecdotal evidence of positive and negative health effects of vitamin C that are widely accepted but have not been substantiated. Only with careful attention to study design and experimental detail can we further our understanding of the possible roles of vitamin C in promoting human health and preventing or treating disease.

Keywords: vitamin C; ascorbic acid; cell culture; animals; human; study design

---

1. Introduction

Ascorbic acid, the reduced form of vitamin C, is an essential component of the human diet. Small amounts of ascorbic acid can prevent the deficiency disease, scurvy, while accumulation of high levels of ascorbate in plasma and tissues may protect against oxidative damage and limit inflammation. However, ascorbic acid is unlike many other vitamins owing in part to its unique redox chemistry. In addition, the "tight control" of vitamin C status and metabolism in the body, along with biological effects of supplementation that may differ between animals that can synthesize ascorbate *versus* species that cannot synthesize ascorbate, like humans, set it apart in the micronutrient field [1–3]. Thus, many common research practices that are sufficient for the study of other vitamins and minerals are often inadequate for the study of vitamin C, leaving the specific challenges to the design and execution of experiments utilizing ascorbic acid underappreciated. Indeed, there are many examples of supplementation studies making poor assumptions and drawing mistaken conclusions that have persisted in the vitamin C literature. Although several landmark discoveries have broadened our understanding of vitamin C's role in human biology, the research is still plagued by a host of myths, artifacts, and flawed scientific reasoning that undermines efforts to determine the roles that vitamin C may play in human health and disease.

As we continue performing vitamin C research in the future, it is worthwhile to periodically review the literature for experimental approaches that may no longer be valid based on contemporary knowledge. The purpose of this article is to closely examine studies where vitamin C research has "failed" due to methodological, experimental, or design flaws and learn from these errors to help improve future studies, rather than to review studies that have found beneficial effects of vitamin C in human health, as has been done previously [1,3–5]. In so doing, we will re-evaluate two common models, cultured cells and experimental animals, and highlight aspects of each system that may contribute to erroneous conclusions. In addition, we will evaluate human research, continuing from previous reviews of the subject [1,2], including an examination of the design and execution of randomized controlled trials (RCTs). Finally, we will explore some of the technical aspects of vitamin C research, in order to promote better awareness of sample handling issues and analytical techniques that are critical for the proper interpretation of study outcomes.

2. Review of Studies Using Ascorbic Acid

2.1. Ascorbic Acid in Human Cell Culture

The conditions found in a typical cell culture environment promote the oxidation and subsequent degradation of ascorbic acid. Therefore, ascorbate is not usually added to cell culture media, as it often leads to the production of deleterious free radicals and reactive oxygen species (ROS). However, such conditions are non-physiological with respect to vitamin C, which is found in all extra- and intracellular, aqueous solutions *in vivo*. The consequences of such "a-scorbic"—or scorbutic—cell culture environment are not fully understood, but it is obvious that any "ascorbate-dependent" enzymatic reactions, the cells' redox "milieu", and antioxidant network must be severely impaired. Furthermore, reintroducing vitamin C to such a cell culture system may give rise to additional artifacts. In this section, we examine the factors that lead to ascorbate oxidation in cell culture media, the artifacts related to the absence of ascorbate in cultured cells or its addition under normal cell culture conditions, and methods that are currently being developed to allow safe addition of ascorbate to cells for physiologically relevant research. Overall, studying vitamin C in cell culture is fraught with many pitfalls and results need to be approached and interpreted with care.

2.1.1. Ascorbate Stability in Cell Culture

The primary concern with the use of ascorbic acid in cell culture is the stability of the molecule under typical incubation conditions. Cell culture incubators use approximately 90%–95% air and 5%–10% CO_2, resulting in oxygen levels approximately 10–100 times greater than those found in the circulation and in tissues. Increased oxygen tension can promote a pro-oxidant environment in cell culture media [6], possibly generating a wide variety of ROS that can react with, and hence deplete, ascorbate [7]. However, high oxygen levels alone are not sufficient to cause substantial ascorbic acid oxidation. Although the reduction potential of the reduced form of vitamin C, the ascorbate mono-anion ($AscH^-$), is sufficient to reduce molecular oxygen to superoxide radicals (Equation 1), the reaction kinetics make this process very slow (estimated second-order rate constant, $k_2 \approx 10^{-4}\ M^{-1}\ s^{-1}$) [8].

$$AscH^- + O_2 \rightarrow Asc^{\bullet -} + O_2^{\bullet -} \quad (1)$$

The stability of the ascorbate mono-anion is apparent in deionized water or simple salt solutions: ascorbate added to phosphate-buffered saline (PBS) shows minimal oxidation over a six-h time period in a cell culture incubator (Figure 1, PBS) or when exposed to ambient air at room temperature (data not shown). In contrast, ascorbate incubated in cell culture media under standard conditions is rapidly oxidized [9,10] (Figure 1, RPMI). The composition of the cell culture media plays an important role in the rate of ascorbate oxidation: in serum-free RPMI medium the half-life of ascorbate is about 1.5 h (Figure 1); however, a more rapid loss of ascorbate has been noted in other cell culture media formulations such as MEM or Williams E media (data not shown), including more complex solutions containing serum [6,11,12].

Figure 1. Ascorbate oxidation in buffer or cell culture medium. Ascorbate (100 μM) was added to RPMI 1640 or phosphate-buffered saline (PBS) and monitored over time. Chelated RPMI was used after overnight treatment with Chelex 100 resin and the addition of diethylenetriaminepentaacetic acid (DTPA, 1 mM) as described in Methods. RPMI RT represents media not incubated under 5% CO_2 but under ambient air at room temperature.

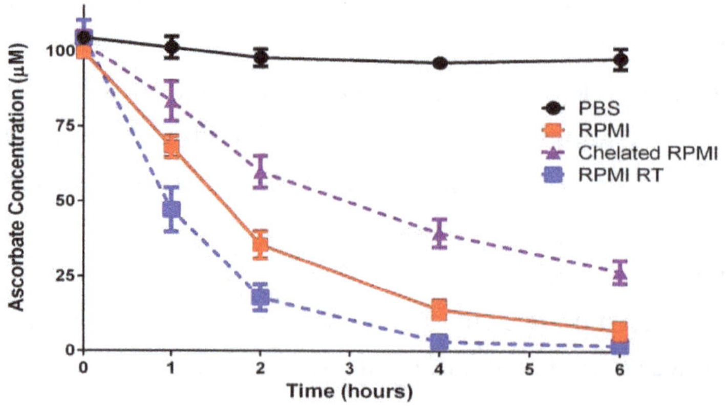

Iron and copper are present in cell culture media, either added as part of the media formulation or appearing fortuitously, as they are required for normal cell growth and function [13,14]. However, the reduced forms of iron (ferrous iron, Fe^{2+}) and copper (cuprous copper, Cu^{+}) are able to reduce molecular oxygen to superoxide and, hence, participate in the production of ROS in cell culture systems. The Haber-Weiss reaction (also known as the superoxide-driven Fenton reaction) involves the reduction of the oxidized forms of iron (ferric iron, Fe^{3+}) or copper (cupric copper, Cu^{2+}) by superoxide (Equation 2) and the subsequent conversion of hydrogen peroxide (formed, e.g., by dismutation of superoxide radicals) to hydroxyl radicals and hydroxide by the reduced metal ions (Fenton reaction, Equation 3) (Scheme 1). Hence, the metal ions act as catalysts and are required only in trace amounts for the Haber-Weiss reaction (Equation 4).

Scheme 1. Metal-dependent and metal-independent production of reactive oxygen species by ascorbate in cell culture media.

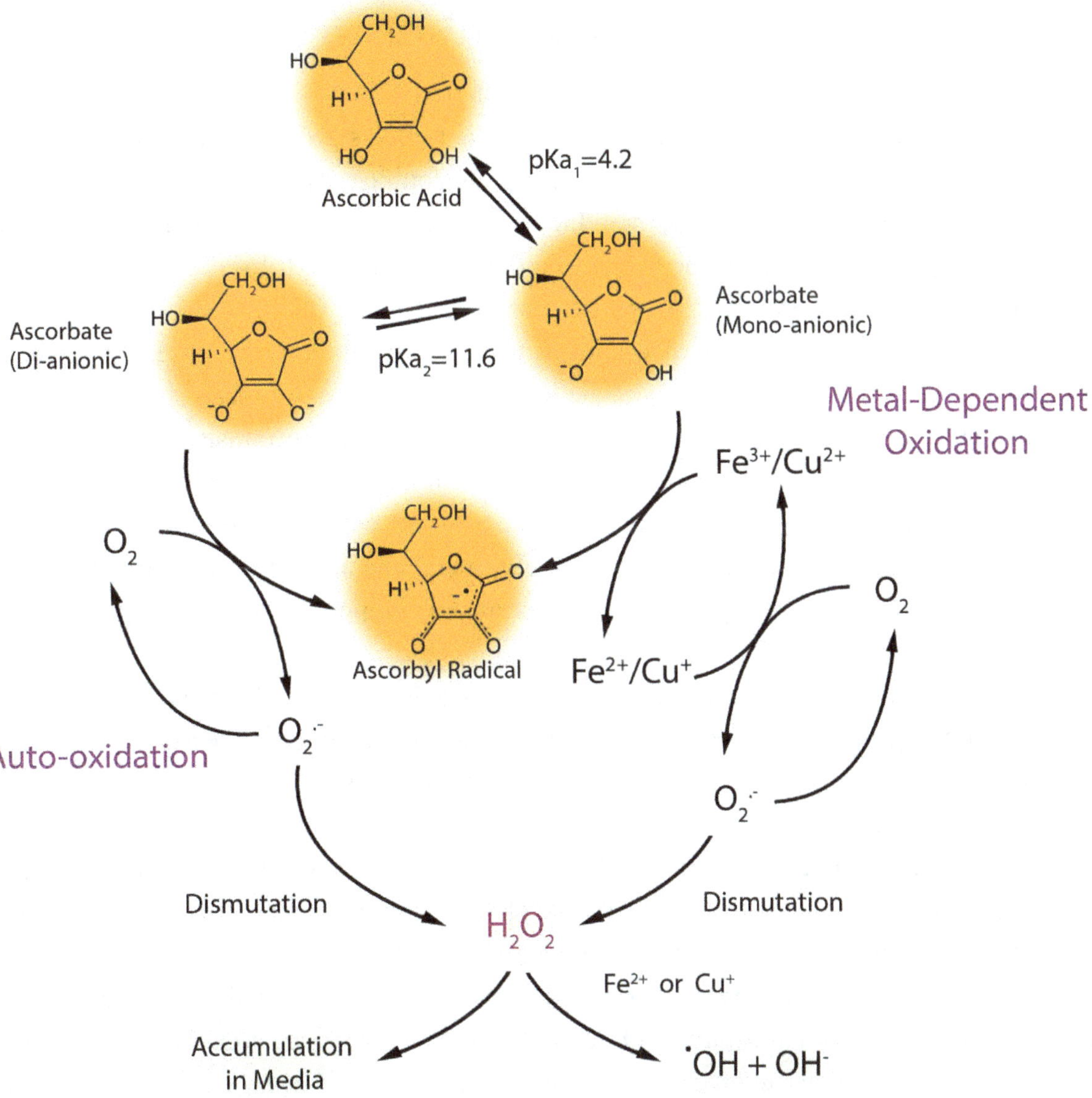

One of the most important biological functions of ascorbate is the reduction of Fe^{3+} or Cu^{2+} in the active site of enzymes, providing electrons used either in the hydroxylation of the enzymes' substrates or the maintenance of the active-site metal ion in the reduced state [3]. In the case of enzyme-bound metals, the transfer of electrons occurs in a controlled manner, which minimizes deleterious side reactions. However, in a solution of non-protein bound iron or copper, added ascorbate will reduce these metal ions (Equation 5); replacing superoxide in Equation 2, leading to superoxide production and facilitating the flow of electrons into the Haber-Weiss reaction (Equation 4). Even if media formulations are carefully controlled, trace amounts of these transition metals may be found on cell culture glassware, plastic dishes, and reagents, fueling ascorbate oxidation and ROS production [8,15].

$$Fe^{3+}/Cu^{2+} + O_2^{\bullet -} \rightarrow Fe^{2+}/Cu^{+} + O_2 \quad (2)$$

$$Fe^{2+}/Cu^{+} + H_2O_2 \rightarrow Fe^{3+}/Cu^{2+} + OH^{\bullet} + OH^{-} \quad (3)$$

$$\text{Sum: } O_2^{\bullet -} + H_2O_2 \xrightarrow{Fe/Cu} O_2 + OH^{\bullet} + OH^{-} \quad (4)$$

$$AscH^{-} + Fe^{3+}/Cu^{2+} \rightarrow Asc^{\bullet -} + Fe^{2+}/Cu^{+} + H^{+} \quad (5)$$

In biological fluids and inside cells *in vivo*, a combination of low oxygen levels and protein-bound metal ions greatly reduce ascorbate-mediated pro-oxidant effects [16–18]. Consequently, ascorbate in human plasma does not get readily oxidized [19]. By contrast, ascorbate addition to cell culture media results in the production of ROS, including superoxide radicals, hydrogen peroxide (from the dismutation of superoxide radicals), and hydroxyl radicals (Scheme 1) [6,15]. For this reason, ascorbic acid is often mistaken for inducing a pro-oxidant environment in cell culture systems [17,20], although the effects of hydrogen peroxide production specifically may be masked by other media components, such as serum proteins, pyruvate, or α-ketoglutarate [6,11,21,22]. A more accurate description may be that ascorbate unmasks the presence of catalytic transition metals in the cell culture environment [15]. Treating cell culture media with metal chelating agents slows the rate of ascorbate oxidation (Figure 1, Chelated RPMI), increasing the half-life from approximately 1.5 h in standard media (RPMI) to about 2.7 h. Interestingly, metal chelation does not completely prevent ascorbate oxidation (Figure 1), suggesting that other media components also contribute to ascorbate loss [6].

One such contributing factor may be ascorbate auto-oxidation: the direct reaction of ascorbate with molecular oxygen [8]. As stated above, the direct interaction between the ascorbate mono-anion and oxygen is highly unfavorable; however, the ascorbate di-anion (Asc^{2-}) rapidly reacts with oxygen (Equation 6). At pH 7.0, the concentration of Asc^{2-} is low, but its contribution to the rate of ascorbate oxidation can become considerable under conditions when pH rises or with increasing concentrations of added ascorbate (Scheme 1) [23]. Cell culture media pH is often stabilized by the addition of sodium bicarbonate to offset the acidic effects of the high CO_2 environment. However, when this media is exposed to air outside the incubator, the pH value can rise rapidly to 8.0 or higher [11]. RPMI media equilibrated to ambient air accelerates ascorbate oxidation when compared to media in a cell culture incubator (Figure 1, RPMI RT *versus* RPMI), decreasing the half-life from about 1.5 h to less than one hour. As the Asc^{2-} present in solution reacts with oxygen to form dehydroascorbic acid, additional Asc^{2-} ions are generated to re-establish the equilibrium driven by the pH (Scheme 1 and Equation 7). This continuous production of Asc^{2-} would fuel auto-oxidation, which is prevalent when supraphysiological levels of ascorbate are added to cell culture media, since the Asc^{2-} concentration would increase proportionally and greatly enhance oxidation effects. Although concentrated ascorbic acid will lower the pH of cell culture media, investigators usually offset this by the addition of sodium hydroxide to limit the impact of the acidic pH on cells. However, any shift toward a neutral or slightly alkaline environment will increase the metal-independent, pH-driven pro-oxidant effects of ascorbate, which may explain the limited effect of metal chelators to reduce the cytotoxicity of millimolar concentrations of ascorbate towards cancer cells [24].

$$Asc^{2-} + O_2 \rightarrow Asc^{\bullet-} + O_2^{\bullet-} \quad (6)$$

$$AscH_2 \leftrightarrow AscH^- + H^+ \leftrightarrow Asc^{2-} + 2H^+ \quad (7)$$

Ascorbate levels can be maintained in cell culture media by frequent addition of vitamin C [9], but the persistent oxidation will continuously generate dehydroascorbic acid [25] and breakdown products, such as oxalate and threonate [26]. Extracellular concentrations of dehydroascorbic acid in excess of 1–2 μM are considered non-physiological, given its short half-life [25] and rapid uptake and by cells [27–29]. Although cells can reduce the dehydroascorbic acid to ascorbic acid, it is currently unclear what effects constant exposure of cells to high levels of dehydroascorbic acid or its breakdown products may have. For example, dehydroascorbic acid exposure has induced stress signaling and cytotoxicity in some cell types, probably due to the loss of NADPH or glutathione needed for dehydroascorbic acid reduction [30]. Oxalate has been shown to exert cytotoxic effects [31], and threonate can impact cell signaling pathways [32]. If anything, these exposures are more likely to generate artifacts as a consequence of the cell culture environment.

2.1.2. "Cellular Scurvy"

Even under conditions of severe vitamin C deficiency, *i.e.*, scurvy, some ascorbate is still present in cells and tissues of humans *in vivo*. As discussed above, cell culture media are not usually supplemented with ascorbic acid, due to its inherent instability in these media. As a consequence, many researchers have reported that cells in culture are devoid of any detectible amounts of ascorbate, even with the use of extremely sensitive HPLC techniques [24,33–38]. Similarly, many complete cell culture media containing fetal bovine serum (FBS) have no detectable amounts of ascorbate [33,34,36,38], and our own analysis of various commercial sources of media and FBS has shown identical results (unpublished observations). The effects of these ascorbate-free conditions are not well defined or understood. However, it should be recognized that many immortalized cell lines likely have been maintained under scorbutic conditions for generations. In this manner, a whole host of cell culture artifacts may be expected when ascorbate is reintroduced into the system.

Cells in culture can be maintained without ascorbic acid because it is not essential to cell growth and division. The biological functions of ascorbate as an electron donor in enzymatic synthesis pathways do not have an absolute requirement for ascorbate [3,39,40]. These enzymes can use other reducing substrates as sources of electrons [39,41], and enzyme activity can still occur in the absence of ascorbate, albeit at a far decreased rate [42]. In particular, the α-ketoglutarate-dependent dioxygenases, such as those involved in collagen synthesis and regulation of hypoxia-inducible factor 1α (HIF-1α), do not require ascorbate as part of the normal catalytic cycle; ascorbate is only needed to rescue the enzyme should an uncoupled enzymatic reaction occur [3]. It has also been suggested that ascorbate may function to maintain intracellular iron in the ferrous state, making it available to replenish or replace ferric iron in the active site of these enzymes [43]. It is possible that cells in culture adapt by increasing ferrous iron uptake and turn-over of iron-containing proteins, partially circumventing the need for ascorbic acid. Regardless of the mechanism, it is evident from cell culture studies that "ascorbate-requiring" enzymes, such as those involved in collagen synthesis [44], degradation of HIF-1α [43], norepinephrine and α-amidated peptide synthesis [45], and histone and DNA demethylase activity [46], still exhibit some residual activity in the absence of ascorbate. However, these enzymes have diverse effects in different tissues, and their activity in an ascorbate-free environment may not be reflective of their roles *in vivo*.

On the other hand, normal physiological functioning of cells can be recapitulated when ascorbate is provided. Ascorbate appears to play an important role in the normal function of cultured endothelial cells, raising antioxidant protection, reducing oxidative stress and damage, and increasing eNOS activity when compared to cells devoid of vitamin C [33,38]. These effects on eNOS, at least, appear dependent on the ability of ascorbate to enhance the stability of tetrahydrobiopterin [34] and influence AMP-activated kinase (AMPK) activity [47]. In addition, ascorbate supplementation of cultured endothelial cells tightens cell-to-cell junctions that are critical for maintaining an endothelial barrier *in vivo* [48] and regulates NADPH oxidase activity [49], a critical component of the inflammatory response.

It is important to note that the effect of ascorbate supplementation may also greatly vary by cell type. Many of the aforementioned effects of ascorbate are observed in primary cell lines. Although propagated in the absence of ascorbate, the response to ascorbate supplementation in these cells reflects responses seen *in vivo*. Cancer cell lines and other immortalized cells, however, often show cytotoxic effects in response to ascorbate addition that are not observed in primary cell lines [24]. This may be the result of adaptations that have accumulated in these cells due to the "culture shock" that alters the normal physiological responses to stimuli [6], possibly involving iron dysregulation or aberrant cell signaling responses.

2.1.3. Proper Use of Ascorbate in Cell Culture

Cell culture study designs may have a large impact on the results obtained with ascorbic acid. To minimize artifacts, cell culture experiments should replicate *in vivo* conditions as closely as possible. Ascorbate levels in media should be maintained within the physiological range of human plasma (about 5–100 μM), and the use of supraphysiological concentrations should be avoided, unless conditions of intravenous vitamin C infusion are being mimicked [24]. When ascorbic acid is added to cell culture, the loss of ascorbate in the media competes with the intracellular accumulation of ascorbate. Although cells may accumulate ascorbate, once the media is depleted of ascorbic acid, intracellular ascorbate levels decline slowly through oxidation or efflux [33–35,38], once again returning cells to a depleted state. Meanwhile, degradation products may accumulate in the media or cells, which would normally be removed under physiological conditions. In addition, cells without ascorbic acid are not a proper control for ascorbate treatment, as some level of ascorbate is always present in all cells of the human body.

Ascorbate should be added to culture media in a way that limits the rate of ascorbate oxidation and the effects of ROS that may be formed. The use of serum-free media that has been supplemented with transferrin to control iron or copper redox chemistry shows great promise in stem cell studies [46]. The stability of ascorbate can be enhanced by low oxygen growth conditions and the use of stabilized derivatives of ascorbate such as ascorbate-2-phosphate (AAP) that cannot participate in redox chemistry outside the cell yet can maintain physiological intracellular ascorbate levels [9]. Furthermore, pyruvate or α-ketoglutarate in cell culture media can be used to blunt the effects of any hydrogen peroxide formed [21,22], although they will not prevent the loss of ascorbic acid.

Due to the inherent instability of the molecule, there is an absolute necessity for monitoring ascorbic acid levels in media and cells during cell culture experiments. As with animal and human studies described below, this is the only method currently available to assess the vitamin C status of cells, and is a valuable tool for understanding the mechanisms of ascorbate's biological actions. Unfortunately, ascorbate levels are rarely measured in cell culture, animal, or human studies, which severely limits their validity and any conclusions that can be drawn.

Despite precautions, conventional cell culture conditions will promote an environment in which ascorbate artifacts are commonplace. Culturing cells with vitamin C requires control over many aspects of the media and culture conditions that has heretofore been lacking. Monitoring ascorbate levels and limiting oxidation may not be sufficient to fully recapitulate the physiological roles of vitamin C. While redesigning cell culture systems to support biologically relevant reactions of ascorbic acid and eliminate artifacts may limit the practicality of experimental designs, these changes are necessary for cell culture models to have continued use in vitamin C research.

2.2. Animal Studies Involving Ascorbic Acid

Since it can be synthesized *de novo* and is not an essential nutrient for most animals, ascorbate should not be referred to as a vitamin in these animals. Conceptually, this questions the use of most experimental animal models, in particular rats and mice, to study the role of ascorbic acid in human health and disease [50]. This echoes recent studies that have cast doubt on the pervasive use of rodent models to mimic human inflammatory responses [51]. Although genetically variant strains incapable of synthesizing ascorbic acid have been established, none of these models fully recapitulate vitamin C transport functions or the effects of vitamin C depletion and repletion observed in humans or guinea pigs [50]. Indeed, there is evidence that regulation of vitamin C transport was altered during the evolutionary loss of L-gulonolactone oxidase (GULO) expression, which does not occur in genetic knockouts. Here, we examine the current issues related to the use of animal models in ascorbate research. Overall, if animals are to be used, the limitations imposed by the model should be well understood. Animal experiments should be avoided if comparable studies can be performed in human subjects.

2.2.1. When a Vitamin in not a Vitamin

Most animal species express a functional copy of L-gulonolactone oxidase, an enzyme with the synthesis of L-ascorbic acid as its only known function. In these animals, the regulation of GULO activity appears to depend primarily on substrate availability, namely the production of gulonolactone as a branch product from glucuronate synthesis [26] derived from UDP-glucose, a product of glycogen breakdown [52,53]. Thus, agents that stimulate glycogenolysis also stimulate ascorbate synthesis when an animal is in a fed state (*i.e.*, when glycogen is present); in contrast, prolonged fasting causes ascorbate synthesis to decline [54]. UDP-glucuronate is also needed for glucuronidation of xenobiotics, and there is a correlation between ascorbate synthesis activity and xenobiotic metabolism [26].

In each of the few mammalian species that do not synthesize ascorbic acid, such as guinea pigs, fruit bats, and primates, the loss of GULO has occurred at a genetic level. Although the mutations accumulated in this gene differ [55], the result is essentially the same: a loss of GULO activity. These species have adapted to the loss of *de novo* synthesis by consuming primarily plant sources of ascorbate. While all non-synthesizing animal species are at risk of developing scurvy and may die when vitamin C intake ceases for an extended period of time, this is a condition that does not occur normally in other animals, including most commonly used experimental animal models, such as mice and rats. Thus, in contrast to ascorbic acid-synthesizing species, in non-synthesizing species, including humans, vitamin C absorption is required to prevent deficiency and maintain health. This represents a fundamental shift from a perspective of diet-health interactions, as the absorption-derived *versus* glycogen-derived source of ascorbic acid may represent differences in ascorbate transport and carbohydrate metabolism that exist in humans and synthesizing animals.

Although evidence in the literature is limited, both rats and mice appear to poorly absorb ascorbate from the diet. Early studies on the small intestine in rats revealed that ascorbate uptake is a passive process, resulting mainly in intestinal mucosa accumulation but not transport to the circulation [56]. Several studies have demonstrated a profound difference in absorption between the rat and guinea pig small intestine [57–59], the latter displaying a robust transepithelial transport system that is sodium-dependent [59–61], similar to the human ileum [61,62]. A recent study in rats monitored the absorption of a single oral dose of ascorbic acid or dehydroascorbic acid given by gavage. The administration of 12 mg of dehydroascorbic acid led to a significant increase in plasma ascorbic acid concentration, but administration of 12 mg of ascorbic acid did not [63]. An inability to efficiently transport vitamin C is also seen in feeding studies, where mice fully capable of synthesizing ascorbate required at least 45 mg of ascorbate per day in their diet to show any significant increases in plasma ascorbate concentration [64]. Although it is difficult to extrapolate these doses to humans, allometric scaling based on calorie consumption suggests that a dose of 45 mg in a 20-g mouse is equivalent to about 3 g in a 70-kg person [65].

Studies on the bioavailability of different forms of ascorbic acid supplements also support the notion that ascorbate is poorly absorbed by rodent models. For example, Ester-C, a calcium ascorbate-threonate mixture, is reported to be more bioavailable in ODS rats than an equivalent dose of ascorbic acid [66]. However, the same comparison of supplements shows that Ester-C has a lower rate of absorption—and certainly no enhanced bioavailability—in human volunteers [67].

Furthermore, work in GULO knockout mice suggested an enhanced bioavailability of vitamin C contained in a kiwifruit puree compared to a pure ascorbic acid supplement gel [68]. However, more recent human data suggest that vitamin C from kiwifruit or a supplement is equally bioavailable [69].

Overall, these data support a species-specific route of ascorbate absorption. While indirect absorption of ascorbate may occur in rats and mice—likely mediated by ascorbic acid oxidation and transient formation and transport of dehydroascorbic acid—there is clear evidence of an active, sodium-dependent transport of vitamin C in guinea pigs and humans. Therefore, the use of rats or mice as a model of human vitamin C absorption and metabolism is ill advised. As indicated above, such studies with experimental animals should be avoided if they can be performed in humans, unless the purpose of the study is to better understand ascorbic acid absorption and metabolism in rodents. More importantly, no conclusions should and can be drawn from such studies for human vitamin C transport or metabolism.

Poor uptake of dietary ascorbate, or complete lack of it, is expected in animals that synthesize ascorbate, as they do not have a need for dietary ascorbate. In addition, high levels of ascorbate in the intestine would likely cause down-regulation of tissue ascorbate synthesis. However, the relationship between absorption and synthesis does not appear to be this simple. Genetically altered rat and mouse models lacking ascorbate synthesis have low tissue levels of ascorbate without supplementation [64,68,70,71]. Although these animals absorb dietary ascorbate, the levels needed to prevent scurvy or saturate tissues are relatively high compared to guinea pigs and humans on a body-weight basis (Table 1). These levels are especially high when contrasted to food sources of ascorbate. As an example, to saturate all tissues, GULO knockout mice need to be supplemented with 3.3 g/L of ascorbate in the drinking water, resulting in an intake of approximately 16.5 mg per day [68,72]. Based on allometric scaling, this dose in mice corresponds to about 1 g per day in a 70-kg person [65]. Although the metabolic rate of these animals likely contributes to high ascorbate requirements, this does not sufficiently explain data supporting an excessive inefficiency of intestinal absorption.

2.2.2. Transporter Troubles

Based on the evidence presented above, animals unable to synthesize vitamin C appear to display an active transport system in the intestine that is both sensitive to varying levels of ascorbic acid and sodium-dependent. This implicates a role of the sodium-dependent vitamin C transport (SVCT) proteins. SVCT1 has been implicated in dietary ascorbate absorption in human enterocytes, as it is found primarily on the luminal side of intestinal cells and involved in trans-epithelial ascorbate transport [73–75]. However, mice genetically modified to remove functional expression of the SVCT1 gene (Slc23a1$^{-/-}$) show similar intestinal ascorbate absorption as wild type mice [76], suggesting SVCT1 is not involved in this process in these animals. Indeed, the concentration of ascorbic acid needed in the drinking water of GULO knockout mice to maintain tissue saturation (3.3g/L or 18.75 mM) far exceeds the transport capacity of SVCT1, which has a measured K_m below 250 μM [77]. On the other hand, the ability of rats to absorb dehydroascorbic acid has been linked to the intestinal expression of glucose transport proteins (GLUTs), namely GLUT2 and GLUT8 that show K_m values of approximately 2–3 mM [63].

Table 1. Animal models for vitamin C research and comparison to humans.

Species/Strain	GULO Status	Maintenance Dose (mg/kg Body Weight) *	Saturation Dose (mg/kg Body Weight)	Comparisons to Humans and Other Models
Mouse (wild-type)	Functional	n/a	n/a	Expresses GLUT4 on erythrocytes [78]
Sfx Mouse	Complete deletion	~20	>100	Spontaneous mutant model that develops spontaneous bone fractures and bone fragility not seen in other GULO knockout mice [71,79]
$GULO^{-/-}$ Mouse	Exon 3 & 4 deleted	~20	~600	Genetically engineered mouse model that displays blood vessel fragility [80] Possible muscle weakness independent of vitamin C status [81]
$SMP30^{-/-}$ mouse	Functional	~20	~240	Not a GULO knockout [82]; may have residual synthesis activity Multiple aging effects independent of vitamin C status [50]
Rat (wild-type)	Functional	n/a	n/a	Expresses GLUT4 on erythrocytes [78] Preferential absorption of dehydroascorbic acid in gut [63] Lack of active ascorbate transport in intestine [49–51]
ODS Rat	GULO point mutation	~10	~200	Spontaneous mutant model that develops hind limb bone disorders [83] Vitamin C deficiency lowers blood pressure [84] Vitamin C deficiency protects from ischemic injury [85] GULO mRNA and protein still expressed [86]
Guinea Pig	Multiple exons lost	~2	~27	GULO gene deletion during evolution [55] Expresses GLUT1 on erythrocytes, similar to humans [78] Active ascorbate absorption in gut, similar to humans [49–51] Vitamin C deficiency exaggerates cardiovascular decline with age, similar to humans [87–89] Other similarities to human vitamin C supplementation [50]
Human	Multiple exons lost	~0.15	~3	

n/a: not applicable or unable to determine due to endogenous ascorbate synthesis; * Approximate dose needed to prevent symptoms of scurvy.

Unfortunately, little is known about differences in expression or regulation of the SVCTs between humans, guinea pigs, rats, and mice. Comparison of the amino acid sequences of mouse, rat, and human SVCT1 shows that seven amino acid residues are missing from the human SVCT1 sequence [90]. This deletion creates a potential protein kinase C (PKC)-binding site in the human sequence not found in rats or mice. Stimulation of PKC has been implicated in membrane trafficking of human SVCT1 [91]. Additionally, the *C*-terminal sequence of rat and mouse SVCT1 has a one-amino acid change in a critical four-amino acid sequence required for apical targeting of the transport protein [92]. SVCT2, responsible for uptake of ascorbate from the blood stream, contains an additional 56 amino acids in the *N*-terminal region of the human protein sequence that are not found in rats and mice [90]. The only study to date on a species difference in SVCT regulation found that buthionine sulfoximine (BSO), a glutathione synthesis inhibitor, reduced the expression of both SVCT1 and SVCT2 in rat liver cell lines, a phenomenon not observed in human hepatoma cells [93].

Although the absorption of dehydroascorbic acid is not considered a major pathway for the maintenance of whole body ascorbic acid levels, it is considered an important scavenger pathway to maintain cellular ascorbate levels if extracellular ascorbate is oxidized to dehydroascorbic acid [94]. Since human erythrocytes do not express SVCT proteins [95], ascorbic acid transport across the plasma membrane is facilitated by dehydroascorbic acid uptake mediated through GLUTs.

Recent evidence suggests that GLUT1 is responsible for dehydroascorbic acid uptake in human red blood cells, enhanced by the co-expression of a protein called stomatin during erythropoiesis [78]. By contrast, mice lose GLUT1 during maturation, and GLUT4 is the predominant glucose transporter expressed in adult mouse erythrocytes [96]. GLUT4, by contrast, has diminished capacity to transport dehydroascorbic acid [97], which is reflected in the transport capacity of murine erythrocytes [78]. Interestingly, GLUT1 expression and the associated dehydroascorbic acid transport in red blood cells are found only in species unable to synthesize ascorbate—lacking from every animal with endogenous ascorbate-synthesis capacity, even in closely related species such as chinchilla and guinea pigs, or lemurs and margot monkeys [78]. Furthermore, this remarkable switch in glucose transport proteins may be indicative of differences in global gene expression patterns between ascorbate synthesizing *versus* non-synthesizing animals.

2.2.3. Choose Models with Care

Although wild-type rat and mice models are still being employed for ascorbate research, the presence of endogenous synthesis alone would suggest that these animals represent a poor model for understanding the role of vitamin C in human health and disease. At the very least, animal models without endogenous ascorbate synthesis should be used. Five rodent models exist, although each with their own limitations (Table 1). Only one of these models, the GULO knockout mouse, was specifically engineered to disable ascorbic acid synthesis [80]. The other mouse and rat models are not genetically engineered and display individual characteristics that poorly recapitulate the effects of human vitamin C deficiency [50]. On the other hand, guinea pigs have lost GULO activity during evolution and likely display compensatory genetic adaptations similar to humans relating to the loss of ascorbate synthesis, such as GLUT1 activity on erythrocytes (see above). Although guinea pigs are currently being employed by some research groups, the lack of molecular and genetic tools for this animal model will likely drive the continued use of rats and mice models instead.

Regardless of the species, experimental conditions, or route of ascorbate administration, it needs to be stressed that measuring ascorbate levels is absolutely necessary for any animal experiment. One of the most frequent assumptions is that dietary ascorbate will always result in a change in tissue and plasma ascorbate levels. However, the relative contributions of *de novo* ascorbate synthesis (if present), absorption of dietary ascorbate, and ascorbate distribution throughout the body are not inherently predictable and must be directly measured. Studies using oral ascorbate administration can be complicated by animals with poor absorptive capacity, and these animals may rely on the production of dehydroascorbic acid in the intestine. Furthermore, stable ascorbate derivatives used in animal diets, such as ascorbate phosphate or ascorbate palmitate, are not well studied and may not distribute throughout the body as ascorbate would if provided by itself. It is also not recommended to rely on intravenous, intraperitoneal, or subcutaneous ascorbate injections, since they may cause the production of hydrogen peroxide in the extracellular space [98].

Since ascorbate is a dietary factor in humans *versus* a product of carbohydrate metabolism in mice and rats, and there are differences in SVCT and GLUT regulation between species, the results of most animal studies with ascorbic acid cannot be extrapolated to humans. Continued evaluation of rodents as relevant models to study ascorbic acid in human health and disease depends on a thorough understanding of the differences between rodents and humans with respect to ascorbate metabolism, regulation, and biological functions. However, it seems apparent that, aside from the guinea pig, animal studies should be avoided as much as possible, with continued focus placed on conducting relevant human studies instead.

2.3. Human Studies with Vitamin C

Randomized controlled trials are considered the "gold standard" by the Institute of Medicine's Food and Nutrition Board for determining efficacy of micronutrients, including vitamin C, in promoting human health and preventing or treating disease [1,2]. However, RCT study designs have serious limitations and pitfalls, and require careful scrutiny to avoid misinterpretation of results and erroneous conclusions. The drive to establish correlations in prospective cohort studies or show a treatment effect in RCTs often ignores assessment of intermediary biomarkers or other biological measures that could provide insights into mechanisms and help establish causation. Indeed, many vitamin C supplementation studies are performed in combination with other supplements, most often "antioxidant vitamins" E and β-carotene, and fail to assess the subjects' vitamin C status at baseline and following supplementation or biomarkers related to vitamin C's proposed mechanism of action, e.g., antioxidant or anti-inflammatory effects [2]. Understanding the study population, limitations of study design, and the nuances of the ascorbic acid chemistry is necessary to avoid many of these pitfalls and artifacts. Furthermore, myths about the health effects of vitamin C supplementation plague the entire body of research and may prompt the spread of misinformation. In this section, we explore the limitations to human research with vitamin C and review the myths surrounding vitamin C supplementation. In the future, it will be necessary to promote a new approach to conducting vitamin C research in humans.

2.3.1. Vitamin C RCTs: Failures in Design

Many, but not all, prospective cohort studies have observed inverse associations between vitamin C intake or plasma levels and the incidence of chronic diseases, including coronary heart disease, ischemic stroke, hypertension, and certain types of cancer [1,15]. However, several large RCTs have shown no benefit of vitamin C supplementation when taken alone or in combination with other micronutrients [28,51]. This apparent failure of vitamin C supplements to affect human health can be attributed to many factors related to study design. The most predominant is the use of the standard RCT study design, which is intended to test the safety and efficacy of a pharmaceutical drug in individuals that are at high risk or are suffering from a condition or illness. By contrast, enrollees in vitamin C supplementation studies, and diet-related RCTs in general, are usually health-conscious individuals who are likely to consume an above-average diet and maintain a healthy body weight [99]. As a consequence, these individuals have a lower disease incidence and a better nutritional status, including vitamin C, than the general population—both of which negatively affect the statistical power of the study. Statistical power is further compromised by the fact that there is no true placebo group in these studies, as even the non-supplemented subjects continue to obtain vitamin C from their diet throughout the duration. These and other serious flaws in study design, including lack of a single supplement (vitamin C only), quality of the methodology employed, and lack of discrimination by genetic polymorphisms, have led some to the unfortunate conclusion that very few well-designed, well-controlled trials of supplemental vitamin C have ever been conducted [2].

One reason previous studies have failed to show health benefits of vitamin C may be the assumption that an individual's plasma or body ascorbate status directly reflects their dietary or supplemental intake of vitamin C. To the contrary, analysis of food frequency questionnaires has revealed that there is little correlation between assessed vitamin C intake and plasma ascorbate levels [100], likely due to inaccuracies in dietary assessment methodology using food frequency questionnaires or food diaries, inaccuracies in the USDA nutrient database, loss of ascorbate during storage, cooking or processing, and large inter-individual differences in vitamin C absorption and metabolism. An example of the latter is the lower plasma ascorbate levels observed in the elderly when compared to younger adults consuming equivalent amounts of vitamin C [101], suggesting changes in absorptive capacity with age. In addition, smoking, chronic aspirin use, high alcohol consumption, high BMI, and low socioeconomic status [102] are all factors that have been associated with lower plasma vitamin C levels. Furthermore, genetic variation in SVCTs, haptoglobin, and glutathione *S*-transferases also may lead to altered plasma ascorbate levels depending on the various single nucleotide polymorphisms involved [103]. In each of these cases, the exact relationship of plasma vitamin C status with vitamin C consumption is unclear. However, this explains why food frequency questionnaires have little predictive value for evaluating the effect vitamin C consumption on disease risk, while plasma ascorbate levels display clear inverse relationship [104]. Therefore, the use of dietary analysis in studies pertaining to vitamin C should be only a secondary measure of vitamin C status, at best. The gold standard must be measurement of plasma ascorbate levels.

Human pharmacokinetic data show that there is a sigmoidal dose-response relationship between plasma ascorbate levels and vitamin C dose for both men [105] and women [106]. Those with frank deficiency have plasma ascorbate values below 11 μM and are at risk for scurvy because corresponding tissue levels are low. Marginal deficiency (<23 μM) and suboptimal concentrations (<50 μM) are levels that exist on the steep part of the dose-response curve, thought to be indicative of increasing levels of ascorbate in most tissues, based on correlations with ascorbate levels in circulating leukocytes. Plasma concentrations start leveling off at doses above 200 mg/day and approach maximal levels in the range of 60–90 μM, when the threshold levels for renal reabsorption are reached and leukocytes also are saturated with vitamin C.

There are limitations to these pharmacokinetic data that must be recognized. First, the studies were performed in a small number of young, healthy individuals and, hence, are limited in their statistical power. As described above, many factors can influence the relationship between plasma and dietary ascorbate, including age and disease status, which may affect vitamin C transport and metabolism. Therefore, vitamin C pharmacokinetics may be substantially different in old or diseased individuals compared to young, healthy subjects. Second, we cannot assume that tissue saturation occurs in every organ along the same continuum of plasma ascorbate levels. Studies in animals show preferential uptake and retention of ascorbate in organs that have high requirements for the vitamin [68,70,107]. Thus, the brain may saturate at lower ascorbate intake and plasma levels than other organs, such as liver or circulating cells. Data in human volunteers suggest that in skeletal muscle ascorbate is more responsive to changes in plasma ascorbate status than in neutrophils or mononuclear cells [108], suggesting different routes of vitamin C transport and levels of tissue saturation. One study showed a continued uptake and no apparent saturation of ascorbate in the human eye lens with increasing plasma ascorbate levels [109]. Thus, the implication here is that transport rate and saturation point in various cells and tissues of the body are variable and may not be directly extrapolated from plasma ascorbate levels.

From the above considerations, three critical issues emerge in relation to RCT design. First, individuals recruited for a research study should have low plasma ascorbate levels at baseline to increase the likelihood of affecting changes in ascorbate status in tissues through vitamin C supplementation. Subjects already consuming enough vitamin C to provide near-maximal or saturating plasma and tissue levels of ascorbate are highly unlikely to demonstrate any further biological or health effects upon vitamin C supplementation. Second, the intervention must be proven effective, demonstrating—at the very least—an elevation in plasma ascorbate steady-state levels. Again, if a research subject's vitamin C status does not change, no changes in health or disease outcomes can be expected unless it can be supported by an alternate mechanism. In many cases, no biological effect can be expected of increasing vitamin C levels if no functional deficit is present. For instance, although studies support the use of vitamin C in improving vascular function and reducing blood pressure [5], continued supplementation of vitamin C when plasma levels are already at saturation will not yield additional vasodilation, and changes in blood pressure are not expected if a subject is already within a healthy blood pressure range. Lastly, in the absence of tissue ascorbate measurements, the study design and endpoints must relate to our knowledge about the distribution of vitamin C in the body. For example, if brain ascorbate levels are near saturation at low vitamin C intake and plasma levels, it is unreasonable to expect an effect on brain function over a wide range of intake and plasma ascorbate levels.

Along with attention to these issues, there needs to be a push toward measurement of mechanism-based endpoints and clinically-relevant, intermediary biomarkers to assess the effects of vitamin C supplementation. As mentioned above, in biological systems vitamin C always acts as a reductant, which may be expressed as antioxidant, anti-inflammatory, enzyme cofactor, or pro-oxidant activity, depending on the specific context. Commonly in clinical trials, vitamin C is assumed to act as an antioxidant or an anti-inflammatory without actual measurements to support such a role, which limits the evaluation of the trial as a successful intervention and the interpretation of the data. Measures of oxidative stress, such as F_2-isoprostanes [110], serve as clinically relevant markers suggesting an antioxidant effect, while changes in circulating levels of inflammatory markers such as C-reactive protein or soluble cellular adhesion molecules can support an anti-inflammatory effect [111]. Without these corroborating data, results from RCTs will continue to be limited in impact and relevance.

With correct study design, it is generally believed that quality research data can be obtained from human subjects. However, the costs of large, tightly controlled RCTs with vitamin C alone are likely to be prohibitive to the implementation of such studies. Therefore, it is likely that smaller, high-quality intervention trials will have to suffice in the future.

2.3.2. Technical Issues of Human Studies

Vitamin C research is heavily dependent on accurate assessment of ascorbate in biological samples. Unfortunately, there is no standard method for measuring vitamin C that has been applied across the field. It is generally acceptable practice to preserve samples in acid or methanol after sample extraction. Furthermore, it is preferred that a direct measure of ascorbic acid be made, such as HPLC separation followed by electrochemical detection (ECD). Other chromatographic methods are generally avoided, especially those that require oxidation of the sample followed by derivatization as these procedures can generate erroneous results. The detection of dehydroascorbic acid cannot be achieved with ECD unless the sample is first treated with a reductant, obtaining total ascorbate levels from which dehydroascorbic acid levels can be inferred [112,113]. However, the value and interpretation of dehydroascorbic acid measurements in biological samples is questionable (see below).

The labile nature of ascorbic acid outside the body underscores the need for controlled conditions during collection, processing, and storage of biological samples. In many human studies, poor standards in obtaining blood or tissues specifically for vitamin C analysis are complicated by a lack of controlled sample handling in many clinical settings. Phlebotomy is common practice, but many factors can contribute to the instability of ascorbic acid in biological samples. Although the use of vacutainers for plasma samples is generally acceptable for vitamin C analysis, the choice of vacutainer type and anticoagulants can influence the results obtained [114]. As an example, plasma ascorbate levels were determined from five individuals using various anticoagulants or no anticoagulant (serum) as a control. Despite individual variability in plasma ascorbate levels reflected in the standard error, the data (Figure 2) suggest that the use of K_2 EDTA vacutainers results in a significant loss of ascorbate compared to both sodium and lithium heparin containers. Consistent with these data, EDTA has been shown to accelerate the oxidation of ascorbate in whole blood and plasma [115,116] and be unable to prevent the loss of ascorbate in the presence of iron or copper [8]. In addition, it has been suggested that fluoride and serum vacutainers should be avoided for vitamin C analysis [114].

Figure 2. Vacutainer effects on plasma ascorbate levels. Plasma ascorbate concentrations were determined from different anticoagulant-containing or untreated vacutainers as described in Materials and Methods. Plasma ascorbate means are the average and standard error from five different subjects. ANOVA analysis shows a significant ($p < 0.05$) decline in plasma ascorbate levels in K_2 EDTA vacutainers when compared to lithium or sodium heparin vacutainers as denoted by asterisk (*).

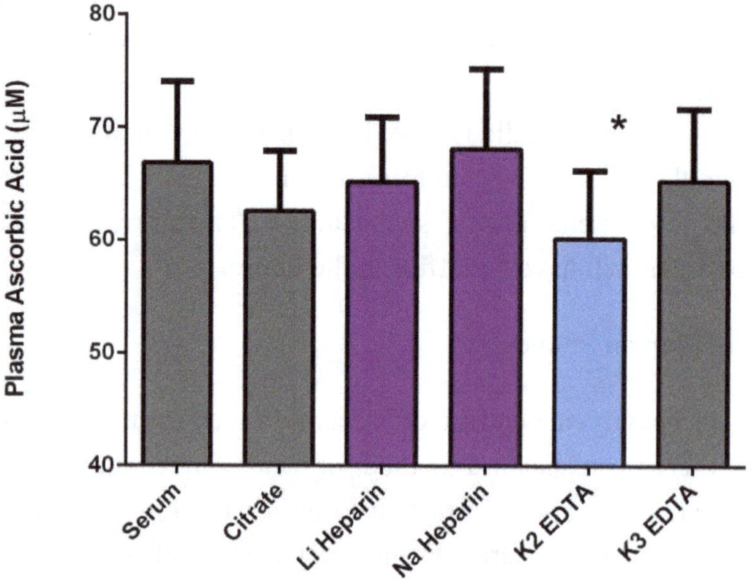

The oxidation of vitamin C in plasma is accelerated by heat, light, and elevated pH, similar to cell culture media as described above. Sample mishandling can cause the aberrant generation of dehydroascorbic acid in the sample and, over time, will cause a loss of total ascorbate. For instance, by careful preparation of the sample under nitrogen and limited exposure to heat and light, dehydroascorbic acid levels can be minimized (Figure 3). More reasonable, standard preparation methods with brief exposures to air, light, and heat result in little change in plasma ascorbate levels (Figure 3b). On the other hand, exposing samples to room temperature for hours not only can result in a significant decline in (reduced) ascorbic acid, but a loss of total ascorbic acid as well (Figure 3a). Not only does this result in an inaccurate estimate of dehydroascorbic acid levels in the exposed sample (Figure 3c) but the loss of total ascorbate suggests degradation of dehydroascorbic acid has also occurred.

The implication of these data (Figure 3) and others [114–116] is that care in sample handling with concern for ascorbate oxidation is crucial for accurate ascorbate analysis. Study designs must incorporate specific handling conditions of samples intended for ascorbate analysis (ideally by immediate plasma isolation, rapid acidification, and freezing below −20 °C) to avoid misinterpretations compounded by the use of poorly preserved samples. Furthermore, it also suggests that the presence of dehydroascorbic acid in clinical samples is more a measure of sample handling than a biologically relevant marker of *in vivo* oxidative stress.

Figure 3. Effects of sample handling on plasma ascorbate and dehydroascorbic acid concentrations. Vacutainers with blood samples were prepared under oxidation controlled, standard and exposed conditions as described in Materials and Methods. Plasma total ascorbate (**a**) and reduced ascorbate (**b**) levels are highest in controlled samples, showing declines under standard and exposed preparations that are reflected in calculated dehydroascorbic acid levels (**c**). Significant changes were observed in the exposed group when compared to controlled or standard samples as determined by ANOVA, and denoted with an asterisk (*).

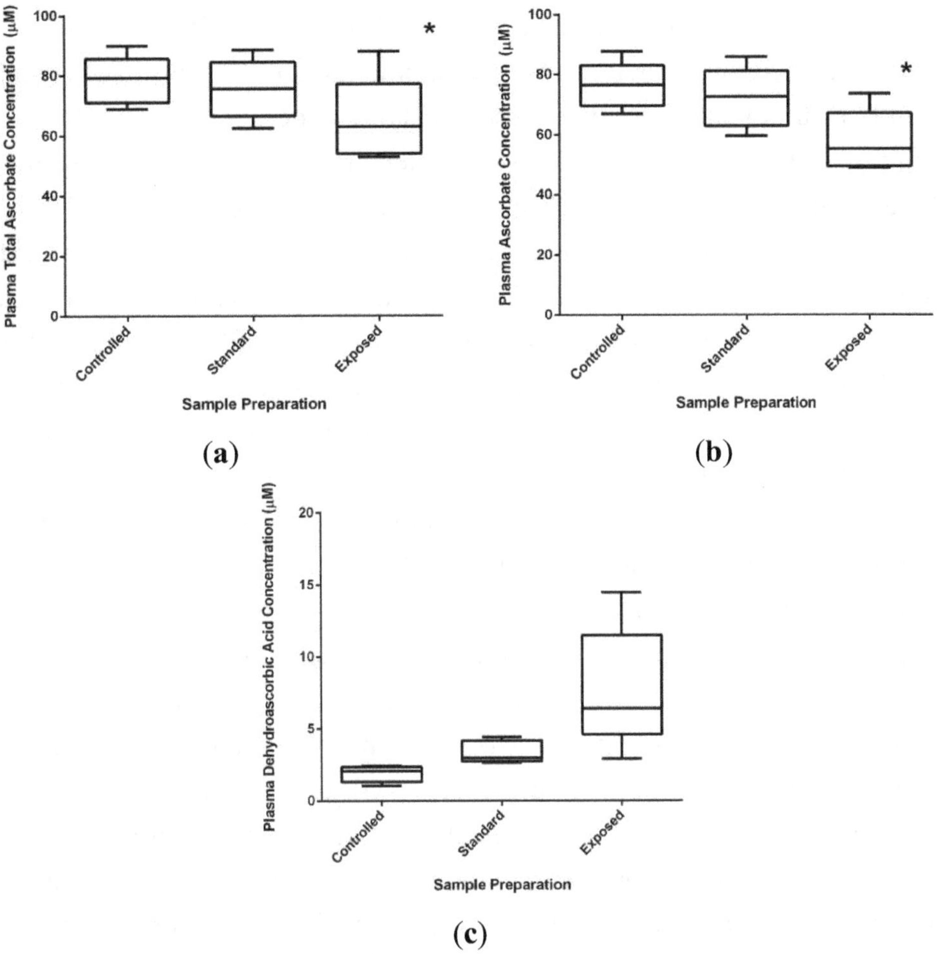

2.3.3. Health Effects of Vitamin C: Reality *versus* Mythology

Many excellent evidence-based reviews have summarized the health effects of vitamin C, focusing on vitamin C's possible role in the prevention or treatment of cardiovascular disease, cancer, diabetes, and other diseases [1,2,4,117]. However, there are a number of health effects attributed to vitamin C supplementation that are not supported by controlled trials with fundamental, mechanism-based endpoints. Opponents of vitamin C supplementation have sensationalized studies that have suggested deleterious health claims, most of which are of little consequence to the general population. For example, since vitamin C promotes iron absorption [118], this led to claims that vitamin C supplements were detrimental in individuals suffering from iron overload and hemochromatosis. On the contrary, in animals and humans with iron overload, high plasma ascorbate levels are protective against oxidative damage induced by excess iron [18,19]. Indeed, the recommendation for these individuals is to not avoid ascorbate, but instead limit dietary iron intake.

Another commonly cited risk of ascorbate supplementation is the formation of kidney stones, as oxalate is a product of dehydroascorbic acid breakdown. The evidence linking ascorbate supplement use and incidence of kidney stones in otherwise healthy individuals is mixed [119–121]. Large amounts of oxalate derived from ascorbate would require excessive vitamin C oxidation, but the mechanism underlying this oxidation has not been explored. Studies that suggest an increased risk observed it in individuals taking more than 1000 mg of vitamin C per day, in far excess of the amount that can be obtained from food sources. Without further study, it is prudent to caution individuals with kidney disease or a history of kidney stones against taking large amounts of vitamin C supplements. Unfortunately, this has also resulted in practitioners to advise individuals undergoing dialysis to severely restrict vitamin C consumption, leading to deficiencies [122].

The consumption of large doses of vitamin C supplements has also been occasionally associated with skin rash, heartburn, nausea, and diarrhea. These are usually the result of the formulation of the vitamin C tablets but may also be caused by excessive consumption of vitamin C in a short period of time. Large doses of vitamin C have been anecdotally associated with vitamin B_{12} deficiency and systemic conditioning (also known as "rebound scurvy"), conditions that have never been documented clinically [123]. Patients with glucose-6-phosphate dehydrogenase (G6PD) deficiency have also been cautioned against taking vitamin C supplements, due to reports of hemolytic anemia that have also not been substantiated [124].

One of the most persistent health claims for vitamin C supplementation is the prevention and treatment of the common cold. Recent meta-analyses of the data from 70 years of placebo-controlled trials demonstrated an overabundance of poorly controlled trials with no apparent focus on the mechanism and biological relevance of vitamin C supplementation [125,126]. Despite the large number of research studies, the evidence supporting the effects of vitamin C supplements on cold incidence and duration has been relatively weak, with the exception of marathon runners, skiers, soldiers in subarctic conditions [125], or individuals with chronic gastritis [127]. A tendency to include older data is a common pitfall for the analysis of vitamin C research, performed when our understanding of vitamin C in biology was limited, and thus allowing for a bias toward poorer designed studies. Our understanding of vitamin C's role in biology has improved over time, leaving a re-analysis of these studies unable to provide any substantial conclusions with respect to the common cold and other proposed health effects of vitamin C supplementation. To resolve the controversies, a modern approach of evaluating rigorously designed, mechanism-based studies is necessary.

2.3.4. Supplementing C: From Formulation to Dose

Vitamin C formulations are as diverse as the recommendations and health claims made in support various marketed supplements. However, there is no data to suggest that any formulation containing ascorbate, alone or in combination with bioflavonoids, liposomes, vitamin C breakdown products, or minerals, has any measurable effect on vitamin C bioavailability in humans. While there are claims that vitamin C from natural *versus* synthetic sources, there is little evidence to support this in human subjects [128].

Pharmacokinetic studies suggest the consumption of at least 200 mg/day of vitamin C in healthy young men and women results in plasma concentrations greater than 50 μM [105,106]. At this dose, nearly complete oral bioavailability is obtained, leukocyte saturation is achieved, and urinary excretion is minimized, suggesting a saturation point has been reached for vitamin C transport. A dose of 200 mg/day can be achieved through a diet rich in fresh fruit and vegetables. Although the limitations of extrapolating this data have been discussed, it has been suggested that 200 mg/day of vitamin C should be set as an optimal intake level for the general population [1]. As mentioned above, it is possible that increased intake of vitamin C is necessary for plasma saturation in some individuals, such as the elderly [101] or individuals with various genetic polymorphisms [103], which would likely necessitate the use of supplements.

Can a case be made for "megadose" levels of vitamin C, or those in excess of 1 g/day? As much as different authors have put forth their own perspectives on the subject, there are few RCTs examining the effect of large daily oral doses of vitamin C. Thus, it is difficult to speculate on the beneficial effect of such doses. Pharmacokinetic data show that daily oral doses of vitamin C up to 2.5 g/day result in higher plasma ascorbate levels than a 200 mg/day dose, despite decreased bioavailability and increased urinary excretion of vitamin C [105,106]; however, the differences are small and biologically most likely of little consequence. It has been speculated that high plasma ascorbate levels can be maintained by frequent dosing with ascorbic acid [129], but it unclear what health effect would be achieved by this regimen. To date, no papers have shown a benefit of achieving greater-than-saturation plasma levels in the long term, and this mechanism would need to be delineated before a recommendation could be made.

One possible effect of megadose levels of vitamin C may be in the gastrointestinal tract, where it may prevent the formation of carcinogenic *N*-nitroso compounds [130] and highly reactive electrophilic compounds from the diet, such as acrolein [131] or lipid peroxidation products [132]. An intriguing idea for a biological role of vitamin C in the digestive tract is an exploration of beneficial changes to microbiota populations in the gut. However, in all of these cases, studies have yet to be performed, currently making it premature to draw any conclusions about the beneficial effects of oral supplementation with high-dose vitamin C. Large doses of intravenous ascorbate are associated with anti-cancer effects [133] and represent a promising area of research in the future that should be a subject of future review.

3. Methods

3.1. Ascorbate in Cell Culture Media

Phosphate Buffered Saline (PBS) solution was prepared from PBS tabs (Sigma Aldrich, St. Louis, MO, USA) dissolved in double deionized, filter sterilized water. Hyclone RPMI 1640 (Thermo Fisher Scientific, Waltam, MA, USA) was either used alone or after overnight chelation with Chelex 100 resin and the addition of 1 mM diethylenetriaminepentaacetic acid (DTPA). PBS or media was placed in 6-well culture dishes in a cell culture incubator (5%/95%: CO_2/air; 37 °C) or at room temperature. Low trace metal ascorbic acid (Sigma Aldrich, St. Louis, MO, USA) was dissolved at a concentration of 10 mM in deionized water before addition to culture dishes. At specified times, aliquots were removed and acidified in 15% perchloric acid (PCA) containing

5 mM DTPA for vitamin C analysis as described below. Cell culture media containing 10% FBS from different commercial sources (Hyclone, Thermo Fisher, Sigma or ATCC) or aliquots of FBS alone were also acidified with an equal amount of PCA, as described above for the analysis of ascorbate content. However, no ascorbate was detected unless ascorbate was added to these solutions.

3.2. Human Subjects and Blood Collection

Five subjects were recruited for blood collection as part of a larger study on vitamin C metabolism approved by the Institutional Review Board for the Protection of Human Subjects at Oregon State University. Subjects were healthy non-smokers taking no prescription or non-prescription drugs that might influence vitamin C metabolism. For the study comparing anticoagulants, blood was collected after an overnight fast in vacutainers containing no additives or sodium heparin, lithium heparin, K2 EDTA, K3 EDTA, or sodium citrate (all from Becton Dickinson, Franklin Lakes, NJ, USA). Immediately after collection, aliquots of blood were collected from vacutainers and centrifuged at 16,000× *g* for 1 min for the separation of plasma from red blood cells. Aliquots of plasma were immediately acidified in 15% PCA containing 5 mM DTPA and placed at 4 °C to limit ascorbate oxidation until analysis, performed immediately, as described below.

For samples collected for the analysis of vitamin C oxidation in plasma, blood was collected in sodium heparin vacutainers from subjects after an overnight fast. Vacutainers were centrifuged in an Allegra X-15R (Beckman Coulter, Brea, CA, USA) at 4000× *g* at 4 °C for the separation of plasma. Vacutainers were then treated in one of three protocols: Oxidation control samples ("Control") were kept on ice with limited light exposure until the vacutainer was opened in a chamber previously purged with nitrogen gas. Plasma was removed and acidified in PCA with DTPA. Vacutainers prepared with the standard protocol ("Standard") were kept at room temperature and opened in ambient air before plasma samples were acidified with PCA. Vacutainers exposed to the environment ("Exposed") were opened under ambient air at room temperature and plasma placed in a clear 2 mL tube. Tubes containing plasma were then incubated at room temperature for two hours before acidification.

3.3. Vitamin C and Urate Analysis

Plasma, media, and FBS samples were prepared for ascorbate analysis using HPLC as previously described [134]. Briefly, acid extracts were diluted in sodium acetate/methanol/water mobile phase (0.3%/7.5%/92% w/v) containing Q12 ion pairing reagent and pH-adjusted with 2.58 M KH_2PO_4 buffer (pH 9.8). Samples were separated on Watters 2695 using an LC-8 column (Supelco) under an applied potential of 600 mV using an electrochemical detector (BSA). Under these conditions, both urate and ascorbate are resolved and quantified by comparisons to authentic standards with a detection limit of approximately 1 nM. For human plasma samples, urate values are used to normalize ascorbate values to minimize any variations within subject samples and to control for volume differences in vacutainer analyses. To obtain total ascorbate, samples were reduced with the addition of tris-2-carboxyethyl phosphine (TCEP) as described elsewhere [113]. Dehydroascorbic acid content is estimated by the difference between TCEP-reduced and standard preparations.

3.4. Statistics

Statistical analysis was performed by GraphPad Prism software, version 6 (GraphPad Software, Inc., La Jolla, CA, USA). Statistical differences between ascorbate samples were determined by two tailed ANOVA using a Tukey post-hoc analysis, with a *p*-value below 0.05 considered significant. Non-linear regression analysis was used to determine the half-life of ascorbate in PBS or media.

4. Conclusions

Performing successful research on vitamin C, especially in the context of human health, requires specific focus and attention to detail. Although this review touched on many of the aspects of cell culture, animal, and human studies that are complicated by the use of ascorbic acid, it is not a complete guide to performing vitamin C research. Each study design is unique, so it must be critically analyzed with respect to ascorbate chemistry and biology to best understand whether and how it will make a contribution in the overall field. As described above, the effects of ascorbic acid within a biological system are potentially multifold, requiring extreme caution in implementation and interpretation.

As we change our view of vitamin C research, we must first address the most prevalent issues in frequently used model systems. The combination of high oxygen tension and the presence of reactive transition metals lead to a rapid oxidation of ascorbic acid in cell culture. The rapid loss of ascorbate in culture media promotes a pro-oxidant environment with the generation of superoxide radicals, hydrogen peroxide, and hydroxyl radicals, as described above. Moreover, depriving cells of ascorbic acid for countless generations produces a cell culture environment that is no longer relevant to human health. Overall, steps must be taken to control ascorbate oxidation if vitamin C research is to continue in cell culture. The use of stable ascorbate derivatives, metal chelation, and low oxygen culture conditions show promise, but much additional work is needed. Understanding the effects of prolonged ascorbate deprivation of cells is also necessary to determine if certain cell lines must be eliminated from use with ascorbic acid.

The continued use of ascorbate-synthesizing animal models also complicates all studies on ascorbic acid *in vivo*. Currently, mouse and rat models that lack ascorbic acid synthesis are available, but show considerable differences from guinea pigs and humans in terms of ascorbic acid bioavailability and metabolism. For example, the apparent lack of intestinal absorption of ascorbic acid in rodent models does not appear related to the synthesis capacity, and must be considered in supplementation studies. Furthermore, the effects of vitamin C deprivation appear to have effects in one model system that are not recapitulated in others, although we do not know if strain differences or dietary factors may have influenced these observations. The use of animal models is especially troubling in light of genetic alterations in the regulation and expression of vitamin C transport proteins in animals without functional ascorbic acid synthesis. Further studies are required to determine if other genetic adaptations have occurred—specifically in primate evolution—that may determine the difference in response of animals and humans to vitamin C supplementation.

Currently, studies involving vitamin C consumption in human subjects are not held to a rigorous standard. Randomized controlled trials, normally considered the benchmark for determining the impact of a compound on human health, have been poorly designed in regard to the chemistry and biology of ascorbic acid. While remaining aware of the effects that different study populations may have on the outcome of vitamin C supplementation, there is a need to determine vitamin C status in subjects before, during, and after a supplementation trial. Evidence shows that methods to record vitamin C intake by using food frequency questionnaires or food diaries are insufficient means of achieving this goal. Therefore study design needs to include assessments of vitamin C status using measurements of plasma, and possibly tissue, ascorbic acid levels. Only with these more precise determinations can we begin to speculate on mechanisms of action and eliminate speculations surrounding the health effects of vitamin C supplementation. Furthermore, eliminating the technical issues surrounding the measurement of vitamin C in clinical settings are additional steps needed to preserve data integrity.

While all study designs deserve higher scrutiny, a note of caution must also be placed in the interpretation of vitamin C research. It is all too common for vitamin C to be assigned a role (as an antioxidant or a pro-oxidant, for instance) without any supporting evidence to validate those claims. It cannot be overemphasized that the primary role of ascorbic acid in biological systems is that of a reductant, and the most established health effects of this reductive power are related to ascorbate's role as an electron-donating enzyme cofactor used, e.g., for pro-collagen, carnitine, and catecholamine biosynthesis [3]. Ascorbic acid has many additional roles in the body beyond these enzyme functions, for example antioxidant protection, and likely more roles will be elucidated in the future. With a critical evaluation of all potential roles of ascorbic acid, the borders of vitamin C research can advance with balanced, evidence-based approaches. Already, emerging roles for vitamin C in various hydroxylase enzymes have recently placed a focus on HIF-1α-dependent gene expression [41,43] and changes in histone and DNA methylation [135,136], suggesting vitamin C may regulate global changes in gene expression. Further innovation has been demonstrated in studies on vitamin C bioavailability [69,108], metabolomics of vitamin C deficiency [137], genetic variation of the vitamin C transporters [103], and intravenous vitamin C infusions in cancer therapy [138,139].

As vitamin C research progresses into the 21st century, it has become clear that much more work still lies ahead of us. The experimental faults, artifacts, and myths currently afflicting vitamin C research limit the impact of many studies, making their contributions to general knowledge of the biological roles of ascorbic acid unremarkable at best, and confusing and detracting from the real issues at worst. This can also stretch beyond the realm of laboratory research, as the persistence of poorly controlled studies within this field often undermines efforts in the medical community to recommend vitamin C as a safe, effective means of promoting health. If nothing else, it weakens efforts to fund additional, well-designed RCTs necessary to establish definitive health claims that are desperately needed. In light of these issues, we must increase scrutiny of vitamin C studies in the past as well as the present, holding them to a higher standard based on the evidence discussed here if we are to make a lasting contribution to our understanding of vitamin C's impact on human health.

References

1. Frei, B.; Birlouez-Aragon, I.; Lykkesfeldt, J. Authors' perspective: What is the optimum intake of vitamin C in humans? *Crit. Rev. Food Sci. Nutr.* **2012**, *52*, 815–829.
2. Lykkesfeldt, J.; Poulsen, H.E. Is vitamin C supplementation beneficial? Lessons learned from randomised controlled trials. *Br. J. Nutr.* **2010**, *103*, 1251–1259.
3. Michels, A.J.; Frei, B.B. Vitamin C. In *Biochemical, Physiological, and Molecular Aspects of Human Nutrition*, 3rd ed.; Stipanuk, M.H., Caudill, M.A., Eds.; Elsevier/Saunders: St. Louis, MO, USA, 2012; pp. 626–654.
4. Carr, A.C.; Frei, B. Toward a new recommended dietary allowance for vitamin C based on antioxidant and health effects in humans. *Am. J. Clin. Nutr.* **1999**, *69*, 1086–1107.
5. Juraschek, S.P.; Guallar, E.; Appel, L.J.; Miller, E.R., III. Effects of vitamin C supplementation on blood pressure: A meta-analysis of randomized controlled trials. *Am. J. Clin. Nutr.* **2012**, *95*, 1079–1088.
6. Halliwell, B. Oxidative stress in cell culture: An under-appreciated problem? *FEBS Lett.* **2003**, *540*, 3–6.
7. Buettner, G.R. The pecking order of free radicals and antioxidants: Lipid peroxidation, α-tocopherol, and ascorbate. *Arch. Biochem. Biophys.* **1993**, *300*, 535–543.
8. Buettner, G.R.; Jurkiewicz, B.A. Catalytic metals, ascorbate and free radicals: Combinations to avoid. *Radiat. Res.* **1996**, *145*, 532–541.
9. Frikke-Schmidt, H.; Lykkesfeldt, J. Keeping the intracellular vitamin C at a physiologically relevant level in endothelial cell culture. *Anal. Biochem.* **2010**, *397*, 135–137.
10. Chepda, T.; Cadau, M.; Girin, P.; Frey, J.; Chamson, A. Monitoring of ascorbate at a constant rate in cell culture: Effect on cell growth. *In Vitro Cell. Dev. Biol. Anim.* **2001**, *37*, 26–30.
11. Wee, L.M.; Long, L.H.; Whiteman, M.; Halliwell, B. Factors affecting the ascorbate- and phenolic-dependent generation of hydrogen peroxide in Dulbecco's Modified Eagles Medium. *Free Radic. Res.* **2003**, *37*, 1123–1130.
12. Clement, M.V.; Ramalingam, J.; Long, L.H.; Halliwell, B. The *in vitro* cytotoxicity of ascorbate depends on the culture medium used to perform the assay and involves hydrogen peroxide. *Antioxid. Redox Signal.* **2001**, *3*, 157–163.
13. Cazzola, M.; Bergamaschi, G.; Dezza, L.; Arosio, P. Manipulations of cellular iron metabolism for modulating normal and malignant cell proliferation: Achievements and prospects. *Blood* **1990**, *75*, 1903–1919.
14. Halliwell, B.; Gutteridge, J.M.C. *Free Radicals in Biology and Medicine*, 4th ed.; Oxford University Press: Oxford, UK, 2007.
15. Buettner, G.R. In the absence of catalytic metals ascorbate does not autoxidize at pH 7: Ascorbate as a test for catalytic metals. *J. Biochem. Biophys. Methods* **1988**, *16*, 27–40.
16. Minetti, M.; Forte, T.; Soriani, M.; Quaresima, V.; Menditto, A.; Ferrari, M. Iron-induced ascorbate oxidation in plasma as monitored by ascorbate free radical formation. No spin-trapping evidence for the hydroxyl radical in iron-overloaded plasma. *Biochem. J.* **1992**, *282*, 459–465.

17. Carr, A.; Frei, B. Does vitamin C act as a pro-oxidant under physiological conditions? *FASEB J.* **1999**, *13*, 1007–1024.
18. Chen, K.; Suh, J.; Carr, A.C.; Morrow, J.D.; Zeind, J.; Frei, B. Vitamin C suppresses oxidative lipid damage *in vivo*, even in the presence of iron overload. *Am. J. Physiol. Endocrinol. Metab.* **2000**, *279*, E1406–E1412.
19. Berger, T.M.; Polidori, M.C.; Dabbagh, A.; Evans, P.J.; Halliwell, B.; Morrow, J.D.; Roberts, L.J., II; Frei, B. Antioxidant activity of vitamin C in iron-overloaded human plasma. *J. Biol. Chem.* **1997**, *272*, 15656–15660.
20. Halliwell, B. Vitamin C: Antioxidant or pro-oxidant *in vivo*? *Free Radic. Res.* **1996**, *25*, 439–454.
21. Long, L.H.; Halliwell, B. Artefacts in cell culture: Pyruvate as a scavenger of hydrogen peroxide generated by ascorbate or epigallocatechin gallate in cell culture media. *Biochem. Biophys. Res. Commun.* **2009**, *388*, 700–704.
22. Long, L.H.; Halliwell, B. Artefacts in cell culture: α-Ketoglutarate can scavenge hydrogen peroxide generated by ascorbate and epigallocatechin gallate in cell culture media. *Biochem. Biophys. Res. Commun.* **2011**, *406*, 20–24.
23. Buettner, G.R.; Jurkiewicz, B.A. Ascorbate free radical as a marker of oxidative stress: An EPR study. *Free Radic. Biol. Med.* **1993**, *14*, 49–55.
24. Chen, Q.; Espey, M.G.; Krishna, M.C.; Mitchell, J.B.; Corpe, C.P.; Buettner, G.R.; Shacter, E.; Levine, M. Pharmacologic ascorbic acid concentrations selectively kill cancer cells: Action as a pro-drug to deliver hydrogen peroxide to tissues. *Proc. Natl. Acad. Sci. USA* **2005**, *102*, 13604–13609.
25. Bode, A.M.; Cunningham, L.; Rose, R.C. Spontaneous decay of oxidized ascorbic acid (dehydro-L-ascorbic acid) evaluated by high-pressure liquid chromatography. *Clin. Chem.* **1990**, *36*, 1807–1809.
26. Linster, C.L.; van Schaftingen, E. Vitamin C. Biosynthesis, recycling and degradation in mammals. *FEBS J.* **2007**, *274*, 1–22.
27. Washko, P.W.; Wang, Y.; Levine, M. Ascorbic acid recycling in human neutrophils. *J. Biol. Chem.* **1993**, *268*, 15531–15535.
28. Rumsey, S.C.; Kwon, O.; Xu, G.W.; Burant, C.F.; Simpson, I.; Levine, M. Glucose transporter isoforms GLUT1 and GLUT3 transport dehydroascorbic acid. *J. Biol. Chem.* **1997**, *272*, 18982–18989.
29. Vera, J.C.; Rivas, C.I.; Fischbarg, J.; Golde, D.W. Mammalian facilitative hexose transporters mediate the transport of dehydroascorbic acid. *Nature* **1993**, *364*, 79–82.
30. Wilson, J.X. The physiological role of dehydroascorbic acid. *FEBS Lett.* **2002**, *527*, 5–9.
31. Pedraza, C.E.; Chien, Y.C.; McKee, M.D. Calcium oxalate crystals in fetal bovine serum: Implications for cell culture, phagocytosis and biomineralization studies *in vitro*. *J. Cell. Biochem.* **2008**, *103*, 1379–1393.
32. Kwack, M.H.; Ahn, J.S.; Kim, M.K.; Kim, J.C.; Sung, Y.K. Preventable effect of L-threonate, an ascorbate metabolite, on androgen-driven balding via repression of dihydrotestosterone-induced dickkopf-1 expression in human hair dermal papilla cells. *BMB Rep.* **2010**, *43*, 688–692.

33. Smith, A.R.; Visioli, F.; Hagen, T.M. Vitamin C matters: Increased oxidative stress in cultured human aortic endothelial cells without supplemental ascorbic acid. *FASEB J.* **2002**, *16*, 1102–1104.
34. Huang, A.; Vita, J.A.; Venema, R.C.; Keaney, J.F., Jr. Ascorbic acid enhances endothelial nitric-oxide synthase activity by increasing intracellular tetrahydrobiopterin. *J. Biol. Chem.* **2000**, *275*, 17399–17406.
35. Bergsten, P.; Amitai, G.; Kehrl, J.; Dhariwal, K.R.; Klein, H.G.; Levine, M. Millimolar concentrations of ascorbic acid in purified human mononuclear leukocytes. Depletion and reaccumulation. *J. Biol. Chem.* **1990**, *265*, 2584–2587.
36. Martin, A.; Frei, B. Both intracellular and extracellular vitamin C inhibit atherogenic modification of LDL by human vascular endothelial cells. *Arterioscler. Thromb. Vas. Biol.* **1997**, *17*, 1583–1590.
37. May, J.M.; Qu, Z.C.; Meredith, M.E. Mechanisms of ascorbic acid stimulation of norepinephrine synthesis in neuronal cells. *Biochem. Biophys. Res. Commun.* **2012**, *426*, 148–152.
38. Visioli, F.; Smith, A.; Zhang, W.; Keaney, J.F., Jr.; Hagen, T.; Frei, B. Lipoic acid and vitamin C potentiate nitric oxide synthesis in human aortic endothelial cells independently of cellular glutathione status. *Redox Rep.* **2002**, *7*, 223–227.
39. Englard, S.; Seifter, S. The biochemical functions of ascorbic acid. *Annu. Rev. Nutr.* **1986**, *6*, 365–406.
40. Bruick, R.K.; McKnight, S.L. A conserved family of prolyl-4-hydroxylases that modify HIF. *Science* **2001**, *294*, 1337–1340.
41. Flashman, E.; Davies, S.L.; Yeoh, K.K.; Schofield, C.J. Investigating the dependence of the hypoxia-inducible factor hydroxylases (factor inhibiting HIF and prolyl hydroxylase domain 2) on ascorbate and other reducing agents. *Biochem. J.* **2010**, *427*, 135–142.
42. Myllyharju, J. Prolyl 4-hydroxylases, the key enzymes of collagen biosynthesis. *Matrix Biol.* **2003**, *22*, 15–24.
43. Knowles, H.J.; Raval, R.R.; Harris, A.L.; Ratcliffe, P.J. Effect of ascorbate on the activity of hypoxia-inducible factor in cancer cells. *Cancer Res.* **2003**, *63*, 1764–1768.
44. Murad, S.; Grove, D.; Lindberg, K.A.; Reynolds, G.; Sivarajah, A.; Pinnell, S.R. Regulation of collagen synthesis by ascorbic acid. *Proc. Natl. Acad. Sci. USA* **1981**, *78*, 2879–2882.
45. Diliberto, E.J., Jr.; Daniels, A.J.; Viveros, O.H. Multicompartmental secretion of ascorbate and its dual role in dopamine β-hydroxylation. *Am. J. Clin. Nutr.* **1991**, *54*, 1163S–1172S.
46. Monfort, A.; Wutz, A. Breathing-in epigenetic change with vitamin C. *EMBO Rep.* **2013**, *14*, 337–346.
47. Ladurner, A.; Schmitt, C.A.; Schachner, D.; Atanasov, A.G.; Werner, E.R.; Dirsch, V.M.; Heiss, E.H. Ascorbate stimulates endothelial nitric oxide synthase enzyme activity by rapid modulation of its phosphorylation status. *Free Radic. Biol. Med.* **2012**, *52*, 2082–2090.
48. May, J.M.; Qu, Z.C.; Qiao, H. Transfer of ascorbic acid across the vascular endothelium: Mechanism and self-regulation. *Am. J. Physiol. Cell Physiol.* **2009**, *297*, C169–C178.
49. Wu, F.; Schuster, D.P.; Tyml, K.; Wilson, J.X. Ascorbate inhibits NADPH oxidase subunit p47phox expression in microvascular endothelial cells. *Free Radic. Biol. Med.* **2007**, *42*, 124–131.

50. Yu, R.; Schellhorn, H.E. Recent applications of engineered animal antioxidant deficiency models in human nutrition and chronic disease. *J. Nutr.* **2013**, *143*, 1–11.

51. Seok, J.; Warren, H.S.; Cuenca, A.G.; Mindrinos, M.N.; Baker, H.V.; Xu, W.; Richards, D.R.; McDonald-Smith, G.P.; Gao, H.; Hennessy, L.; *et al.* Genomic responses in mouse models poorly mimic human inflammatory diseases. *Proc. Natl. Acad. Sci. USA* **2013**, *110*, 3507–3512.

52. Braun, L.; Csala, M.; Poussu, A.; Garzo, T.; Mandl, J.; Banhegyi, G. Glutathione depletion induces glycogenolysis dependent ascorbate synthesis in isolated murine hepatocytes. *FEBS Lett.* **1996**, *388*, 173–176.

53. Chan, T.S.; Wilson, J.X.; O'Brien, P.J. Glycogenolysis is directed towards ascorbate synthesis by glutathione conjugation. *Biochem. Biophys. Res. Commun.* **2004**, *317*, 149–156.

54. Banhegyi, G.; Braun, L.; Csala, M.; Puskas, F.; Mandl, J. Ascorbate metabolism and its regulation in animals. *Free Radic. Biol. Med.* **1997**, *23*, 793–803.

55. Yang, H. Conserved or lost: Molecular evolution of the key gene GULO in vertebrate vitamin C biosynthesis. *Biochem. Genet.* **2013**, *51*, 413–425.

56. Spencer, R.P.; Purdy, S.; Hoeldtke, R.; Bow, T.M.; Markulis, M.A. Studies on intestinal absorption of L-ascorbic acid-1-C-14. *Gastroenterology* **1963**, *44*, 768–773.

57. Hornig, D.; Weber, F.; Wiss, O. Site of intestinal absorption of ascorbic acid in guinea pigs and rats. *Biochem. Biophys. Res. Commun.* **1973**, *52*, 168–172.

58. Hornig, D. Distribution of ascorbic acid, metabolites and analogues in man and animals. *Ann. N. Y. Acad. Sci.* **1975**, *258*, 103–118.

59. Stevenson, N.R.; Brush, M.K. Existence and characteristics of Na positive-dependent active transport of ascorbic acid in guinea pig. *Am. J. Clin. Nutr.* **1969**, *22*, 318–326.

60. Bianchi, J.; Wilson, F.A.; Rose, R.C. Dehydroascorbic acid and ascorbic acid transport systems in the guinea pig ileum. *Am. J. Physiol.* **1986**, *250*, G461–G468.

61. Mellors, A.J.; Nahrwold, D.L.; Rose, R.C. Ascorbic acid flux across mucosal border of guinea pig and human ileum. *Am. J. Physiol.* **1977**, *233*, E374–E379.

62. Stevenson, N.R. Active transport of L-ascorbic acid in the human ileum. *Gastroenterology* **1974**, *67*, 952–956.

63. Corpe, C.P.; Eck, P.; Wang, J.; Al-Hasani, H.; Levine, M. Intestinal dehydroascorbic acid (DHA) transport mediated by the facilitative sugar transporters, GLUT2 and GLUT8. *J. Biol. Chem.* **2013**, *288*, 9092–9101.

64. Tsao, C.S.; Leung, P.Y.; Young, M. Effect of dietary ascorbic acid intake on tissue vitamin C in mice. *J. Nutr.* **1987**, *117*, 291–297.

65. Rucker, R.B. Allometric scaling, metabolic body size and interspecies comparisons of basal nutritional requirements. *J. Anim. Physiol. Anim. Nutr.* **2007**, *91*, 148–156.

66. Bush, M.J.; Verlangieri, A.J. An acute study on the relative gastro-intestinal absorption of a novel form of calcium ascorbate. *Res. Commun. Chem. Pathol. Pharmacol.* **1987**, *57*, 137–140.

67. Johnston, C.S.; Luo, B. Comparison of the absorption and excretion of three commercially available sources of vitamin C. *J. Am. Diet. Assoc.* **1994**, *94*, 779–781.

68. Vissers, M.C.; Bozonet, S.M.; Pearson, J.F.; Braithwaite, L.J. Dietary ascorbate intake affects steady state tissue concentrations in vitamin C-deficient mice: Tissue deficiency after suboptimal intake and superior bioavailability from a food source (kiwifruit). *Am. J. Clin. Nutr.* **2011**, *93*, 292–301.
69. Carr, A.C.; Bozonet, S.M.; Pullar, J.M.; Simcock, J.W.; Vissers, M.C. A randomized steady-state bioavailability study of synthetic *versus* natural (Kiwifruit-Derived) vitamin C. *Nutrients* **2013**, *5*, 3684–3695.
70. Iwama, M.; Shimokado, K.; Maruyama, N.; Ishigami, A. Time course of vitamin C distribution and absorption after oral administration in SMP30/GNL knockout mice. *Nutrition* **2011**, *27*, 471–478.
71. Mohan, S.; Kapoor, A.; Singgih, A.; Zhang, Z.; Taylor, T.; Yu, H.; Chadwick, R.B.; Chung, Y.S.; Donahue, L.R.; Rosen, C.; *et al.* Spontaneous fractures in the mouse mutant sfx are caused by deletion of the gulonolactone oxidase gene, causing vitamin C deficiency. *J. Bone Miner. Res.* **2005**, *20*, 1597–1610.
72. Meredith, M.E.; Harrison, F.E.; May, J.M. Differential regulation of the ascorbic acid transporter SVCT2 during development and in response to ascorbic acid depletion. *Biochem. Biophys. Res. Commun.* **2011**, *414*, 737–742.
73. Boyer, J.C.; Campbell, C.E.; Sigurdson, W.J.; Kuo, S.M. Polarized localization of vitamin C transporters, SVCT1 and SVCT2, in epithelial cells. *Biochem. Biophys. Res. Commun.* **2005**, *334*, 150–156.
74. Maulen, N.P.; Henriquez, E.A.; Kempe, S.; Carcamo, J.G.; Schmid-Kotsas, A.; Bachem, M.; Grunert, A.; Bustamante, M.E.; Nualart, F.; Vera, J.C. Up-regulation and polarized expression of the sodium-ascorbic acid transporter SVCT1 in post-confluent differentiated CaCo-2 cells. *J. Biol. Chem.* **2003**, *278*, 9035–9041.
75. MacDonald, L.; Thumser, A.E.; Sharp, P. Decreased expression of the vitamin C transporter SVCT1 by ascorbic acid in a human intestinal epithelial cell line. *Br. J. Nutr.* **2002**, *87*, 97–100.
76. Corpe, C.P.; Tu, H.; Eck, P.; Wang, J.; Faulhaber-Walter, R.; Schnermann, J.; Margolis, S.; Padayatty, S.; Sun, H.; Wang, Y.; *et al.* Vitamin C transporter Slc23a1 links renal reabsorption, vitamin C tissue accumulation, and perinatal survival in mice. *J. Clin. Investig.* **2010**, *120*, 1069–1083.
77. Savini, I.; Rossi, A.; Pierro, C.; Avigliano, L.; Catani, M.V. SVCT1 and SVCT2: Key proteins for vitamin C uptake. *Amino Acids* **2008**, *34*, 347–355.
78. Montel-Hagen, A.; Kinet, S.; Manel, N.; Mongellaz, C.; Prohaska, R.; Battini, J.L.; Delaunay, J.; Sitbon, M.; Taylor, N. Erythrocyte Glut1 triggers dehydroascorbic acid uptake in mammals unable to synthesize vitamin C. *Cell* **2008**, *132*, 1039–1048.
79. Beamer, W.G.; Rosen, C.J.; Bronson, R.T.; Gu, W.; Donahue, L.R.; Baylink, D.J.; Richardson, C.C.; Crawford, G.C.; Barker, J.E. Spontaneous fracture (sfx): A mouse genetic model of defective peripubertal bone formation. *Bone* **2000**, *27*, 619–626.
80. Maeda, N.; Hagihara, H.; Nakata, Y.; Hiller, S.; Wilder, J.; Reddick, R. Aortic wall damage in mice unable to synthesize ascorbic acid. *Proc. Natl. Acad. Sci. USA* **2000**, *97*, 841–846.
81. Ward, M.S.; Lamb, J.; May, J.M.; Harrison, F.E. Behavioral and monoamine changes following severe vitamin C deficiency. *J. Neurochem.* **2013**, *124*, 363–375.

82. Kondo, Y.; Inai, Y.; Sato, Y.; Handa, S.; Kubo, S.; Shimokado, K.; Goto, S.; Nishikimi, M.; Maruyama, N.; Ishigami, A. Senescence marker protein 30 functions as gluconolactonase in L-ascorbic acid biosynthesis, and its knockout mice are prone to scurvy. *Proc. Natl. Acad. Sci. USA* **2006**, *103*, 5723–5728.
83. Horio, F.; Ozaki, K.; Yoshida, A.; Makino, S.; Hayashi, Y. Requirement for ascorbic acid in a rat mutant unable to synthesize ascorbic acid. *J. Nutr.* **1985**, *115*, 1630–1640.
84. Horio, F.; Hayashi, K.; Mishima, T.; Takemori, K.; Oshima, I.; Makino, S.; Kakinuma, A.; Ito, H. A newly established strain of spontaneously hypertensive rat with a defect of ascorbic acid biosynthesis. *Life Sci.* **2001**, *69*, 1879–1890.
85. Vergely, C.; Perrin, C.; Laubriet, A.; Oudot, A.; Zeller, M.; Guilland, J.C.; Rochette, L. Postischemic myocardial recovery and oxidative stress status of vitamin C deficient rat hearts. *Cardiovasc. Res.* **2001**, *51*, 89–99.
86. Nishikimi, M.; Koshizaka, T.; Kondo, K.; Ozawa, T.; Yagi, K. Expression of the mutant gene for L-gulono-gamma-lactone oxidase in scurvy-prone rats. *Experientia* **1989**, *45*, 126–129.
87. Fernandez, M.L.; McNamar, D.J. Dietary fat-mediated changes in hepatic apoprotein B/E receptor in the guinea pig: Effect of polyunsaturated, monounsaturated, and saturated fat. *Metabolism* **1989**, *38*, 1094–1102.
88. Bell, J.P.; Mosfer, S.I.; Lang, D.; Donaldson, F.; Lewis, M.J. Vitamin C and quinapril abrogate LVH and endothelial dysfunction in aortic-banded guinea pigs. *Am. J. Physiol. Heart Circ. Physiol.* **2001**, *281*, H1704–H1710.
89. Wolkart, G.; Wenzl, M.V.; Beretta, M.; Stessel, H.; Schmidt, K.; Mayer, B. Vascular tolerance to nitroglycerin in ascorbate deficiency. *Cardiovasc. Res.* **2008**, *79*, 304–312.
90. Liang, W.J.; Johnson, D.; Jarvis, S.M. Vitamin C transport systems of mammalian cells. *Mol. Membr. Biol.* **2001**, *18*, 87–95.
91. Liang, W.J.; Johnson, D.; Ma, L.S.; Jarvis, S.M.; Wei, J.L. Regulation of the human vitamin C transporters expressed in COS-1 cells by protein kinase C [corrected]. *Am. J. Physiol. Cell Physiol.* **2002**, *283*, C1696–C1704.
92. Subramanian, V.S.; Marchant, J.S.; Boulware, M.J.; Said, H.M. A *C*-terminal region dictates the apical plasma membrane targeting of the human sodium-dependent vitamin C transporter-1 in polarized epithelia. *J. Biol. Chem.* **2004**, *279*, 27719–27728.
93. Mardones, L.; Zuniga, F.A.; Villagran, M.; Sotomayor, K.; Mendoza, P.; Escobar, D.; Gonzalez, M.; Ormazabal, V.; Maldonado, M.; Onate, G.; *et al*. Essential role of intracellular glutathione in controlling ascorbic acid transporter expression and function in rat hepatocytes and hepatoma cells. *Free Radic. Biol. Med.* **2012**, *52*, 1874–1887.
94. Nualart, F.J.; Rivas, C.I.; Montecinos, V.P.; Godoy, A.S.; Guaiquil, V.H.; Golde, D.W.; Vera, J.C. Recycling of vitamin C by a bystander effect. *J. Biol. Chem.* **2003**, *278*, 10128–10133.
95. May, J.M.; Qu, Z.C.; Qiao, H.; Koury, M.J. Maturational loss of the vitamin C transporter in erythrocytes. *Biochem. Biophys. Res. Commun.* **2007**, *360*, 295–298.
96. Montel-Hagen, A.; Blanc, L.; Boyer-Clavel, M.; Jacquet, C.; Vidal, M.; Sitbon, M.; Taylor, N. The Glut1 and Glut4 glucose transporters are differentially expressed during perinatal and postnatal erythropoiesis. *Blood* **2008**, *112*, 4729–4738.

97. Rumsey, S.C.; Daruwala, R.; Al-Hasani, H.; Zarnowski, M.J.; Simpson, I.A.; Levine, M. Dehydroascorbic acid transport by GLUT4 in Xenopus oocytes and isolated rat adipocytes. *J. Biol. Chem.* **2000**, *275*, 28246–28253.
98. Chen, Q.; Espey, M.G.; Sun, A.Y.; Pooput, C.; Kirk, K.L.; Krishna, M.C.; Khosh, D.B.; Drisko, J.; Levine, M. Pharmacologic doses of ascorbate act as a prooxidant and decrease growth of aggressive tumor xenografts in mice. *Proc. Natl. Acad. Sci. USA* **2008**, *105*, 11105–11109.
99. Roberts, L.J., II; Traber, M.G.; Frei, B. Vitamins E and C in the prevention of cardiovascular disease and cancer in men. *Free Radic. Biol. Med.* **2009**, *46*, 1558.
100. Dehghan, M.; Akhtar-Danesh, N.; McMillan, C.R.; Thabane, L. Is plasma vitamin C an appropriate biomarker of vitamin C intake? A systematic review and meta-analysis. *Nutr. J.* **2007**, *6*, 41.
101. Brubacher, D.; Moser, U.; Jordan, P. Vitamin C concentrations in plasma as a function of intake: A meta-analysis. *Int. J. Vitam. Nutr. Res.* **2000**, *70*, 226–237.
102. Schleicher, R.L.; Carroll, M.D.; Ford, E.S.; Lacher, D.A. Serum vitamin C and the prevalence of vitamin C deficiency in the United States: 2003–2004 National Health and Nutrition Examination Survey (NHANES). *Am. J. Clin. Nutr.* **2009**, *90*, 1252–1263.
103. Michels, A.J.; Hagen, T.M.; Frei, B. Human genetic variation influences vitamin C homeostasis by altering vitamin C transport and antioxidant enzyme function. *Annu. Rev. Nutr.* **2013**, *33*, 45–70.
104. Harding, A.H.; Wareham, N.J.; Bingham, S.A.; Khaw, K.; Luben, R.; Welch, A.; Forouhi, N.G. Plasma vitamin C level, fruit and vegetable consumption, and the risk of new-onset type 2 diabetes mellitus: The European prospective investigation of cancer—Norfolk prospective study. *Arch. Intern. Med.* **2008**, *168*, 1493–1499.
105. Levine, M.; Conry-Cantilena, C.; Wang, Y.; Welch, R.W.; Washko, P.W.; Dhariwal, K.R.; Park, J.B.; Lazarev, A.; Graumlich, J.F.; King, J.; *et al.* Vitamin C pharmacokinetics in healthy volunteers: Evidence for a recommended dietary allowance. *Proc. Natl. Acad. Sci. USA* **1996**, *93*, 3704–3709.
106. Levine, M.; Wang, Y.; Padayatty, S.J.; Morrow, J. A new recommended dietary allowance of vitamin C for healthy young women. *Proc. Natl. Acad. Sci. USA* **2001**, *98*, 9842–9846.
107. Kim, H.; Bae, S.; Yu, Y.; Kim, Y.; Kim, H.R.; Hwang, Y.I.; Kang, J.S.; Lee, W.J. The analysis of vitamin C concentration in organs of gulo$^{-/-}$ mice upon vitamin C withdrawal. *Immune Netw.* **2012**, *12*, 18–26.
108. Carr, A.C.; Bozonet, S.M.; Pullar, J.M.; Simcock, J.W.; Vissers, M.C. Human skeletal muscle ascorbate is highly responsive to changes in vitamin C intake and plasma concentrations. *Am. J. Clin. Nutr.* **2013**, *97*, 800–807.
109. Taylor, A.; Jacques, P.F.; Nowell, T.; Perrone, G.; Blumberg, J.; Handelman, G.; Jozwiak, B.; Nadler, D. Vitamin C in human and guinea pig aqueous, lens and plasma in relation to intake. *Curr. Eye Res.* **1997**, *16*, 857–864.
110. Dietrich, M.; Block, G.; Benowitz, N.L.; Morrow, J.D.; Hudes, M.; Jacob, P., III; Norkus, E.P.; Packer, L. Vitamin C supplementation decreases oxidative stress biomarker

f2-isoprostanes in plasma of nonsmokers exposed to environmental tobacco smoke. *Nutr. Cancer* **2003**, *45*, 176–184.

111. Block, G.; Jensen, C.D.; Dalvi, T.B.; Norkus, E.P.; Hudes, M.; Crawford, P.B.; Holland, N.; Fung, E.B.; Schumacher, L.; Harmatz, P. Vitamin C treatment reduces elevated C-reactive protein. *Free Radic. Biol. Med.* **2009**, *46*, 70–77.
112. Dhariwal, K.R.; Washko, P.W.; Levine, M. Determination of dehydroascorbic acid using high-performance liquid chromatography with coulometric electrochemical detection. *Anal. Biochem.* **1990**, *189*, 18–23.
113. Lykkesfeldt, J. Determination of ascorbic acid and dehydroascorbic acid in biological samples by high-performance liquid chromatography using subtraction methods: Reliable reduction with tris[2-carboxyethyl]phosphine hydrochloride. *Anal. Biochem.* **2000**, *282*, 89–93.
114. Lykkesfeldt, J. Ascorbate and dehydroascorbic acid as biomarkers of oxidative stress: Validity of clinical data depends on vacutainer system used. *Nutr. Res.* **2012**, *32*, 66–69.
115. Karlsen, A.; Blomhoff, R.; Gundersen, T.E. Stability of whole blood and plasma ascorbic acid. *Eur. J. Clin. Nutr.* **2007**, *61*, 1233–1236.
116. Chung, W.Y.; Chung, J.K.; Szeto, Y.T.; Tomlinson, B.; Benzie, I.F. Plasma ascorbic acid: Measurement, stability and clinical utility revisited. *Clin. Biochem.* **2001**, *34*, 623–627.
117. Tveden-Nyborg, P.; Lykkesfeldt, J. Does Vitamin C deficiency increase lifestyle-associated vascular disease progression? Evidence based on experimental and clinical studies. *Antioxid. Redox Signal.* **2013**, doi:10.1089/ars.2013.5382.
118. Cook, J.D.; Reddy, M.B. Effect of ascorbic acid intake on nonheme-iron absorption from a complete diet. *Am. J. Clin. Nutr.* **2001**, *73*, 93–98.
119. Taylor, E.N.; Stampfer, M.J.; Curhan, G.C. Dietary factors and the risk of incident kidney stones in men: New insights after 14 years of follow-up. *J. Am. Soc. Nephrol.* **2004**, *15*, 3225–3232.
120. Thomas, L.D.; Elinder, C.G.; Tiselius, H.G.; Wolk, A.; Akesson, A. Ascorbic acid supplements and kidney stone incidence among men: A prospective study. *JAMA Intern. Med.* **2013**, *173*, 386–388.
121. Taylor, E.N.; Fung, T.T.; Curhan, G.C. DASH-style diet associates with reduced risk for kidney stones. *J. Am. Soc. Nephrol.* **2009**, *20*, 2253–2259.
122. Singer, R.F. Vitamin C supplementation in kidney failure: Effect on uraemic symptoms. *Nephrol. Dial. Transpl.* **2011**, *26*, 614–620.
123. Hathcock, J.N.; Azzi, A.; Blumberg, J.; Bray, T.; Dickinson, A.; Frei, B.; Jialal, I.; Johnston, C.S.; Kelly, F.J.; Kraemer, K.; *et al.* Vitamins E and C are safe across a broad range of intakes. *Am. J. Clin. Nutr.* **2005**, *81*, 736–745.
124. Rees, D.C.; Kelsey, H.; Richards, J.D. Acute haemolysis induced by high dose ascorbic acid in glucose-6-phosphate dehydrogenase deficiency. *BMJ* **1993**, *306*, 841–842.
125. Hemila, H.; Chalker, E. Vitamin C for preventing and treating the common cold. *Cochrane Database Syst. Rev.* **2013**, *1*, CD000980.
126. Douglas, R.M.; Hemila, H. Vitamin C for preventing and treating the common cold. *PLoS Med.* **2005**, *2*, e168.

127. Sasazuki, S.; Sasaki, S.; Tsubono, Y.; Okubo, S.; Hayashi, M.; Tsugane, S. Effect of vitamin C on common cold: Randomized controlled trial. *Eur. J. Clin. Nutr.* **2006**, *60*, 9–17.
128. Carr, A.C.; Vissers, M.C. Synthetic or food-derived vitamin C—Are they equally bioavailable? *Nutrients* **2013**, *5*, 4284–4304.
129. Padayatty, S.J.; Sun, H.; Wang, Y.; Riordan, H.D.; Hewitt, S.M.; Katz, A.; Wesley, R.A.; Levine, M. Vitamin C pharmacokinetics: Implications for oral and intravenous use. *Ann. Intern. Med.* **2004**, *140*, 533–537.
130. Tannenbaum, S.R. Preventive action of vitamin C on nitrosamine formation. *Int. J. Vitam. Nutr. Res. Suppl.* **1989**, *30*, 109–113.
131. Kesinger, N.G.; Stevens, J.F. Covalent interaction of ascorbic acid with natural products. *Phytochemistry* **2009**, *70*, 1930–1939.
132. Miranda, C.L.; Reed, R.L.; Kuiper, H.C.; Alber, S.; Stevens, J.F. Ascorbic acid promotes detoxification and elimination of 4-hydroxy-2(*E*)-nonenal in human monocytic THP-1 cells. *Chem. Res. Toxicol.* **2009**, *22*, 863–874.
133. Du, J.; Cullen, J.J.; Buettner, G.R. Ascorbic acid: Chemistry, biology and the treatment of cancer. *Biochim. Biophys. Acta* **2012**, *1826*, 443–457.
134. Frei, B.; England, L.; Ames, B.N. Ascorbate is an outstanding antioxidant in human blood plasma. *Proc. Natl. Acad. Sci. USA* **1989**, *86*, 6377–6381.
135. Yin, R.; Mao, S.Q.; Zhao, B.; Chong, Z.; Yang, Y.; Zhao, C.; Zhang, D.; Huang, H.; Gao, J.; Li, Z.; *et al.* Ascorbic acid enhances Tet-mediated 5-methylcytosine oxidation and promotes DNA demethylation in mammals. *J. Am. Chem. Soc.* **2013**, *135*, 10396–10403.
136. Chung, T.L.; Brena, R.M.; Kolle, G.; Grimmond, S.M.; Berman, B.P.; Laird, P.W.; Pera, M.F.; Wolvetang, E.J. Vitamin C promotes widespread yet specific DNA demethylation of the epigenome in human embryonic stem cells. *Stem Cells* **2010**, *28*, 1848–1855.
137. Kirkwood, J.S.; Lebold, K.M.; Miranda, C.L.; Wright, C.L.; Miller, G.W.; Tanguay, R.L.; Barton, C.L.; Traber, M.G.; Stevens, J.F. Vitamin C deficiency activates the purine nucleotide cycle in zebrafish. *J. Biol. Chem.* **2012**, *287*, 3833–3841.
138. Monti, D.A.; Mitchell, E.; Bazzan, A.J.; Littman, S.; Zabrecky, G.; Yeo, C.J.; Pillai, M.V.; Newberg, A.B.; Deshmukh, S.; Levine, M. Phase I evaluation of intravenous ascorbic acid in combination with gemcitabine and erlotinib in patients with metastatic pancreatic cancer. *PLoS One* **2012**, *7*, e29794.
139. Welsh, J.L.; Wagner, B.A.; van't Erve, T.J.; Zehr, P.S.; Berg, D.J.; Halfdanarson, T.R.; Yee, N.S.; Bodeker, K.L.; Du, J.; Roberts, L.J., II; *et al.* Pharmacological ascorbate with gemcitabine for the control of metastatic and node-positive pancreatic cancer (PACMAN): Results from a phase I clinical trial. *Cancer Chemother. Pharmacol.* **2013**, *71*, 765–775.

8

Vitamin C: A Novel Regulator of Neutrophil Extracellular Trap Formation

Bassem M. Mohammed [1,2], Bernard J. Fisher [3], Donatas Kraskauskas [3], Daniela Farkas [3], Donald F. Brophy [1], Alpha A. Fowler III [3] and Ramesh Natarajan [3,*]

1 Department of Pharmacotherapy and Outcomes Science, Virginia Commonwealth University, Richmond, VA 23298, USA; E-Mails: mohammedbm@vcu.edu (B.M.M.); dbrophy@vcu.edu (D.F.B.)

2 Department of Clinical Pharmacy, Faculty of Pharmacy, Cairo University, Cairo 11562, Egypt

3 Division of Pulmonary Disease and Critical Care Medicine, Virginia Commonwealth University, Richmond, VA 23298, USA; E-Mails: bjfisher@vcu.edu (B.J.F.); dkraskauskas@vcu.edu (D.K.); dfarkas3@vcu.edu (D.F.); afowler@mcvh-vcu.edu (A.A.F.)

* Author to whom correspondence should be addressed; E-Mail: rnataraj@vcu.edu;

Abstract: Introduction: Neutrophil extracellular trap (NET) formation was recently identified as a novel mechanism to kill pathogens. However, excessive NET formation in sepsis can injure host tissues. We have recently shown that parenteral vitamin C (VitC) is protective in sepsis. Whether VitC alters NETosis is unknown. **Methods**: We used Gulo$^{-/-}$ mice as they lack the ability to synthesize VitC. Sepsis was induced by intraperitoneal infusion of a fecal stem solution (abdominal peritonitis, FIP). Some VitC deficient Gulo$^{-/-}$ mice received an infusion of ascorbic acid (AscA, 200 mg/kg) 30 min after induction of FIP. NETosis was assessed histologically and by quantification for circulating free DNA (cf-DNA) in serum. Autophagy, histone citrullination, endoplasmic reticulum (ER) stress, NFκB activation and apoptosis were investigated in peritoneal PMNs. **Results**: Sepsis produced significant NETs in the lungs of VitC deficient Gulo$^{-/-}$ mice and increased circulating cf-DNA. This was attenuated in the VitC sufficient Gulo$^{-/-}$ mice and in VitC deficient Gulo$^{-/-}$ mice infused with AscA. Polymorphonuclear neutrophils (PMNs) from VitC deficient Gulo$^{-/-}$ mice demonstrated increased activation of ER stress, autophagy, histone citrullination, and NFκB activation, while apoptosis was inhibited. VitC also significantly attenuated PMA induced NETosis in PMNs from healthy human volunteers. **Conclusions**: Our *in vitro* and *in vivo* findings identify VitC as a novel regulator of NET formation in sepsis. This study complements the notion that VitC is protective in sepsis settings.

Keywords: vitamin C; sepsis; neutrophils; NETosis; cell free DNA; nuclear factor κB

---

1. Introduction

Polymorphonuclear neutrophils (PMN) play key roles in the host response to pathogens by regulating innate host defenses and modulating inflammation. PMN combat pathogens by multiple mechanisms including phagocytosis, followed by exposure to reactive oxygen intermediates (short-lived and long-lived) in phagolysosomes [1], degranulation, which involves release of anti-bacterial peptides and proteases to kill pathogens [2], as well as production of cytokines and other inflammatory mediators. Aside from these traditional mechanisms, another mechanism for pathogen killing, the formation of neutrophil extracellular traps (NETs) by NETosis, a novel cell death pathway different from apoptosis and necrosis, was recently identified [3,4]. Although NETosis plays a crucial role in host defense during local infection by trapping and killing pathogens, excessive NET formation during systemic infections becomes self-defeating by promoting tissue injury and organ damage [5].

Sepsis, a leading cause of death with high mortality rates, is characterized by excessive inflammation and exuberant immune responses that lead to increased circulating PMN levels and extensive PMN sequestration in the lung. This massive influx of PMNs to the lungs often leads to acute lung injury (ALI) [6]. One postulated mechanism by which PMNs cause ALI is NETosis [7]. In sepsis, NETs are formed in response to pro-inflammatory stimuli such as lipopolysaccharide (LPS) and interleukin-8 (IL-8) [8,9] by expulsion of genomic DNA into web-like extracellular structures that display antimicrobial proteins such as histones, neutrophil elastase, and myeloperoxidase [10]. During NETosis, various signaling pathways lead to dissolution of nuclear envelope, thus allowing the mixing of nuclear chromatin with granular antimicrobial proteins from cytoplasmic granules, and then, by releasing the DNA into lattice-like structures, NETs concentrate proteases and antimicrobial proteins in the vicinity of trapped pathogens. However, in sepsis, exposure to NETs also produces organ injury. Indeed, Dwivedi *et al.* recently showed that NETosis, as determined by the circulating cell free DNA (cf-DNA) content, could predict ICU mortality in severe sepsis better than existing severity of illness or organ dysfunction scoring systems and was also better than IL-6, thrombin, and protein C [11]. While effective targeting or inhibition of NET structures has been suggested as therapy to benefit sepsis [8], identification of agents with the potential to alter NET formation remains elusive.

Vitamin C (VitC) is an essential vitamin for humans. While its role as an endogenous antioxidant is well recognized, our recent research suggests that VitC beneficially impacts multiple pathways associated with sepsis [12]. Its pleiotropic mechanisms including attenuation of the pro-inflammatory response, enhancement of epithelial barrier function, increasing alveolar fluid clearance, and prevention of coagulation abnormalities constitute a primary line of defense that is protective in sepsis syndromes [13]. Intracellular levels of VitC in various tissues differ significantly from circulating plasma levels with high cellular concentrations considered to be indicative of essential metabolic function [14]. In particular, VitC accumulates in millimolar quantities in PMNs where it regulates neutrophil apoptosis [14,15]. We recently showed that VitC attenuated neutrophiliccapillaritis and improved survival in murine sepsis models [12,13]. However, whether VitC alters NETosis in sepsis settings remains unknown. Humans lack functional L-gulono-γ-lactone oxidase (Gulo), the final enzyme in the biosynthesis of VitC [16]. In contrast, mice express functional Gulo, resulting in tissues generally maintaining high levels of VitC. In order to translate data from VitC studies in mice to humans we have examined NETosis in septic mice lacking Gulo ($Gulo^{-/-}$). Our studies show that VitC sufficiency attenuated NETosis in septic mice. Importantly, at a cellular level, we show that VitC deficient PMN were more susceptible to undergo NETosis through increased activation of endoplasmic reticulum (ER) stress and autophagy, processes considered vital for NETosis [17]. VitC deficient PMNs displayed increased expression of peptidylargininedeiminase 4 (PAD4), the key enzyme required for hypercitrullination of histones and chromatin decondensation [18]. Moreover, our studies show that the pro-survival transcription factor nuclear factor kappa B (NFκB) was augmented in the VitC deficient PMNs while apoptosis was suppressed. The inhibitory effect of VitC on NETosis was recapitulated in phorbolmyristate acetate (PMA) activated human PMN.

2. Experimental Section

2.1. Animals

$Gulo^{-/-}$ mice were bred in-house from an established homozygous colony as previously described [19]. Vitamin C *sufficient* mice were fed *ad libitum* with regular chow and water supplemented with vitamin C (0.330 g/L) renewed twice per week. Vitamin C *deficient* mice were generated by reducing vitamin C supplementation (0.033 g/L) for one week, followed by complete removal of dietary vitamin C for an additional two weeks. Others have shown that this reduced supplementation significantly decreases the concentration of VitC in immune cells, plasma and organs [20,21].

2.1.1. Feces Induced Peritonitis

Polymicrobial sepsis (peritonitis) was induced by intraperitoneal (i.p.) introduction of fecal stem solution into the peritoneum as described previously [13,19]. Thirty minutes after fecal challenge (45 mg/mL), some mice received i.p. injection of VitC as ascorbic acid (200 mg/kg in saline). Untreated mice received i.p. saline instead of VitC. Blood was collected 16 h later by cardiac puncture, and lungs harvested. Blood was allowed to coagulate, spun to separate serum, and stored at −80 °C for batch analysis of cell-free DNA (see below).

All animal studies were performed in accordance to the Virginia Commonwealth University Animal Care and Use Committee's approved protocols (Protocol # AM10100, approved 15 March, 2011).

2.1.2. $Gulo^{-/-}$ Mice Were Divided into Five Groups

(1) (+): vitamin C *sufficient* mice received saline alone (0.4 mL, i.p.)

(2) **FIP(+)**: vitamin C *sufficient* mice received fecal stem solution (0.4 mL, i.p.) followed 30 min later by saline (0.1 mL, i.p.)
(3) (−): vitamin C *deficient* mice received saline alone (0.4 mL, i.p.)
(4) **FIP(−)**: vitamin C *deficient* mice received fecal stem solution (0.4 mL, i.p.) followed 30 min later by saline (0.1 mL, i.p.)
(5) **FIP(−) + AscA**: vitamin C *deficient* mice received fecal stem solution (0.4 mL, i.p.) followed 30 min later by ascorbic acid (0.1 mL, i.p.)

2.2. Isolation of Mouse Peritoneal Neutrophils

Induction of an enriched exudate of leukocytes in the peritoneal cavity of mice was performed by i.p. injection of 1 mL of aged, sterile 3% thioglycollate solution [16]. After 16 h, mice were euthanized, and the peritoneal cavity was flushed with 5 mL sterile Hanks' balanced salt solution containing 1% BSA (HBSS). The leukocyte pellet containing ~80% neutrophils and ~20% macrophages was washed with HBSS and resuspended in RPMI-1640 medium. Total cell counts were determined with a hemacytometer. Leukocyte viability was assessed by trypan blue exclusion (>99%). PMNs were then purified by adherence to a plastic dish as described by Tsurubuchi *et al.* [22]. Briefly, cells from peritoneal exudate were plated into a 35-mm plastic dish and incubated at 37 °C in 5% CO_2 in air for 10 min in HBSS. The cells were washed twice with fresh HBSS to remove non-adherent cells. Although there was loss of some PMNs, which did not adhere to the dish, this procedure eliminated most of the macrophages. Cytochemical staining of adherent cells using HARLECO® Hemacolor® Solution (EMD Millipore, EMD Millipore) revealed that >95% of the adherent cells were PMNs.

2.3. Immunofluorescence and Differential Interference Contrast Imaging of Lung NETs

Formalin fixed paraffin embedded mouse lung sections (3 μm) were rehydrated and heat induced antigen retrieval performed in 0.01 M citrate buffer pH 6.0 for 20 min. Sections were blocked with 1% normal swine serum (NSS, DAKO, Carpinteria, CA, USA) and incubated with primary antibody #1, rat anti-mouse CD41 (MWReg30, ab33661, Abcam, Cambridge, MA, USA), 1:10 diluted in 1% NSS/PBS overnight at 4 °C. Sections were then incubated with goat anti-rat Alexa Fluor® 488 1:50 (Abcam) in PBS for 4 h followed by incubation with primary antibody #2, rabbit anti-myeloperoxidase (ab45977, Abcam) 1:10 diluted in PBS overnight at 4 °C. Sections were then incubated with chicken anti-rabbit Alexa Fluor® 647 (Invitrogen, Life Technologies, Grand Island, NY, USA) 1:50 in PBS for 4 h followed by incubation with primary antibody #3, mouse anti-histone H2A (L88A6, Cell Signaling, Danvers, MA, USA) 1:200 in PBS overnight at 4 °C, and then finally incubated with goat anti-mouse IgG1 Alexa Fluor® 594 (Invitrogen) 1:50 in PBS for 4 h. Nuclear counterstain was performed with DAPI (Invitrogen) 1:500 for 5 min and sections mounted with Slow Fade Gold (Invitrogen). Negative controls were run in parallel with nonspecific IgG or specific isotype. Confocal microscopy was performed with a Leica TCS SP2 laser scanning confocal microscopy system of the VCU Department of Anatomy and Neurobiology Microscope Facility. Separate images of optical sections were acquired with filters for Alexa Fluor® (AF) 488, 594, 647 and DAPI. Images were assembled with ImageJ software.

2.4. RNA Isolation and Real-Time Quantitative PCR (QPCR) Analysis

Isolation of total RNA and real-time QPCR analyses were performed as described previously [12]. Primers used for QPCR are listed in Table 1.

Table 1. Murine primers used for Quantitative PCR (QPCR).

Name	Sequence 5′ to 3′
ATF4 forward	CCTAGGTCTCTTAGATGACTATCTGGAGG
ATF4 reverse	CCAGGTCATCCATTCGAAACAGAGCATCG
BiP forward	GTGCAGCAGGACATCAAGTTCTTGCC
BiP reverse	TTCCCAAATACGCCTCAGCAGTCTCC
CHOP forward	CACCTATATCTCATCCCCAGGAAACG
CHOP reverse	TTCCTTGCTCTTCCTCCTCTTCCTCC
EDEM forward	GCCCTTTGGTGACATGACAATTGAGG
EDEM reverse	TCATTATTGCTGTCAGGAGGAACACC
XBP-1s forward	TGAGTCCGCAGCAGGTGC
XBP-1s reverse	CAACTTGTCCAGAATGCCCAAAAGG
XBP-1un forward	AAGAACACGCTTGGGAATGGACACGC
XBP-1un reverse	ACCTGCTGCAGAGGTGCACATAGTC
PAD4 forward	ACAGGTGAAAGCAGCCAGC
PAD4 reverse	AGTGATGTAGATCAGGGCTTGG
ATG3 forward	CACCACTGTCCAACATGGC
ATG3 reverse	GTTTACACCGCTTGTAGCATGG
ATG5 forward	ACAAGCAGCTCTGGATGGG
ATG5 reverse	GGAGGATATTCCATGAGTTTCCG
ATG6 forward	CACGAGCTTCAAGATCCTGG
ATG6 reverse	TCCTGAGTTAGCCTCTTCCTCC
ATG7 forward	ACGATGACGACACTGTTCTGG
ATG7 reverse	AGGTTACAGGGATCGTACACACC
ATG8 forward	ACAAAGAGTGGAAGATGTCCG
ATG8 reverse	GGAACTTGGTCTTGTCCAGG
TNFα forward	GATGAGAAGTTCCCAAATGGC
TNFα reverse	TTGGTGGTTTGCTACGACG
IL-1β forward	CTGAACTCAACTGTGAAATGCC
IL-1β reverse	CAGGTCAAAGGTTTGGAAGC
18S forward	GATAGCTCTTTCTCGATTCCG
18S reverse	AGAGTCTCGTTCGTTATCGG

2.5. Western Blot Analysis

Neutrophil whole-cell and nuclear extracts were isolated for Western blot analysis as described previously [13]. Nuclear extracts were isolated using the NE-PER kit (Pierce Biotechnology, Rockford, IL, USA). Proteins were resolved by SDS polyacrylamide gel electrophoresis (4%–20%) and electrophoretically transferred to polyvinylidene fluoride membranes (0.2 μm pore size). Immunodetection was performed using chemiluminescent detection with the Renaissance Western Blot Chemiluminescence Reagent Plus (Perkin Elmer Life Sciences Inc., Boston, MA, USA). Blots were stripped using the Restore™ Western Blot Stripping Buffer (Pierce Biotechnology Inc., Rockford, IL, USA) as described by the manufacturer. Purified rabbit polyclonal antibodies to LC3B (L7543, Sigma-Aldrich), cleaved caspase-3 (#9661, Cell Signaling), caspase-3 (#9662, Cell Signaling), p62/SQSTM1 (NBP1-48320, Novus Biologicals), NFκB p65 (sc-109, Santa Cruz Biotechnology), Lamin B (sc-6216, Santa Cruz Biotechnology), and actin (sc-1616, Santa Cruz Biotechnology) were used in this study. Optical densities of antibody-specific bands were determined using Quantity One acquisition and analysis software (Bio-Rad, Hercules, CA, USA).

2.6. Isolation of Human Neutrophils and NETs Release

Human neutrophils were isolated by density gradient centrifugation and hypotonic lysis [23]. Cells were adjusted to 2 × 10^6/mL in RPMI-1640, seeded onto 8-well IbiTreat μ-slides (Ibidi #80826), 0.3 mL per well, and allowed to adhere for 15 min. PMNs were VitC loaded by incubating for 1 h with 0.3 mM or 3 mM buffered ascorbic acid (Mylan Institutional LLC, Rockville, IL, USA). Neutrophils were stimulated with 50 nM PMA for three hours at 37 °C. Neutrophil conditioned media were centrifuged at 400× *g* for 5 min and the supernatants used for quantification of cf-DNA [24].

2.7. Immunofluorescence Staining of Human NETs

PMNs were fixed with 4% paraformaldehyde, permeabilized with 0.15% Triton X-100 in PBS, and blocked with 5% normal chicken serum (Sigma) in PBS. To stain NETs, slides were incubated with a mouse monoclonal anti-myeloperoxidase antibody (1:200; Santa Cruz sc-52707) and a secondary Alexa Fluor® 488-conjugated chicken anti-mouse IgG antibody (1:200; Molecular Probes A-21200). After staining of DNA with DAPI, neutrophil-derived NET formation was visualized by immunofluorescence microscopy performed on an Olympus model IX70 inverted microscope outfitted with an IX-FLA fluorescence observation system equipped with a FITC and DAPI filter cubes (Chroma Technology, Brattleboro, VT, USA) through Uplan FI objectives (20×, 60×). Images were captured by an Olympus XM10 digital camera using CellSens imaging software (Olympus America, Melville, NY, USA).

2.8. Quantification of Cell Free DNA

The levels of cf-DNA in human neutrophil supernatants and mouse serum were quantified using the Invitrogen Quant-iTPicoGreendsDNA assay kit according to the manufacturer's instructions (Life Technologies, Grand Island, NY, USA). Fluorescence intensity was measured on a SpectraMax Gemini XPS microplate reader with excitation at 490 nm and emission at 525 nm, with a 515 nm emission cutoff filter (Molecular Devices, Sunnyvale, CA, USA).

2.9. Statistical Analysis

Statistical analysis was performed using SAS 9.3 and GraphPad Prism 6.0 (GraphPad Software, San Diego, CA, USA). Data are expressed as mean ± SE. Results were compared using Student-Newman-Keuls test or one-way ANOVA and the *post hoc* Tukey test to identify specific differences between groups. Statistical significance was confirmed at a p value of <0.05.

Figure 1. Vitamin C sufficient Gulo$^{-/-}$ mice demonstrate reduced lung NETs and lower cf-DNA following peritonitis-induced sepsis. Representative immunofluorescence and differential interference contrast imaging of lung NETs (**A**–**E**): (**A**) VitC sufficient Gulo$^{-/-}$ mice (+) received saline alone (0.4 mL, i.p.); (**B**) FIP exposed VitC sufficient Gulo$^{-/-}$ mice [**FIP**(+)] received fecal stem solution (45 mg/mL, i.p.) followed 30 min later by saline (0.1 mL, i.p.); (**C**) VitC deficient Gulo$^{-/-}$ mice (−) received saline alone (0.4 mL, i.p.); (**D**) FIP exposed VitC deficient Gulo$^{-/-}$ mice [**FIP**(−)] mice received fecal stem solution (45 mg/mL, i.p.) followed 30 min later by saline (0.1 mL, i.p.). (**E**) AscA treated FIP exposed VitC deficient Gulo$^{-/-}$ mice [**FIP**(−) + **AscA**] mice received fecal stem solution (45 mg/mL, i.p.) followed 30 min later by AscA (200 mg/kg, i.p.). Platelet CD-41 (green), histones (red), and myeloperoxidase (grey) are seen in the merged images. Arrowheads indicate NET formation shown by co-staining for platelet CD-41 (green), histones (red), myeloperoxidase (grey), and DAPI (blue) in the vascular and alveolar spaces. Arrows indicate extensive extra-nuclear histones (red); (10× magnification, $N = 3$ for each group). (**F**) Serum levels of cf-DNA were quantified using the Quant-iTPicoGreen dsDNA assay kit ($N = 5$–11 for each group, $p < 0.05$).

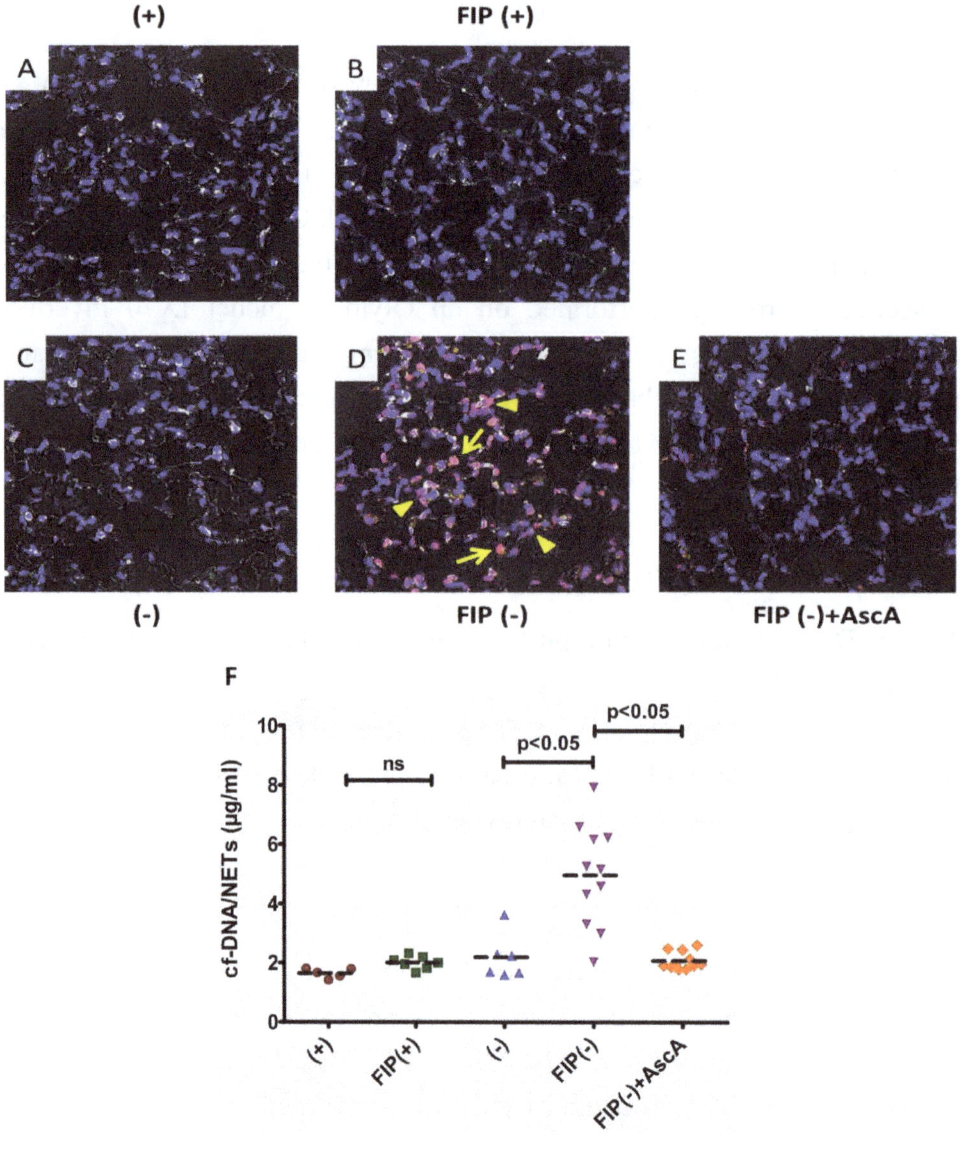

3. Results

3.1. Vitamin C Sufficient Mice Demonstrate Reduced Lung NETs and Lower cf-DNA Following Peritonitis-Induced Sepsis

We have previously shown that fecal peritonitis promotes PMN infiltration of the lungs in VitC deficient mice [19]. Here we used immunofluorescence staining and DIC microscopy to examine the extent of NETs in lungs of mice following FIP induced sepsis. Immuno-positive staining for platelet CD-41 (green), nuclear histones (red), and myeloperoxidase (grey) are visible in the lungs of saline exposed mice (Figure 1A). No appreciable immuno-positive staining differences were seen in the lungs of saline exposed VitC deficient mice (Figure 1C). FIP induced a mild increase in CD-41 immuno-positivity as well as some cytosolic histone staining (Figure 1B). However, no significant histological changes were evident in the VitC sufficient septic mice. In contrast, FIP induced significant NETs in VitC deficient mice as evidenced by dramatically increased co-staining for platelet CD-41 (green), histones (red), and myeloperoxidase (grey) in the vascular and alveolar spaces of septic mice (arrowheads, Figure 1D). Moreover, extensive extra-nuclear staining of histones (arrows) is also evident in this representative section along with thickened alveolar walls. Importantly, FIP exposed vitamin C deficient mice treated with ascorbic acid exhibited significant attenuation of NETs (Figure 1E).

In order to quantify NETs we determined levels of cf-DNA in the serum of VitC sufficient and deficient mice 16 h after sham treatment or FIP. Levels of serum cf-DNA were significantly elevated in the FIP exposed VitC deficient mice (Figure 1F, 5-fold, $p < 0.05$). Treatment of septic VitC deficient mice with ascorbic acid significantly lowered the cf-DNA values to control levels ($p < 0.05$). In addition peritoneal neutrophils from vitamin C deficient mice were more susceptible to NETosis than those from vitamin C deficient mice (Supplementary Material, Figure S1).

3.2. Vitamin C Deficient Neutrophils Show Increased PAD4 mRNA

Unlike apoptosis, rapid intracellular decondensation of nuclear chromatin is a hallmark of NETosis [19,25]. Decondensation of nuclear chromatin requires the removal of positively charged arginine residues on histones by deimination or citrullination, which is carried out by a family of peptidylargininedeiminases (PAD). Of these, only PAD4 is expressed by neutrophils [26] and possesses a classical nuclear localization signal [27]. Importantly Wang *et al.* have shown that PAD4 is indispensable for NETosis [18]. Therefore, we examined mRNA expression of PAD4 in PMNs from VitC sufficient and deficient mice. As seen in Figure 2, PAD4 mRNA expression was significantly higher in thioglycollate elicited peritoneal PMNs from VitC deficient mice ($p < 0.05$).

3.3. Autophagy Signaling Is Induced in Vitamin C Deficient Neutrophils

Autophagy is a vital process for the catabolism of cytosolic proteins and organelles, but has also been shown to be required for NETosis [17,28]. To examine whether VitC regulates autophagy in PMNs we assessed the expression of several autophagy genes in thioglycollate elicited PMNs from VitC sufficient and deficient mice. As seen in Figure 3A, the expression of autophagy related signaling molecules (except for ATG6) were significantly elevated in the VitC *deficient* PMNs ($p < 0.05$).

Figure 2. Vitamin C deficient neutrophils show increased PAD4 mRNA. Real time QPCR for PAD4 shows two-fold increase in mRNA expression from peritoneal PMNs of VitC deficient Gulo$^{-/-}$ mice when compared to PMNs from VitC sufficient Gulo$^{-/-}$ mice ($N = 6$ for each group, * $p < 0.05$).

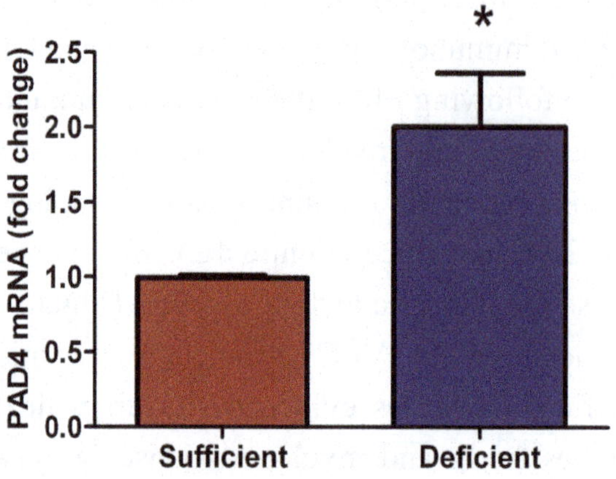

Activation of the autophagic process causes lipidation of ATG8/LC3B (LC3B-I to LC3B-II conversion) and the lipid-modified LC3B-II translocates to autophagosomes. This LC3B-I to LC3B-II conversion is considered a critical marker of autophagy activation [29]. We observed significantly enhanced LC3B-I to LC3B-II conversion in cell lysates of VitC *deficient* PMNs by immunoblotting (Figure 3B, $p < 0.05$).

Figure 3. Autophagy signaling is induced in Vitamin C deficient neutrophils. (**A**) Real time QPCR for ATG3, ATG5, ATG6, ATG7, and ATG8 mRNA from peritoneal PMNs of VitC sufficient and deficient Gulo$^{-/-}$ mice, ($N = 6$ for each group, * $p < 0.05$). (**B**) Representative Western blot for expression of LC3B-I and LC3B-II from peritoneal PMNs of VitC sufficient and deficient Gulo$^{-/-}$ mice. Densitometry of LC3B-II/actin from peritoneal PMNs of VitC sufficient and deficient Gulo$^{-/-}$ mice ($N = 6$ for each group, * $p < 0.05$). (**C**) Representative Western blot for expression of p62 and actin from peritoneal PMNs of VitC sufficient and deficient Gulo$^{-/-}$ mice. Densitometry of normalized p62 expression from peritoneal PMNs of VitC sufficient and deficient Gulo$^{-/-}$ mice ($N = 6$ for each group, ns $p = 0.3$).

A

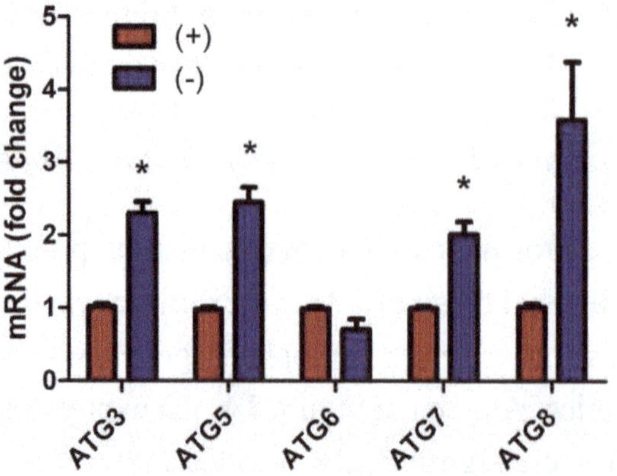

Figure 3. *Cont.*

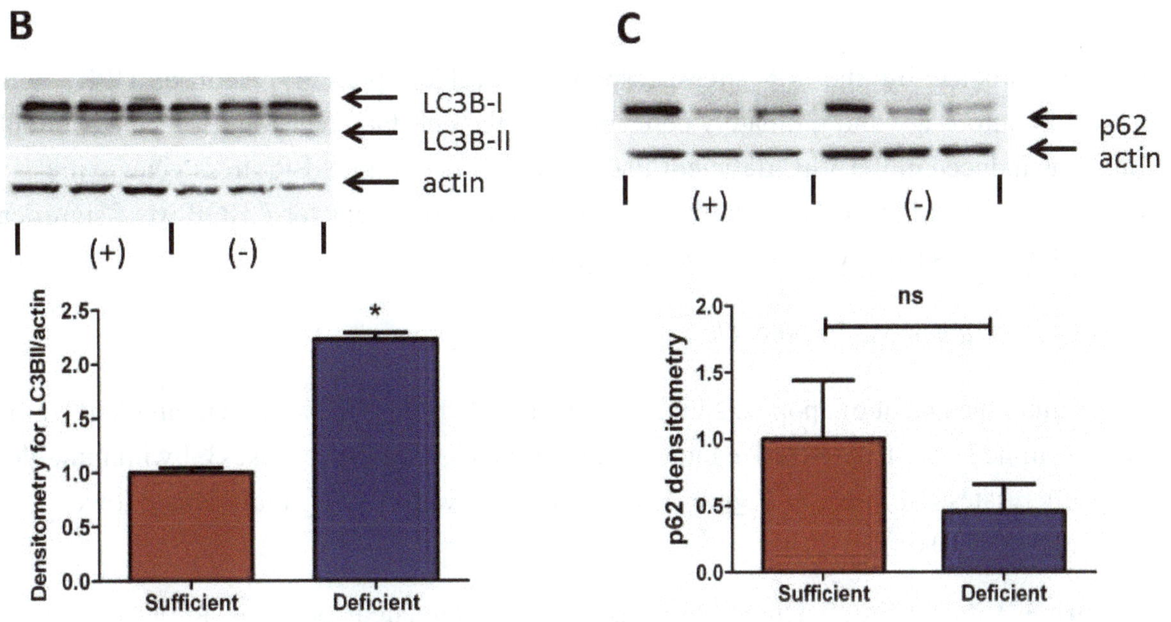

To further investigate the regulation of autophagy signaling by VitC in PMNs we examined the accumulation of p62/sequestosome I in these cell lysates. The loss of p62 in cells is typically indicative of increased autophagic activity [30]. Detection of p62 by immunoblotting showed a trend towards decreases p62 levels in the VitC *deficient* PMNs (Figure 3C). However this decline did not reach statistical significance ($p = 0.3$).

Figure 4. Endoplasmic reticulum stress associated gene expression in up-regulated in vitamin C deficient neutrophils. Real time QPCR for activating transcription factor 4 (ATF4), glucose-regulated protein 78 (Grp78, BiP), C/EBP homologous protein (CHOP), ER degradation-enhancing α-mannosidase-like protein (EDEM), X-box binding protein-1 spliced (XBP-1s), and unspliced (XBP-1un) mRNA from peritoneal PMNs of VitC sufficient and deficient Gulo$^{-/-}$ mice, ($N = 6$ for each group, * $p < 0.05$).

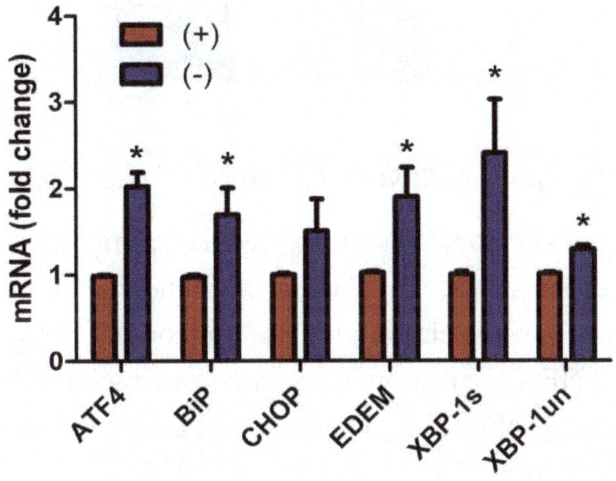

3.4. Endoplasmic Reticulum Stress Associated Gene Expression Is Up-Regulated in Vitamin C Deficient Neutrophils

Signaling initiated by the ER stress response (unfolded protein response, UPR) actively participates in autophagy and ultimately contributes to the cell fate decision [31]. Since autophagy signaling was induced in the VitC deficient PMNs, we next examined ER stress gene expression in the PMNs. As seen in Figure 4, all the UPR genes examined except for CHOP were significantly up-regulated in PMNs from VitC *deficient* mice ($p < 0.05$).

3.5. Vitamin C Deficient Neutrophils Undergo Attenuated Apoptosis

To determine the extent of apoptosis in peritoneal PMNs from VitC sufficient and VitC deficient mice, we examined a well characterized marker of apoptosis, cleaved caspase-3, by immunoblotting of PMN cell lysates. As seen in Figure 5, caspase-3 activation was significantly lower in VitC *deficient* PMNs ($p < 0.05$).

Figure 5. Vitamin C deficient neutrophils undergo attenuated apoptosis. Representative Western blot for expression of caspase-3 and cleaved caspase-3 from peritoneal PMNs of VitC sufficient and deficient Gulo$^{-/-}$ mice. Densitometry of cleaved caspase-3/caspase-3 from peritoneal PMNs of VitC sufficient and deficient Gulo$^{-/-}$ mice ($N = 6$ for each group, * $p < 0.05$).

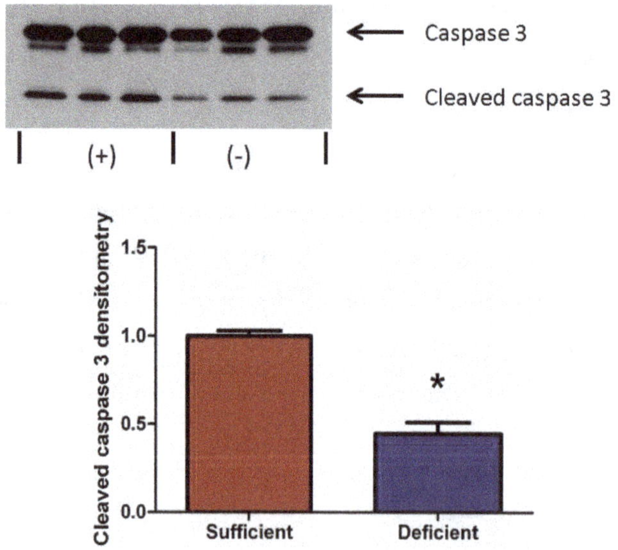

3.6. Vitamin C Deficient Neutrophils Exhibit Increased NFκB Activation

The transcription factor NFκB modulates the expression of many immuno-regulatory mediators in the acute inflammatory response in sepsis. Yang *et al.* found that diminished nuclear translocation of NFκB in peripheral PMNs was associated with less time on the ventilator and improved survival in critically ill patients [32]. NFκB activation is also associated with increased ROS production and endoplasmic reticulum stress signaling [33]. Therefore, we examined nuclear translocation of NFκB in peritoneal PMNs isolated from VitC sufficient and deficient mice. As seen in Figure 6A, significantly increased NFκB translocation was observed in nuclei of VitC *deficient* PMNs ($p < 0.05$).

Increased nuclear NFκB translocation was associated with induction of the NFκB dependent pro-inflammatory genes for TNFα and IL-1β (Figure 6B, $p < 0.05$).

Figure 6. Vitamin C deficient neutrophils exhibit increased NFκB activation. (**A**) Representative Western blot for nuclear expression of NFκBp65 and Lamin B from peritoneal PMNs of VitC sufficient and deficient Gulo$^{-/-}$ mice. Densitometry of NFκBp65/Lamin B from peritoneal PMNs of VitC sufficient and deficient Gulo$^{-/-}$ mice ($N = 4$ for each group, * $p < 0.05$). (**B**) Real time QPCR for TNFα and IL-1β mRNA from peritoneal PMNs of VitC sufficient and deficient Gulo$^{-/-}$ mice, ($N = 6$ for each group, * $p < 0.05$).

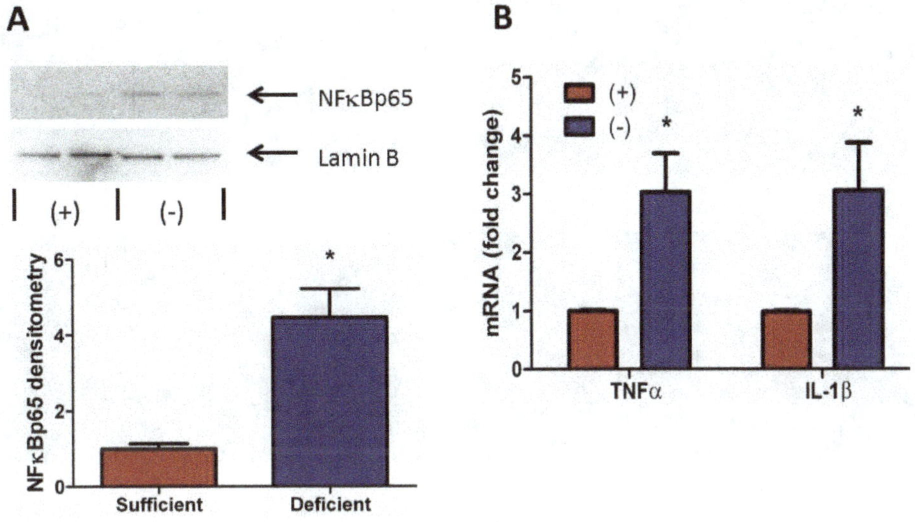

3.7. Vitamin C Attenuates NET Formation in Activated Human Neutrophils

Freshly isolated human PMNs formed NETs following activation by PMA (50 nM) for three hours as seen by immunofluorescence staining (Figure 7B,E). Loading the cells with VitC (3 mM) prior to PMA stimulation greatly reduced NET formation by human PMN (Figure 7C,F). Further, quantification of cf-DNA from the supernatants showed VitC (3 mM) loading significantly reduced NETs release from activated PMN (Figure 7G, $p < 0.05$).

4. Discussion

In this study we show that VitC could play a critical role in regulating the ultimate fate of PMNs in sepsis. Activated PMNs undergo extensive NETosis in septic mice lungs, resulting in potential damage to lung alveolar and endothelial cells. This effect was predominant in PMNs from VitC deficient mice and could be rescued by VitC infusion after the onset of sepsis. In contradistinction, PMNs from VitC sufficient mice underwent attenuated NETosis. Importantly, at a molecular level, VitC deficient peritoneal PMNs were likely to be more pro-inflammatory, to resist apoptosis, and to preferentially undergo NETosis.

Figure 7. Vitamin C attenuates NET formation in activated human neutrophils. Representative image of immunofluorescent staining for NETs in human neutrophils: DNA (blue); myeloperoxidase (green). **Upper Panels**: Control PMNs (**A**, 20×); PMNs exposed to PMA (50 nM) for 3 h (**B**, 20×); PMNs loaded with VitC (3 mM) for 1 h and then exposed to PMA (50 nM) for 3 h (**C**, 20×). **Lower Panels**: Control PMNs (**D**, 60×); PMNs exposed to PMA (50 nM) for 3 h (**E**, 60×); PMNs loaded with VitC (3 mM) for 1 h and then exposed to PMA (50 nM) for 3 h (**F**, 60×). (N = 3 for each group, Magnification: upper panel 20×, lower panel 60×). (**G**) Quantification of cf-DNA in the supernatants above ($N = 3$ for each group, $p < 0.05$).

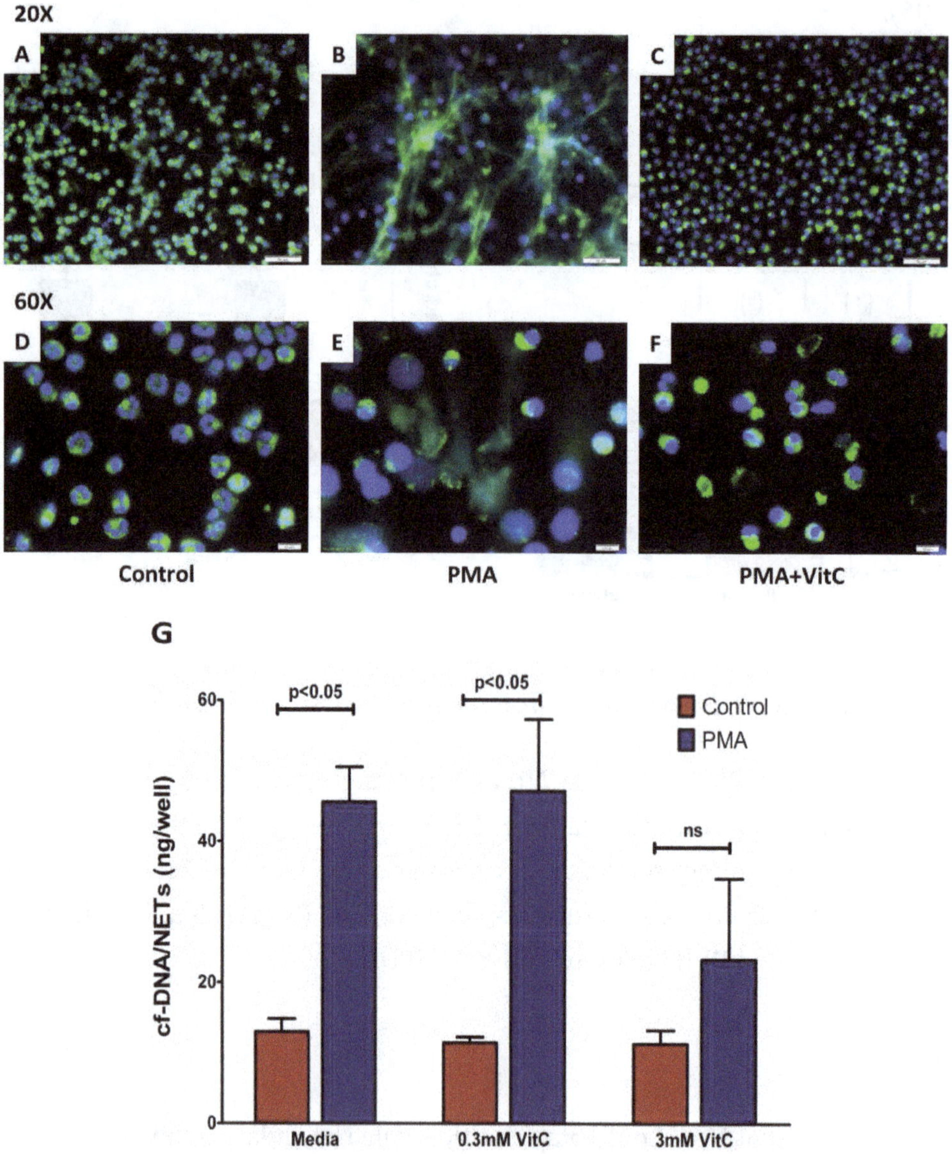

Although several signaling mechanisms responsible for NET formation have been reported, critical regulatory elements remain unidentified. This study advances our understanding of PMN function and NET biology by identifying a novel regulatory mechanism for NET formation in both murine and human PMNs. Using our previously well-characterized model of abdominal peritonitis induced sepsis we show that sepsis promotes NET formation in lungs of VitC deficient mice (Figure 1). NETosis in this model was accompanied by increased circulating cf-DNA (Figure 1F). VitC sufficiency or infusion of VitC after initiation of sepsis significantly decreased NETosis in lungs and circulating cf-DNA content (Figure 1). NET formation in VitC deficient peritoneal PMNs required activation of well characterized signaling pathways including ROS generation (data not shown), activation of the peptidylargininedeiminase PAD4 (Figure 2), autophagy (Figure 3), endoplasmic reticulum stress (Figure 4), and inhibition of apoptosis (Figure 5). NFκB, a pro-inflammatory, pro-survival transcription factor was activated in the VitC deficient peritoneal PMNs (Figure 6). VitC sufficiency or treatment with VitC attenuated these signaling pathways in PMNs.

Intracellular chromatin decondensation is essential for NET formation. Chromatin decondensation is brought about by peptidylargininedeiminase 4 (PAD4), a nuclear enzyme that deiminates arginine residues on histone tails thereby converting positively charged arginines to uncharged citrullines [17,18]. The importance of PAD4 is that many NET forming stimuli including PMA, LPS, and IL-8 as well as various bacterial and fungal species converge to its activation. While PAD4 is expressed in PMNs and is localized to the nucleus [26,27], little is known about its mechanism of action or its transcriptional regulation. Ying *et al.* have shown that PAD1, which belongs to the same family of enzymes as PAD4, is transcriptionally regulated by NFκB [34]. We have previously shown that VitC blocks NFκB activation in septic mouse lungs [12]. Cárcamo *et al.* also demonstrated that VitC blocks IκB kinase activity and NFκB activation [35]. In this study we observed that nuclear NFκB levels were higher in the VitC deficient PMNs (Figure 6A). Further, PAD4 mRNA expression was also significantly higher in PMNs from VitC deficient mice (Figure 2). Therefore, we hypothesize that VitC decreases PAD4 expression by suppressing NFκB activation in PMNs. Further, by decreasing PAD4 expression VitC could decrease histone citrullination activity and therefore chromatin decondensation in VitC sufficient PMNs.

Autophagy has been identified as a well-conserved, homeostatic mechanism that clears damaged organelles or proteins and plays an essential role in cell survival during periods of nutrient depletion [36]. Despite the view that it might not occur in neutrophils, autophagy was recently shown to occur both in murine and human PMNs [37,38]. While Mitroulis *et al.* reported that autophagy occurs in human PMNs in response to PMA activation [39]. Remijsen *et al.* have shown that autophagy is necessary for the induction of intracellular chromatin decondensation during PMA-induced NETosis [17]. In our study, we found increased expression of autophagy genes (Figure 3A) as well as significantly enhanced LC3B-I to LC3B-II conversion in VitC deficient PMNs (Figure 3B) indicative of the presence of more autophagosomes in VitC deficient PMNs. However, LC3B-I to LC3B-II conversion is a static measure of autophagosome number, and does not measure the actual activity of the pathway. The increased LC3B-II could be interpreted as either high autophagic activity or a downstream block in the system that results in an accumulation of LC3B-II protein, even though autophagic degradation itself is diminished. To supplement our observations we examined levels of p62/sequestosome I, a cytosolic chaperone protein with an LC3B binding domain [40]. The normal function of p62 protein is to carry polyubiquitinated proteins to the autphagolysosome where it binds to LC3B before getting degraded. Thus, the loss of p62 protein is a measure of the flux of autophagy and indicative of increased autophagy [41]. In our studies we found a trend towards decreased p62 levels in the VitC deficient PMNs (Figure 3C). While this decline did not reach statistical significance, in combination with the increased autophagy gene expression and increased LC3B conversion, our data imply increased autophagy in VitC deficient PMNs.

The unfolded protein response (UPR) and autophagic machinery have been shown to be critically linked to each other. It is well established that activation of the UPR genes transcriptionally up-regulates several autophagy related genes required for induction and construction of the autophagy machinery [42]. However, it is not known whether activation of the UPR drives autophagy and eventually leads to NET formation in PMNs. Our study shows that most of the UPR genes examined except for CHOP were significantly up-regulated in PMNs from VitC deficient mice (Figure 4). This implies that VitC deficient PMNs could be actively undergoing ER stress, which in turn could drive autophagy genes and increase their susceptibility to undergo NETosis.

The transcription factor NFκB is central to pro-inflammatory/pro-survival responses in sepsis. It is normally sequestered to IκB in the cytosol. Upon appropriate stimulation, IκB is degraded allowing NFκB to migrate to the nucleus and drives transcription of numerous genes that regulate the immune response in sepsis. Moine *et al.* have demonstrated increased NFκB translocation in the lungs of patients with ALI [43]. Yang *et al.* found that increased nuclear levels of NFκB in unstimulated neutrophils were associated with a worse clinical outcome [32]. As discussed above, NFκB likely drives expression of PAD4 in PMNs. NFκB activation also drives expression of pro-survival genes [44]. In this study we found that nuclear NFκB translocation was higher in VitC deficient PMNs (Figure 6A). Further, NFκB translocation in these VitC deficient PMNs increased expression of the pro-inflammatory genes TNFα and IL-1β (Figure 6). NFκB activation also inhibited apoptosis as seen by the reduced activation of caspase 3 in VitC deficient PMNs (Figure 5). These results suggest that NFκB may play a critical role in modulating cell signaling pathways that eventually regulate the fate of PMNs. By activating PAD4 (chromatin decondensation), inducing ER stress and subsequent autophagy, and inhibiting apoptosis, NFκB may drive the cellular machinery of VitC deficient PMNs towards NET formation (Figure 8). VitC sufficiency or infusion of VitC allows PMNs to increase intracellular levels of VitC and attenuate NFκB activation. This could dampen the pathways required for NETosis and may allow PMNs to undergo apoptosis instead. While the decreased apoptosis rate in VitC deficient PMNs may benefit the host by giving more time for PMNs to perform their innate immune functions, studies show that it could also be detrimental in sepsis due to the PMN-dependent inflammation and tissue damage that could be heightened by a prolonged lifespan. Recent reports in the literature have implicated NETs in transfusion-related acute lung injury (TRALI), the leading cause of death after transfusion therapy [45,46]. NETs were shown to be present during TRALI both in mice and humans and so it was suggested that targeting NET formation may be a new approach for the treatment of acute lung injury. While we did not examine TRALI in our studies, it is conceivable that VitC infusion could be a useful adjunct for the prevention/treatment of TRALI or other disease states involving exuberant formation of NETs particularly in the lungs.

Our study has several limitations: (1) It is possible that the PMNs isolated within the peritoneal cavity by thioglycollate could be partially activated; (2) We examined PMN function *ex vivo*. Further *in vivo* studies are needed to characterize the fate of PMNs; (3) others have performed studies with PMNs isolated from bone marrow instead of thioglycollate elicitation. These PMNs would be less "activated" when compared to thioglycollate elicited PMNs, but would also have a large component of immature PMNs which have been shown to behave somewhat differently from mature PMNs [47].

Figure 8. Schematic hypothesis of regulation of signaling pathways that leads to NETosis by VitC. Septic stimuli activate NFκB in PMNs with increased activation observed in VitC deficient PMNs. NFκB nuclear translocation drives expression of PAD4, ER stress and autophagy signaling genes while inhibiting caspase 3 in activated PMNs. This drives the fate of activated PMN away from apoptosis and enhances NETosis. VitC likely blocks up-regulation of PAD4, ER stress and autophagy signaling genes by decreasing NFκB activation. Activated PMNs now undergo apoptosis while NETosis is attenuated.

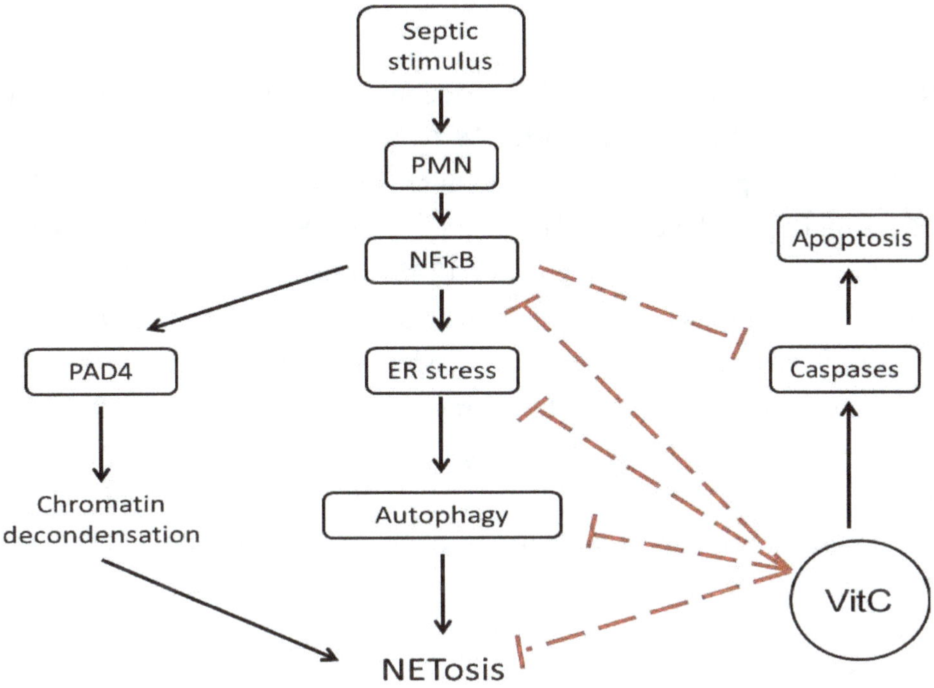

5. Conclusions

In the past few years circulating cf-DNA has been identified as a prognostic marker in severe sepsis [11,48,49]. Indeed cf-DNA was shown to have better discriminatory power than IL-6, thrombin or protein C to predict ICU mortality in sepsis [11]. The cellular origin of cf-DNA from host cells was shown by Dwivedi *et al.* [11] who confirmed that the release of cf-DNA was independent of the infecting organism and was likely mediated by inflammatory mediators generated during the exacerbated host immune response. Our study showed attenuated NET formation and reduced cf-DNA in the serum of septic VitC sufficient mice and in VitC deficient mice treated with ascorbic acid (Figure 1). Our study did not examine the origin of cf-DNA in the serum of these mice. It is possible that some of this DNA could be non-neutrophilic in origin since mast cells, eosinophils, and basophils have also been shown to expel their DNA in a manner similar to PMNs [50]. However, a detailed examination of the origin of cf-DNA in these septic mice is beyond the scope of this study. Nevertheless, data from our study implies that attenuation of NETs maybe crucial for resolution of sepsis in mice.

Overall, our *in vitro* and *in vivo* findings identify a novel regulatory mechanism that limits NET formation in sepsis. These findings implicate VitC as a previously unrecognized layer of regulation that prevents generation of excessive NETs.

Acknowledgments

This research was supported by grants from the Aubery Sage Mac Farlane Endowment for Acute Lung Injury Research, the AD Williams Research Foundation (NR), the Jeffress Memorial Trust (NR) and the Victoria Johnson Center for Lung Research.

Microscopy was performed at the VCU Department of Anatomy and Neurobiology Microscopy Facility, supported in part with funding from NIH-NINDS Center core grant (5P30NS047463).

References

1. Winterbourn, C.C.; Kettle, A.J. Redox reactions and microbial killing in the neutrophil phagosome. *Antioxid. Redox Signal.* **2013**, *18*, 642–660.
2. Borregaard, N. Neutrophils, from marrow to microbes. *Immunity* **2010**, *33*, 657–670.
3. Takei, H.; Araki, A.; Watanabe, H.; Ichinose, A.; Sendo, F. Rapid killing of human neutrophils by the potent activator phorbol 12-myristate 13-acetate (PMA) accompanied by changes different from typical apoptosis or necrosis. *J. Leukoc. Biol.* **1996**, *59*, 229–240.
4. Brinkmann, V.; Reichard, U.; Goosmann, C.; Fauler, B.; Uhlemann, Y.; Weiss, D.S.; Weinrauch, Y.; Zychlinsky, A. Neutrophil extracellular traps kill bacteria. *Science* **2004**, *303*, 1532–1535.
5. Narasaraju, T.; Yang, E.; Samy, R.P.; Ng, H.H.; Poh, W.P.; Liew, A.A.; Phoon, M.C.; van Rooijen, N.; Chow, V.T. Excessive neutrophils and neutrophil extracellular traps contribute to acute lung injury of influenza pneumonitis. *Am. J. Pathol.* **2011**, *179*, 199–210.
6. Grommes, J.; Soehnlein, O. Contribution of neutrophils to acute lung injury. *Mol. Med.* **2011**, *17*, 293–307.
7. Saffarzadeh, M.; Juenemann, C.; Queisser, M.A.; Lochnit, G.; Barreto, G.; Galuska, S.P.; Lohmeyer, J.; Preissner, K.T. Neutrophil extracellular traps directly induce epithelial and endothelial cell death: A predominant role of histones. *PLoS One* **2012**, *7*, e32366.
8. Douda D.N.; Jackson, R.; Grasemann, H.; Palaniyar, N. Innate immune collectin surfactant protein D simultaneously binds both neutrophil extracellular traps and carbohydrate ligands and promotes bacterial trapping. *J. Immunol.* **2011**, *187*, 1856–1865.
9. Gupta, A.K.; Hasler, P.; Holzgreve, W.; Gebhardt, S.; Hahn, S. Induction of neutrophil extracellular DNA lattices by placental microparticles and IL-8 and their presence in preeclampsia. *Hum. Immunol.* **2005**, *66*, 1146–1154.
10. Papayannopoulos, V.; Zychlinsky, A. NETs: A new strategy for using old weapons. *Trends Immunol.* **2009**, *30*, 513–521.
11. Dwivedi, D.J.; Toltl, L.J.; Swystun, L.J.; Pogue, J.; Liaw, K.L.; Weitz, J.I.; Cook, D.J.; Fox-Robichaud, A.E.; Liaw, P.C.; Canadian Critical Care Translational Biology Group. Prognostic utility and characterization of cell-free DNA in patients with severe sepsis. *Crit. Care* **2012**, *16*, R151.
12. Fisher, B.J.; Seropian, I.M.; Kraskauskas, D.; Thakkar, J.N.; Voelkel, N.F.; Fowler, A.A.; Natarajan, R. Ascorbic acid attenuates lipopolysaccharide-induced acute lung injury. *Crit. Care Med.* **2011**, *39*, 1454–1460.

13. Fisher, B.J.; Kraskauskas, D.; Martin, E.J.; Farkas, D.; Wegelin, J.A.; Brophy, D.; Ward, K.R.; Voelkel, N.F.; Fowler, A.A.; Natarajan, R. Mechanisms of attenuation of abdominal sepsis induced acute lung injury by ascorbic acid. *Am. J. Physiol. Lung Cell. Mol. Physiol.* **2012**, *303*, L20–L32.
14. Padayatty, S.J.; Katz, A.; Wang, Y.; Eck, P.; Kwon, O.; Lee, J.H.; Chen, S.; Corpe, C.; Dutta, A.; Dutta, S.K.; *et al.* Vitamin C as an antioxidant: evaluation of its role in disease prevention. *J. Am. Coll. Nutr.* **2003**, *22*, 18–35.
15. Vissers, M.C.; Wilkie, R.P. Ascorbate deficiency results in impaired neutrophil apoptosis and clearance and is associated with up-regulation of hypoxia-inducible factor 1α. *J. Leukoc. Biol.* **2007**, *81*, 1236–1244.
16. Nishikimi, M.; Fukuyama, R.; Minoshima, S.; Shimizu, N.; Yagi, K. Cloning and chromosomal mapping of the human nonfunctional gene for L-gulono-γ-lactone oxidase, the enzyme for L-ascorbic acid biosynthesis missing in man. *J. Biol. Chem.* **1994**, *269*, 13685–13688.
17. Remijsen, Q.; Vanden Berghe, T.; Wirawan, E.; Asselbergh, B.; Parthoens, E.; de Rycke, R.; Noppen, S.; Delforge, M.; Willems, J.; Vandenabeele, P. Neutrophil extracellular trap cell death requires both autophagy and superoxide generation. *Cell Res.* **2011**, *21*, 290–304.
18. Wang, Y.; Li, M.; Stadler, S.; Correll, S.; Li, P.; Wang, D.; Hayama, R.; Leonelli, L.; Han, H.; Grigoryev, S.A.; *et al.* Histone hypercitrullination mediates chromatin decondensation and neutrophil extracellular trap formation. *J. Cell Biol.* **2009**, *184*, 205–213.
19. Fisher, B.J.; Kraskauskas, D.; Martin, E.J.; Farkas, D.; Puri, P.; Massey, H.D.; Idowu, M.O.; Brophy, D.; Voelkel, N.F.; Fowler, A.A.; *et al.* Attenuation of sepsis induced organ injury by vitamin C. *J. Parenter. Enter. Nutr.* **2013**, in press.
20. Kim, H.; Bae, S.; Yu, Y.; Kim, Y.; Kim, H.R.; Hwang, Y.I.; Kang, J.S.; Lee, W.J. The analysis of vitamin C concentration in organs of gulo($^{-/-}$) mice upon vitamin C withdrawal. *Immune Netw.* **2012**, *12*, 18–26.
21. Vissers, M.C.; Bozonet, S.M.; Pearson, J.F.; Braithwaite, L.J. Dietary ascorbate intake affects steady state tissue concentrations in vitamin C-deficient mice: Tissue deficiency after suboptimal intake and superior bioavailability from a food source (kiwifruit). *Am. J. Clin. Nutr.* **2011**, *93*, 292–301.
22. Tsurubuchi, T.; Aratani, Y.; Maeda, N.; Koyama, H. Retardation of early-onset PMA-induced apoptosis in mouse neutrophils deficient in myeloperoxidase. *J. Leukoc. Biol.* **2001**, *70*, 52–58.
23. Fowler, A.A.; Fisher, B.J.; Centor, R.M.; Carchman R.A. Development of the adult respiratory distress syndrome: Progressive alteration of neutrophil chemotactic and secretory processes. *Am. J. Pathol.* **1984**, *116*, 427–435.
24. Meng, W.; Paunel-Görgülü, A.; Flohé, S.; Witte, I.; Schädel-Höpfner, M.; Windolf, J.; Lögters T.T. Deoxyribonuclease is a potential counter regulator of aberrant neutrophil extracellular traps formation after major trauma. *Mediat. Inflamm.* **2012**, *2012*, doi:10.1155/2012/149560.
25. Fuchs, T.A.; Abed, U.; Goosmann, C.; Hurwitz, R.; Schulze, I.; Wahn, V.; Weinrauch, Y.; Brinkmann, V.; Zychlinsky, A. Novel cell death program leads to neutrophil extracellular traps. *J. Cell Biol.* **2007**, *176*, 231–241.

26. Asaga, H.; Nakashima, K.; Senshu, T.; Ishigami, A.; Yamada, M. Immunocytochemical localization of peptidylargininedeiminase in human eosinophils and neutrophils. *J. Leukoc. Biol.* **2001**, *70*, 46–51.
27. Mastronardi, F.G.; Wood, D.D.; Mei, J.; Raijmakers, R.; Tseveleki, V.; Dosch, H.M.; Probert, L.; Casaccia-Bonnefil, P.; Moscarello, M.A. Increased citrullination of histone H3 in multiple sclerosis brain and animal models of demyelination: A role for tumor necrosis factor-induced peptidylargininedeiminase 4 translocation. *J. Neurosci.* **2006**, *26*, 11387–11396.
28. Cheng, O.Z.; Palaniyar, N. NET balancing: A problem in inflammatory lung diseases. *Front. Immunol.* **2013**, *4*, 1–13.
29. Klionsky, D.J.; Abeliovich, H.; Agostinis, P.; Agrawal, D.K.; Aliev, G.; Askew, D.S.; Baba, M.; Baehrecke, E.H.; Bahr, B.A.; Ballabio, A.; *et al.* Guidelines for the use and interpretation of assays for monitoring autophagy in higher eukaryotes. *Autophagy* **2008**, *4*, 151–175.
30. Bjorkoy, G.; Lamark, T.; Pankiv, S.; Overvatn, A.; Brech, A.; Johansen, T. Monitoring autophagic degradation of p62/SQSTM1. *Methods Enzymol.* **2009**, *452*, 181–197.
31. Deegan, S.; Saveljeva, S.; Gorman, A.M.; Samali, A. Stress-induced self-cannibalism: On the regulation of autophagy by endoplasmic reticulum stress. *Cell. Mol. Life Sci.* **2013**, *70*, 2425–2441.
32. Yang, K.Y.; Arcaroli, J.J.; Abraham, E. Early alterations in neutrophil activation are associated with outcome in acute lung injury. *Am. J. Respir. Crit. Care Med.* **2003**, *167*, 1567–1574.
33. Clarke, R.; Cook, K.L.; Hu, R.; Facey, C.O.; Tavassoly, I.; Schwartz, J.L.; Baumann, W.T.; Tyson, J.J.; Xuan, J.; Wang, Y.; *et al.* Endoplasmic reticulum stress, the unfolded protein response, autophagy, and the integrated regulation of breast cancer cell fate. *Cancer Res.* **2012**, *72*, 1321–1331.
34. Ying, S.; Kojima, T.; Kawada, A.; Nachat, R.; Serre, G.; Simon, M.; Takahara, H. An intronic enhancer driven by NF-κB contributes to transcriptional regulation of peptidylargininedeiminase type I gene in human keratinocytes. *J. Investig. Dermatol.* **2010**, *130*, 2543–2552.
35. Cárcamo, J.M.; Pedraza, A.; Bórquez-Ojeda, O.; Golde, D.W. Vitamin C suppresses TNFα-induced NFκB activation by inhibiting IκBα phosphorylation. *Biochemistry* **2002**, *41*, 12995–13002.
36. Klionsky, D.J.; Emr, S.D. Autophagy as a regulated pathway of cellular degradation. *Science* **2000**, *290*, 1717–1721.
37. Beertsen, W.; Willenborg, M.; Everts, V.; Zirogianni, A.; Podschun, R.; Schröder, B.; Eskelinen, E.L.; Saftig, P. Impaired phagosomal maturation in neutrophils leads to periodontitis in lysosomal-associated membrane protein-2 knockout mice. *J. Immunol.* **2008**, *180*, 475–482.
38. Huang, J.; Canadien, V.; Lam, G.Y.; Steinberg, B.E.; Dinauer, M.C.; Magalhaes, M.A.; Glogauer, M.; Grinstein, S.; Brumell, J.H. Activation of antibacterial autophagy by NADPH oxidases. *Proc. Natl. Acad. Sci. USA* **2009**, *106*, 6226–6231.
39. Mitroulis, I.; Kourtzelis, I.; Kambas, K.; Rafail, S.; Chrysanthopoulou, A.; Speletas, M.; Ritis, K. Regulation of the autophagic machinery in human neutrophils. *Eur. J. Immunol.* **2010**, *40*, 1461–1472.

40. Pankiv, S.; Clausen, T.H.; Lamark, T.; Brech, A.; Bruun, J.A.; Outzen, H.; Overvatn, A.; Bjorkoy, G.; Johansen, T. P62/SQSTM1 binds directly to Atg8/LC3 to facilitate degradation of ubiquitinated protein aggregates by autophagy. *J. Biol. Chem.* **2007**, *282*, 24131–24145.
41. Patel, A.S.; Morse, D.; Choi, A.M. Regulation and functional significance of autophagy in respiratory cell biology and disease. *Am. J. Respir. Cell Mol. Biol.* **2013**, *48*, 1–9.
42. Rouschop, K.M.; van den Beucken, T.; Dubois, L.; Niessen, H.; Bussink, J.; Savelkouls, K.; Keulers, T.; Mujcic, H.; Landuyt, W.; Voncken, J.W.; *et al.* The unfolded protein response protects human tumor cells during hypoxia through regulation of the autophagy genes MAP1LC3B and ATG5. *J. Clin. Investig.* **2012**, *120*, 127–141.
43. Moine, P.; McIntyre, R.; Schwartz, M.D.; Kaneko, D.; Shenkar, R.; Le Tulzo, Y.; Moore, E.E.; Abraham, E. NF-κB regulatory mechanisms in alveolar macrophages from patients with acute respiratory distress syndrome. *Shock* **2000**, *13*, 85–91.
44. Burstein, E.; Duckett, C.S. Dying for NF-κB? Control of cell death by transcriptional regulation of the apoptotic machinery. *Curr. Opin. Cell Biol.* **2003**, *15*, 732–737.
45. Caudrillier, A.; Kessenbrock, K.; Gilliss, B.M.; Nguyen, J.X.; Marques, M.B.; Monestier, M.; Toy, P.; Werb, Z.; Looney, M.R. Platelets induce neutrophil extracellular traps in transfusion-related acute lung injury. *J. Clin. Investig.* **2012**, *122*, 2661–2671.
46. Thomas, G.M.; Carbo, C.; Curtis, B.R.; Martinod, K.; Mazo, I.B.; Schatzberg, D.; Cifuni, S.M.; Fuchs, T.A.; von Andrian, U.H.; Hartwig, J.H.; *et al.* Extracellular DNA traps are associated with the pathogenesis of TRALI in humans and mice. *Blood* **2012**, *119*, 6335–6343.
47. Drifte, G.; Dunn-Siegrist, I.; Tissières, P.; Pugin, J. Innate immune functions of immature neutrophils in patients with sepsis and severe systemic inflammatory response syndrome. *Crit. Care Med.* **2013**, *41*, 820–832.
48. Rhodes, A.; Wort, S.J.; Thomas, H.; Collinson, P.; Bennett, E.D. Plasma DNA concentration as a predictor of mortality and sepsis in critically ill patients. *Crit. Care* **2006**, *10*, R60.
49. Saukkonen, K.; Lakkisto, P.; Pettila, V.; Varpula, M.; Karlsson, S.; Ruokonen, E.; Pulkki, K. Cell-free plasma DNA as a predictor of outcome in severe sepsis and septic shock. *Clin. Chem.* **2008**, *54*, 1000–1007.
50. Guimarães-Costa, A.B.; Nascimento, M.T.; Wardini, A.B.; Pinto-da-Silva, L.H.; Saraiva, E.M. ETosis: A Microbicidal Mechanism beyond Cell Death. *J. Parasitol. Res.* **2012**, *2012*, 929743.

9

Vitamin C in Cultured Human (HeLa) Cells: Lack of Effect on DNA Protection and Repair

Amaya Azqueta [1,2,*], Solange Costa [2,3], Yolanda Lorenzo [2], Nasser E. Bastani [2] and Andrew R. Collins [2]

[1] Department of Pharmacology and Toxicology, University of Navarra, C/Irunlarrea 1, 31009 Pamplona, Spain

[2] Department of Nutrition, Institute of Basic Medical Sciences, University of Oslo, PB 1046 Blindern, 0316 Oslo, Norway; E-Mails: solange.costa2@gmail.com (S.C.); y.c.lorenzo@medisin.uio.no (Y.L.); n.e.bastani@medisin.uio.no (N.E.B.); a.r.collins@medisin.uio.no (A.R.C.)

[3] Environmental Health Department, National Institute of Health, Rua Alexandre Herculano 321, 4000-055 Porto, Portugal

* Author to whom correspondence should be addressed; E-Mail: amazqueta@unav.es;

Abstract: Aims: Dietary antioxidants, including vitamin C, may be in part responsible for the cancer-preventive effects of fruits and vegetables. Human intervention trials with clinical endpoints have failed to confirm their protective effects, and mechanistic studies have given inconsistent results. Our aim was to investigate antioxidant/pro-oxidant effects of vitamin C at the cellular level. Experimental approach: We have used the comet assay to investigate effects of vitamin C on DNA damage, antioxidant status, and DNA repair, in HeLa (human tumor) cells, and HPLC to measure uptake of vitamin C into cells. Results: Even at concentrations in the medium as high as 200 μM, vitamin C did not increase the background level of strand breaks or of oxidized purines in nuclear DNA. Vitamin C is taken up by HeLa cells and accumulates to mM levels. Preincubation of cells with vitamin C did not render them resistant to strand breakage induced by H_2O_2 or to purine oxidation by photosensitizer plus light. Vitamin C had no effect on the rate of repair of strand breaks or oxidized bases by HeLa cells. However, vitamin C at a concentration of less than 1 μM, or extract from cells preincubated for 6 h with vitamin C, was able to induce damage (strand breaks) in lysed, histone-depleted nuclei (nucleoids). Conclusion: In these cultured human cells, vitamin C displays neither antioxidant nor pro-oxidant properties; nor does it affect DNA strand break or base excision repair.

Keywords: DNA damage; DNA protection; DNA repair; vitamin C

---

1. Introduction

Vitamin C (ascorbic acid) is one of the best known and most studied dietary antioxidants. Its antioxidant credentials are well-established *in vitro*, since it can readily be demonstrated to prevent oxidation of lipids, DNA and other biological molecules. However, it is also possible for vitamin C to act as a pro-oxidant, through its ability to reduce transition metal ions, thus promoting the Fenton reaction which, acting on peroxides, produces highly reactive hydroxyl radicals [1]. The effect of vitamin C *in vivo* has been investigated in human trials with DNA oxidation as the measured endpoint. They include single dose intervention and longer trials, typically of a few weeks with daily supplementation. The first single-dose study was carried out by Green *et al.* [2], who administered 35 mg/kg of vitamin C to six healthy volunteers after an overnight fast and found a protection against γ radiation-induced DNA breaks in white blood cells, using the comet assay (described below). Since then, more than 20 intervention studies with vitamin C have been carried out, and they have been critically reviewed by Duarte and Lunec [3] who find that most of the studies show either a decrease in DNA oxidation or no effect, while there are some that show an increase in DNA lesions. Møller and Loft [4] also describe conflicting results with vitamin C, concluding that more studies with better designs to avoid bias should be made in order to understand the role of vitamin C in protecting against DNA oxidation. In a subsequent supplementation trial, Møller *et al.* [5] found that a slow release formulation of vitamin C had a more pronounced and sustained protective effect on the steady state level of DNA base oxidation than did a normal release formulation.

Herbert *et al.* [6] carried out a double-blind placebo-controlled trial giving different doses of vitamin C (0, 80, 200 and 400 mg/day) to four groups of 40 healthy volunteers over a period of 15 weeks (plus a 10 week washout period). They showed that vitamin C did not affect the intracellular level of 8-oxodGuo measured by HPLC. (This challenged an earlier report that vitamin C caused oxidation of bases in DNA [7]).

Sram *et al.* [8] recently reviewed human studies based on measurement of a variety of biomarkers of genetic damage—including some trials aimed at specific groups with occupational/environmental exposure to genotoxins. Generally either a protective effect or no effect was seen, depending—they suggest—on factors such as individual diet-derived vitamin C concentrations, levels of exposure to xenobiotics, and oxidative stress.

Bjelakovic *et al.* [9] published a meta-analysis of randomized trials of antioxidant supplements aimed at primary and secondary prevention of various diseases, with mortality as the endpoint. They concluded that antioxidant supplements have no beneficial effects on mortality, though in the case of vitamin C the number of individuals sampled is still relatively small and a definitive statement cannot be made.

Reviews of this subject conclude that we still need more studies to clarify the effect of vitamin C in humans [1,8–10]. We considered that it would be useful to investigate effects of vitamin C on genetic stability in cell culture, and so have examined, in the human tumor cell line HeLa, potential pro-oxidant, DNA-damaging effects of the vitamin; protection against DNA breakage caused by H_2O_2; and protection against base oxidation induced by photosensitizer plus visible light. In addition, we investigate the possibility that vitamin C might influence the capacity of cells for DNA repair.

We applied the comet assay, as used in many human biomonitoring studies, to the measurement of DNA damage, both strand breaks (SBs) and oxidized bases (employing the enzyme formamidopyrimidine DNA glycosylase (FPG) which converts 8-oxoGua and breakdown products of damaged purines to SBs). We used two approaches to measure repair of DNA damage [11]. If cells are subjected to damage (SBs or base oxidation), and then incubated to allow cellular repair, the residual lesions can be measured at intervals to show the kinetics of damage removal. Alternatively, in an *in vitro* assay, a cell extract is incubated with substrate DNA containing specific damage. The ability of the extract to introduce DNA breaks in the substrate cells reflects the activity of the enzymes responsible for the initial steps of repair, *i.e.*, removing the lesion.

2. Materials and Methods

2.1. Cell Culture

HeLa cells (derived from human cervical cancer) were grown in DMEM supplemented with 10% fetal bovine serum and antibiotics (100 U/mL penicillin and 100 μg/mL streptomycin). According to the formulation for DMEM it does not contain vitamin C. Vitamin C was not detectable in the batch of serum used. Cells were maintained as monolayer cultures at 37 °C in a humidified atmosphere with 5% CO_2 and routinely passaged by trypsinization when nearly confluent.

2.2. Cell Treatment for DNA Damage and Protection

HeLa cells in culture medium were incubated with 0, 5, 25, 50, 100 or 200 μM vitamin C (ascorbic acid) for 30 min or 6 h (3 h incubation, followed by a wash with PBS and a further 3 h incubation with vitamin C at the same concentration) at 37 °C in the dark. The two consecutive 3 h treatments were designed to allow for the possible instability of vitamin C in solution. Vitamin C was dissolved in PBS in the dark just before use in each experiment. After treatment the comet assay was performed as described below. To check for DNA protection, after vitamin C treatment, cells were washed with PBS and then treated on ice with 25 μM H_2O_2 for 5 min to induce SBs, or with 1 μM of the photosensitizer Ro (Ro-19-8022, from F. Hoffmann-La Roche) plus 1.5 min visible light (500 W tungsten halogen lamp, at 33 cm on ice) to induce oxidized purines, mostly 8-oxoGua. After treatment the comet assay was performed (see below). Three independent experiments were carried out.

2.3. Measuring Uptake of Vitamin C

Near-confluent cultures of HeLa cells in 60 mm dishes were incubated for 6 h (3 h + wash + 3 h, as above) with vitamin C at 50 or 200 μM. At the end of this incubation, or after a further 24 h incubation in fresh medium without vitamin C, cells were washed with PBS and scraped with a silicone rubber scraper into suspension in PBS. A cell count was carried out. The suspension was centrifuged (400× *g*, 5 min) and the pellet resuspended in 250 μL of PBS to which an equal volume of 10% metaphosphoric acid was added before storing at −20 °C.

The frozen, acidified samples were thawed, and centrifuged (3500× *g* at 4 °C for 10 min). A volume of 100 μL clear supernatant was mixed with 400 μL of the mobile phase (2% acetonitrile in 2.5 mM NaH_2PO_4, 2.5 mM dodecyltrimethyl ammonium chloride and 1.25 mM Na_2EDTA in Milli-Q water) for direct determination of vitamin C by high-performance liquid chromatography (HPLC). For separation of vitamin C from interfering sample constituents, a Chromolith Performance RP18-e, 4.6 mm × 100 mm column was used, with a Chromolith Performance RP18-e, 4.6 mm × 10 mm guard column (Phenomenex, Torrance, USA). The injection volume was 5 μL and the flow rate was 6.0 mL/min. A variable wavelength ultraviolet (UV) detector was used at 264 nm.

2.4. Treatment of Cells for Cellular Repair Assay

Repair of DNA damage can be studied by treating cells with a DNA-damaging agent, incubating, and measuring the damage remaining at intervals. Using this cellular repair assay we investigated the kinetics of DNA SB rejoining and base excision repair (BER). To check the influence of vitamin C on the repair of SBs, HeLa cells were pre-incubated with 0, 50 or 100 μM vitamin C overnight. Then cells were washed with PBS, treated with 0 or 100 μM H_2O_2 for 5 min on ice, and incubated for 10, 30 or 60 min in culture medium. To check the influence of vitamin C on the repair of oxidized bases, pre-incubation overnight with 0, 50 or 100 μM vitamin C was followed by a wash with PBS, treatment with 0 or 1 μM Ro plus 5 min of light, and incubation for 1, 2, 4, 6, 8, or 24 h in culture medium. In another experimental design, HeLa cells in culture medium were pre-incubated with a higher concentration (200 μM) of vitamin C but for only 30 min. Then cells were washed with PBS, treated with 1 μM Ro plus 2.5 min of light, and incubated for 3 h in culture medium including 0 or 200 μM vitamin C. They were then washed with PBS and incubated again in culture medium with the same concentration of vitamin C for a further 3 h. The comet assay was performed after each time of incubation. The concentration of vitamin C used in these experiments was not genotoxic. Three independent experiments were performed.

2.5. Comet Assay

Just after treatment (or after incubation for repair), HeLa cells were trypsinized and resupended in PBS (1×10^6 cells/mL). Thirty μL of each cell suspension were mixed with 140 μL of 1% low melting point agarose, and two drops of 70 μL were spread onto microscope slides precoated with 1% of normal melting point agarose. Glass cover slips were placed on the drops of agarose, which were allowed to set at 4 °C. Then the cover slips were removed and the cells embedded in agarose were lysed for 1 h by immersion in 2.5 M NaCl, 0.1 M Na_2EDTA, 0.1 M Tris base, pH 10 and 1% Triton X-100 at 4 °C (lysis solution). For measurement of SBs, the slides were then placed in a horizontal gel electrophoresis tank and the DNA was allowed to unwind for 40 min in freshly prepared alkaline electrophoresis solution (0.3 M NaOH and 1 mM Na_2EDTA, pH > 13).

For measurement of oxidized purines, after lysis, slides were washed three times (5 min each time) with buffer F (0.1 M KCl, 0.5 mM Na_2EDTA, 40 mM HEPES, 0.2 mg/mL BSA, pH 8.0) and incubated for 30 min at 37 °C with FPG in buffer F, or with buffer F alone, in a moist box. After incubation the slides were placed in the electrophoresis solution.

Electrophoresis was carried out in the alkaline solution for 30 min at 1.1 V/cm and approximately 300 mA at 4 °C. The slides were washed in 0.4 M Tris base (pH 7.5) for 10 min at 4 °C to neutralize the excess alkali and 10 min in water at 4 °C. Then they were left to dry overnight.

Gels were stained with 25 µL of DAPI (4′,6-diamidine-2-phenylindol dihydrochloride, 1 µg/mL), covered with a cover slip and coded before microscopic analysis. DAPI-stained nuclei were evaluated with a Nikon Eclipse TS-100 fluorescence microscope. A total of 50 comets on each gel were visually scored as belonging to one of five classes according to the tail intensity. Each comet class was given a value between 0 and 4: (0) = undamaged and (4) = maximum damage [12]. The total score in arbitrary units (AU) was calculated by the following equation:

$$(\text{percentage of cells in class } 0 \times 0) + (\text{percentage of cells in class } 1 \times 1) + (\text{percentage of cells in class } 2 \times 2) + (\text{percentage of cells in class } 3 \times 3) + (\text{percentage of cells in class } 4 \times 4).$$

Consequently, the total score was in the range from 0 to 400 arbitrary units. Net H_2O_2-induced damage was calculated by subtracting the comet score for non-H_2O_2-treated cells from the score + H_2O_2. Net FPG-sensitive sites were calculated by subtracting the score for the slide incubated with buffer from the score for the slide incubated with enzyme. Net Ro-induced damage was calculated as the difference in net FPG-sensitive sites between Ro-treated cells and cells not treated with Ro.

2.6. In Vitro *Assay for DNA Repair*

The *in vitro* repair assay is used to check the ability of cell extracts to carry out the first steps of BER. Gel-embedded nucleoids from HeLa cells carrying oxidized bases (substrate) were incubated with extracts from HeLa cells pre-incubated with/without vitamin C and with different concentrations of vitamin C directly.

2.6.1. Preparation of Substrate Cells

HeLa cells were grown to 80% confluence, washed with PBS and treated with 1 µM Ro plus 4 min of light. Then they were washed with cold PBS, detached by trypsinization, centrifuged for 5 min at 800× *g* at 4 °C and resuspended in freezing medium (DMEM supplemented with 20% fetal bovine serum, and 10% DMSO) at a concentration of 1×10^6 cells per mL. Aliquots of 0.7 mL were frozen slowly and stored at −80 °C.

2.6.2. Preparation of Cell Extracts

Extracts were prepared from HeLa cells incubated with 0, 50, 100 or 200 µM vitamin C for 6 h (3 h + wash + 3 h). They were washed with cold PBS, trypsinized, centrifuged at 800× *g* for 5 min at 4 °C and resuspended in cold PBS at a concentration of 1.25×10^6 cells per mL. Then the cell suspension was split into aliquots of 1 mL and centrifuged at 14,000× *g* for 5 min at 4 °C. The supernatant of each aliquot was completely discarded and the dry pellets were frozen in liquid nitrogen and stored at −80 °C. After thawing the pellets were resuspended in 32 μL of extraction buffer A (45 mM HEPES, 0.4 M KCl, 1 mM EDTA, 0.1 mM dithiothreitol and 10% glycerol, pH 7.8) containing 0.25% of Triton X-100, mixed using vortex at high speed for 5–10 s, incubated for 5 min on ice and centrifuged at 14,000× *g* for 5 min at 4 °C. Then 27 μL of the supernatant was mixed with 110 μL of cold reaction buffer F.

2.6.3. The Reaction

The substrate cells were thawed, diluted in cold PBS, centrifuged at 800× *g* for 5 min at 4 °C and resuspended in PBS at a concentration of 1×10^6 cells per mL. As described in section 2.4 gels were made, put in lysis for 1 h and washed 3 times (5 min each time) with buffer F. Then 30 μL of extract (experimental treatment), FPG (positive control), or buffer F (negative control) were placed on each gel (two gels per condition) and covered with a cover slip. Slides were placed in a moist box and incubated for 10 and 20 min. Afterwards the rest of the comet assay was performed as described above.

2.6.4. Treatment of Nucleoids with Vitamin C

In order to check the direct effect of vitamin C on DNA, non-damaged HeLa cell nucleoids, or substrate nucleoids prepared as described in Section 2.6.1, were treated for 10 or 20 min with vitamin C dissolved in buffer A at 0, 1, 5 or 25 μM and diluted with buffer F, as described in Section 2.6.2. The reaction was carried out as described in Section 2.6.3. The final concentrations of vitamin C were therefore 0, 0.25, 1.25, and 6.25 μM.

2.7. Statistical Analysis

The statistical analysis was performed by using the software SPSS 11.0. Data are presented with descriptive analysis (mean ± SD for 3 independent experiments). The comparisons between total comet scores of the different groups were performed by the non-parametric Kruskal-Wallis test followed by Mann-Whitney U test when the first one showed the presence of differences. Probability $p \leq 0.05$ was accepted as the level of significance.

3. Results

3.1. Direct Induction of DNA Damage

We evaluated DNA damage, *i.e.*, SBs and oxidized bases, just after incubating HeLa cells with different concentrations of vitamin C for 30 min or 6 h, using the comet assay with and without FPG. Treatment with different concentrations of vitamin C (5–200 μM) did not cause or decrease SBs or base oxidation in HeLa cells (Figure 1A,B).

Figure 1. Effect of different concentrations of vitamin C on DNA integrity (SBs and net formamidopyrimidine DNA glycosylase (FPG)-sensitive sites) of HeLa cells treated for 30 min (**A**) and 6 h (**B**) and measured using the comet assay. Bars: SD calculated from the results of 3 independent experiments. No significant effects were seen.

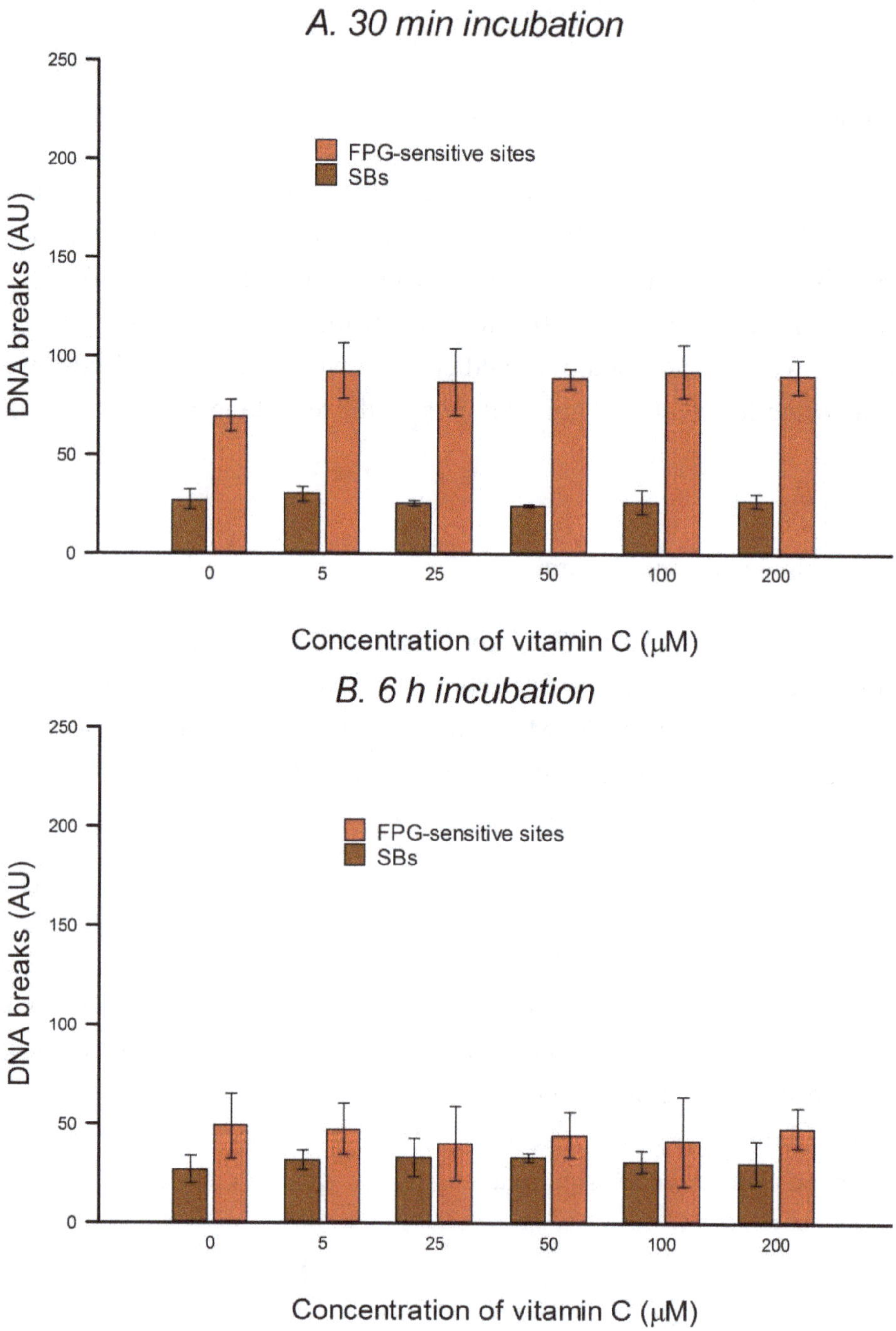

3.2. Protection against H_2O_2- and Ro-Induced DNA Damage

Using the comet assay we investigated the possible protective effect of vitamin C against DNA damage caused by H_2O_2 or Ro plus light after pre-incubating HeLa cells with vitamin C (5–200 μM) for 30 min or 6 h. In HeLa cells the yield of damage, net H_2O_2-induced breaks or net Ro-induced FPG-sensitive sites, was unchanged by the vitamin C incubation (Figures 2A,B and 3A,B).

Figure 2. Effect of pre-incubation of HeLa cells with different concentrations of vitamin C for 30 min (**A**) or 6 h (**B**) on damage induced by H_2O_2. Net H_2O_2-induced damage was calculated by subtracting comet score without H_2O_2 (as in Figure 1) from the total comet score with H_2O_2. Bars: SD calculated from the results of 3 independent experiments. No significant effects were seen.

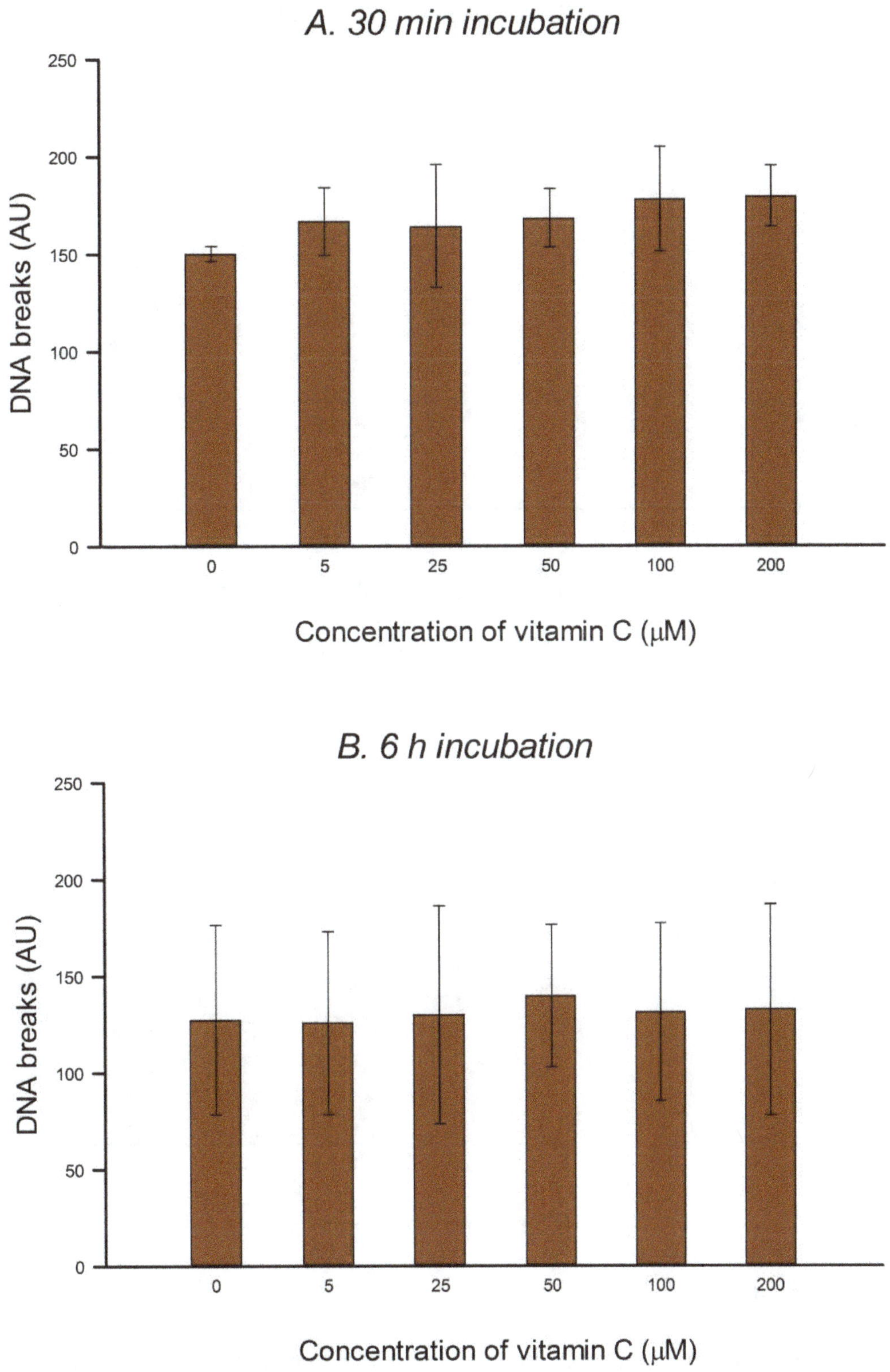

Figure 3. Effect of pre-incubation of HeLa cells with different concentrations of vitamin C for 30 min (**A**) or 6 h (**B**) on FPG-sensitive sites induced by Ro plus light. Net Ro-induced damage was calculated by subtracting the FPG-sensitive sites without Ro plus light (as in Figure 1) from the FPG-sensitive sites with Ro plus light. Bars: SD calculated from the results of 3 independent experiments. No significant effects were seen.

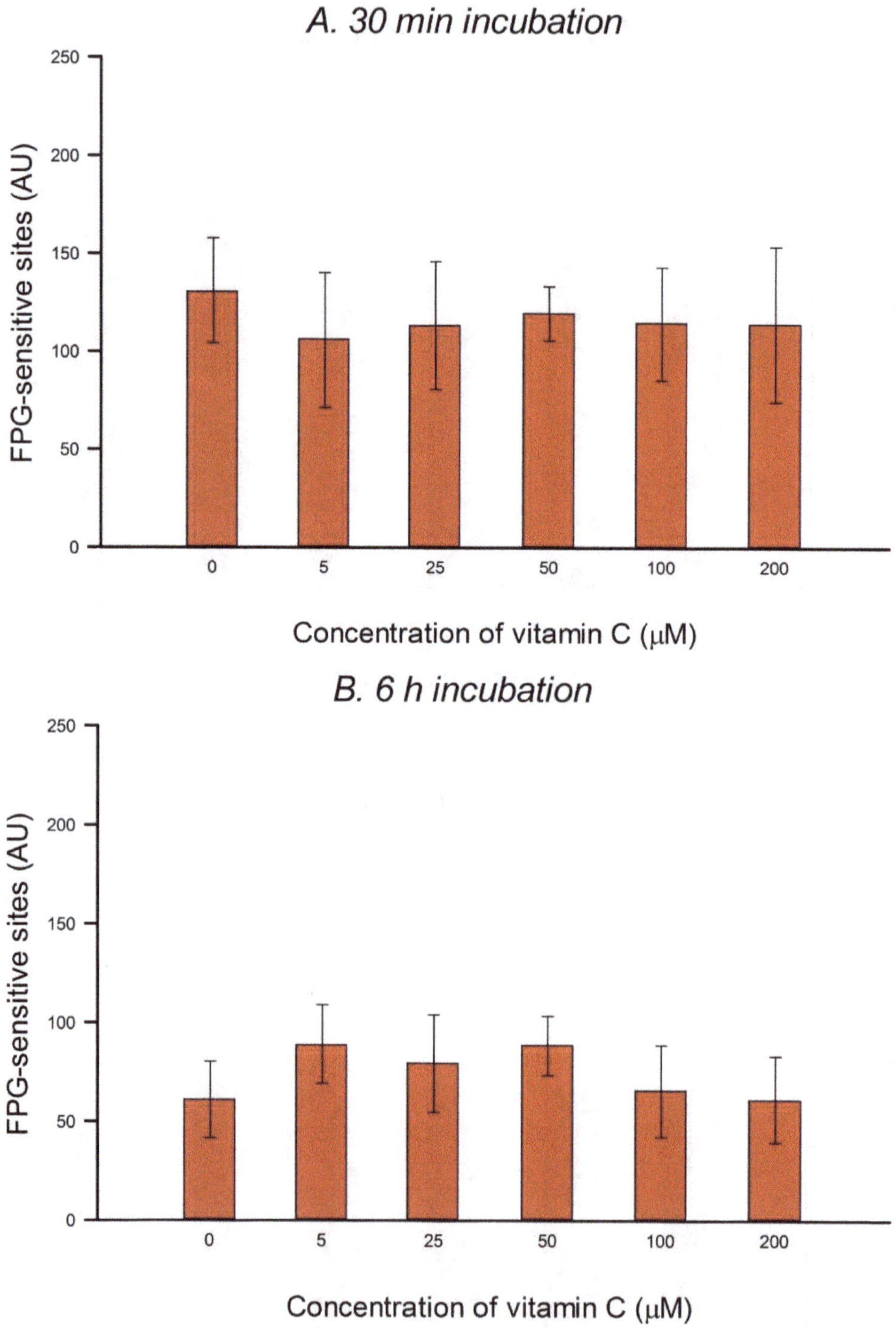

3.3. Cellular Repair of SBs

We studied the effect of vitamin C on the kinetics of repair of SBs induced by H_2O_2 after pre-incubating HeLa cells with different concentrations of vitamin C overnight. After H_2O_2

treatment cells were incubated and SBs remaining were measured at intervals. As is seen in Figure 4, rejoining of SBs is rapid, with a $t_{1/2}$ of about 20 min and complete repair by 60 min. Pre-incubation of cells with 50 or 100 μM vitamin C overnight did not affect the repair of the SBs induced by H_2O_2.

Figure 4. Effect of overnight pre-incubation of HeLa cells with different concentrations of vitamin C on the kinetics of repair of SBs: residual SBs were measured after different times of incubation after H_2O_2 treatment. C-: control cells without any kind of treatment. Bars: SD calculated from the results of 3 independent experiments. No significant effects were seen.

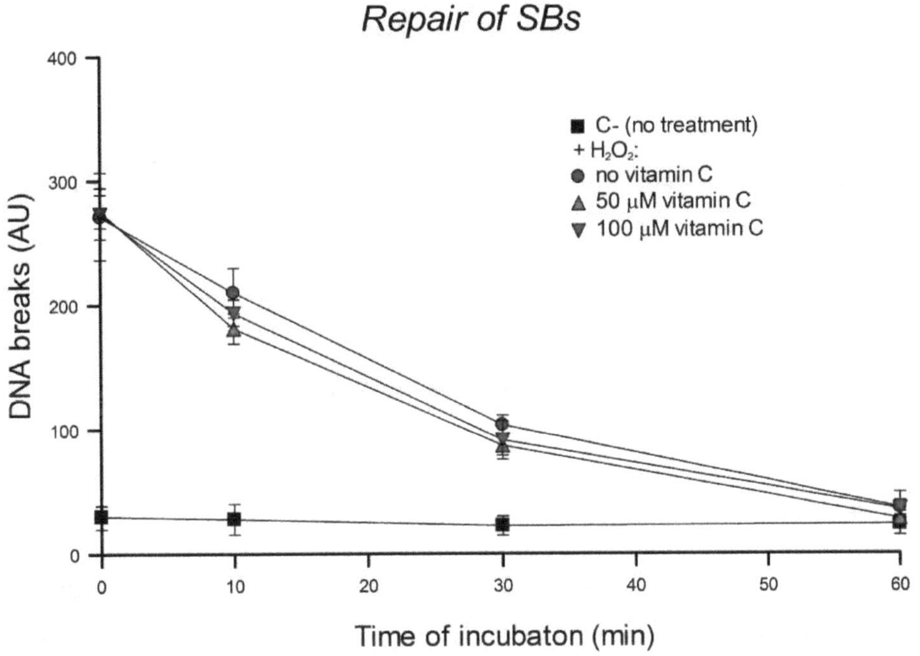

3.4. Cellular Repair of Oxidized Purines

We next investigated the effect of vitamin C on the kinetics of BER after pre-incubating HeLa cells with different concentrations of vitamin C overnight. We induced oxidized purines, mostly 8-oxoGua, using Ro plus light. The comet assay was performed after different times of incubation of the treated cells up to 6 h. The pre-incubation of cells with 50 or 100 μM vitamin C overnight did not affect the removal of the FPG-sensitive sites induced by Ro plus light (data not shown). We modified the protocol by pre-incubating HeLa cells with 200 μM of vitamin C for 30 min, and adding the same concentration of vitamin C also during the 6 h incubation period after inducing the damage. Figure 5 shows that the repair of oxidized bases is much slower than SB rejoining, and the presence of vitamin C during the incubation period after damaging the cells still did not influence the repair of the FPG-sensitive sites induced by Ro plus light.

Figure 5. Effect of incubation of HeLa cells with 200 μM of vitamin C before and during the repair of oxidized bases induced by Ro plus light; residual FPG-sensitive sites were measured at different time points. Bars: SD calculated from the results of 3 independent experiments. No significant effects were seen.

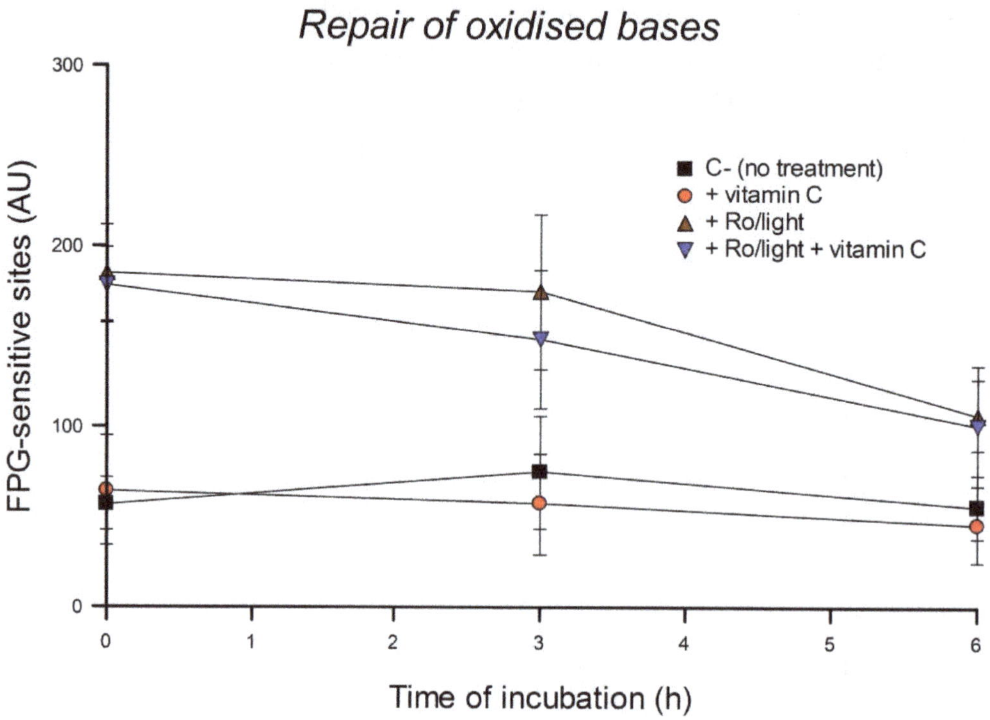

3.5. In Vitro *Repair Assay*

As a final check as to whether vitamin C has any effect on DNA repair activity we used an *in vitro* approach, measuring the ability of extracts of vitamin C-preincubated cells to recognize and incise oxidized bases in substrate nucleoids. HeLa cells were treated with 200 μM vitamin C for 6 h. Extracts were prepared and incubated for 10 or 20 min with gel-embedded HeLa nucleoid DNA containing oxidized purines. (Previous experiments [13] have shown no significant breaks induced in undamaged substrate.) Then the comet assay was performed to measure the breaks induced by the extracts, as an indicator of repair activity. Extracts from HeLa cells preincubated with 200 μM vitamin C produced a significant increase in SBs in substrate nucleoids (compared with extracts from non-vitamin C-treated cells) at both reaction incubation times (Figure 6A). Lower concentrations of vitamin C (50 or 100 μM) did not have any effect. However, when we checked the possibility that vitamin C was having a direct effect on the DNA, we found that breaks were in fact induced in HeLa nucleoid DNA containing oxidized purines or in undamaged DNA (Figure 6B,C). A significant effect is seen at a concentration as low as 1 μM. This concentration relates to the concentration as prepared in buffer A, before 5× dilution with buffer F. Therefore the concentration capable of damaging DNA is actually as low as 0.2 μM.

Figure 6. (**A**) Effect of extracts from HeLa cells pre-treated with 0 and 200 μM of vitamin C for 6 h on a DNA substrate containing oxidized purines. (**B**) Effect of different concentrations of vitamin C on a DNA substrate containing oxidized purines. (**C**) Effect of different concentrations of vitamin C on a non-damaged DNA substrate. In (**A**), Buffer F was used as a negative control. In (**A**) and (**B**), where nucleoids contained oxidized bases, FPG was employed as a positive control. Concentrations of vitamin C displayed in the box on panels (**B**) and (**C**) refer to concentrations in buffer A: final concentrations were 4× less. Bars: SD calculated from the results of 3 independent experiments. Statistical comparisons (* $p < 0.05$): vitamin C (different concentrations) *vs.* 0 μM.

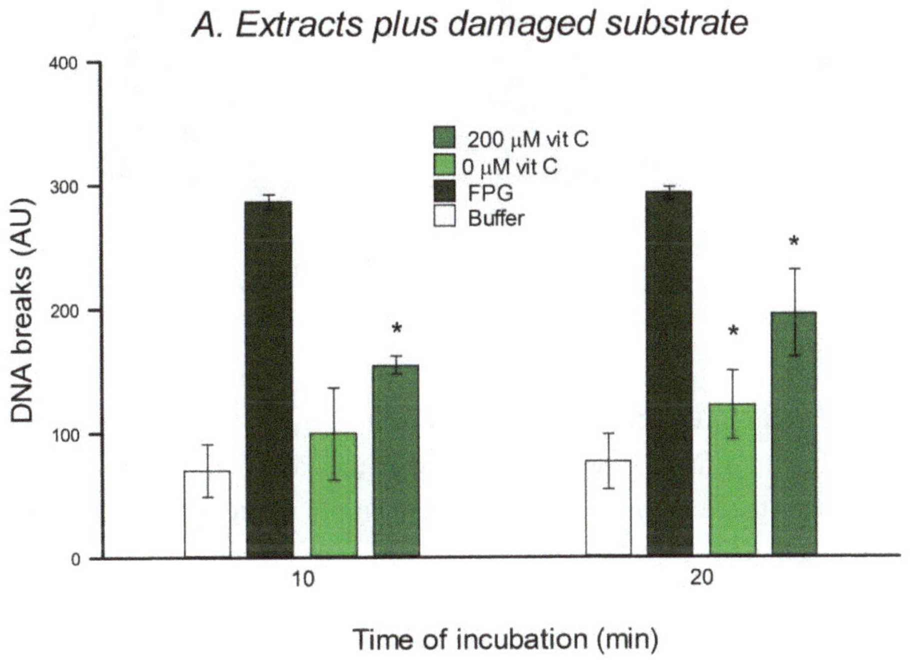

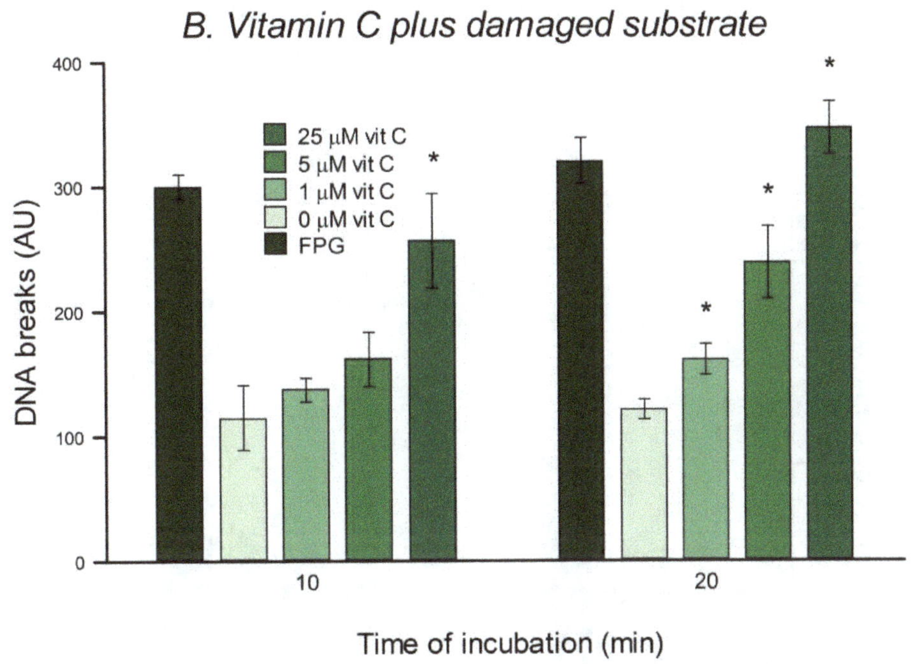

Figure 6. *Cont.*

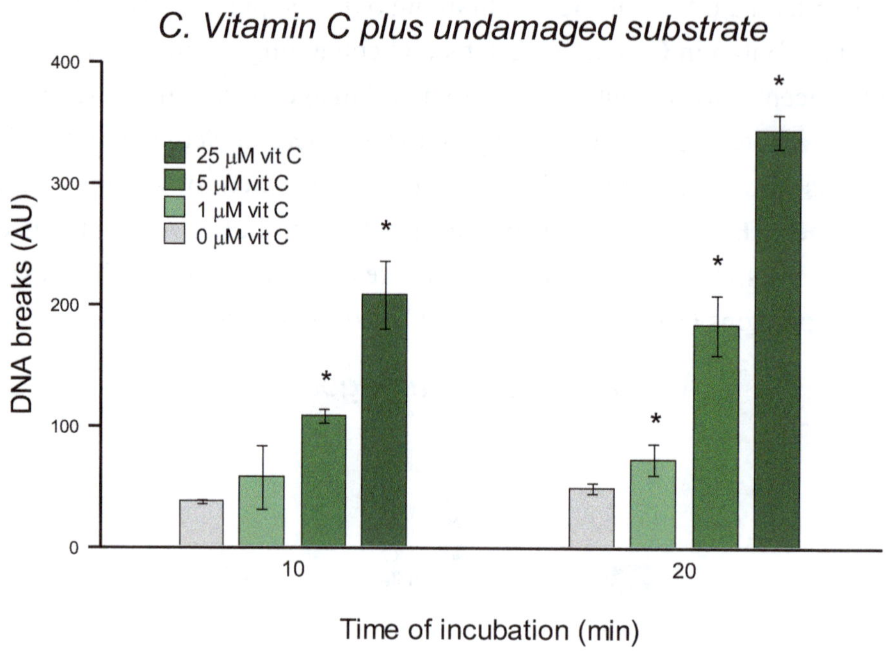

3.6. Uptake of Vitamin C

Concentrations of vitamin C measured in cell pellets after 6 h or 24 h incubation are shown in Figure 7. The concentration within the cells is estimated on the basis of a volume of 5 µL per 10^6 cells. It is clear that vitamin C is taken up by HeLa cells and accumulates to a concentration far higher than that provided in the medium.

Figure 7. Uptake of vitamin C by HeLa cells. Cells were incubated for 6 h in medium containing vitamin C at 50 µM (light shading) or 200 µM (dark shading). Intracellular vitamin C was measured by HPLC at the end of this incubation or after a further 24 h incubation.

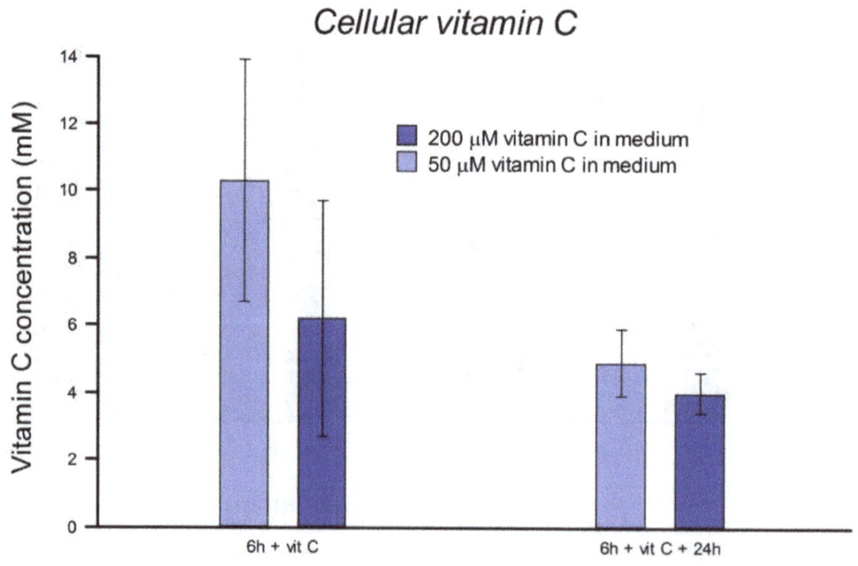

4. Discussion

In vitro, vitamin C is capable of acting as a pro-oxidant, particularly in combination with metal ions [14], and there are concerns that it might lead to excessive DNA oxidation in humans. There are reports of increases in oxidized bases in the DNA of white blood cells after supplementation of normal subjects with vitamin C [7] or with vitamin C plus ferrous sulfate [15]. However, these studies were carried out using GC-MS to measure oxidized bases—a technique now recognized as being particularly prone to artifact and therefore unsuitable for determining low level base oxidation [16].

The saturation plasma level for vitamin C in humans is around 80 μM, and this concentration is approached with daily intake of 200 mg/day [17]—an intake that can feasibly be attained by a recommended intake of several portions of fruits and vegetables each day. The justification for exceeding in our experiments the maximum vitamin C concentration found in plasma is that vitamin C is reportedly not stable in cell culture medium; 40% depletion was detected after 2 h of incubation [18], and only about 30% remained at 6 h.

In vivo, in subjects supplemented with 200 mg of vitamin C per day, active accumulation by lymphocytes results in intracellular levels saturating at 3.5 mM [17]. Welch *et al.* [19] reported a linear accumulation of vitamin C up to about 0.5 mM in 4 h in human fibroblasts incubated in 50 μM vitamin C. We found that the concentration of vitamin C inside HeLa cells after culture in medium with the vitamin was in the mM range, and was still high after 24 h. Although they have undergone many changes in their several decades of continuous culture from their origin in tumor tissue, HeLa cells evidently retain the active transport mechanisms responsible in normal cells for uptake of vitamin C [19], and so we regard them as suitable for an investigation of intracellular effects of vitamin C.

In the present study, in spite of the high intracellular concentration of vitamin C, there was no increase in SBs or FPG-sensitive sites. Others have reported no increase in SBs and/or oxidized bases in various cell types after incubation with vitamin C—in human HepG2 liver-derived cells with 10 μM vitamin C [20], in primary human fibroblasts incubated with 100 μM vitamin C [21], and most recently in HL-60 cells (human leukemic cell line) incubated with concentrations of 50–250 μM vitamin C [22,23].

In our experiments, preincubation with up to 200 μM vitamin C had no significant effect on the level of H_2O_2-induced breaks or 8-oxoGua induced by treatment with Ro plus light. There are mixed reports on the effect of pre-incubation with vitamin C on the DNA damage inflicted by genotoxic agents. Vitamin C pre-incubation (30 min, 10 or 50 μM) decreased the SBs caused by streptozotocin in lymphocytes or HeLa cells [24], and protected against the effect of $NiCl_2$ in lymphocytes [25]. Duarte and Jones [21] preincubated primary human fibroblasts for 12 h with 20, 100 or 500 μM vitamin C, and—also using the comet assay—found an increase in H_2O_2-induced damage. Carbofuran-induced damage to human lymphocyte DNA was decreased by preincubation with 30 μM vitamin C [26]. Similar protection was afforded by 10–50 μM vitamin C pretreatment against damage induced by 2-hydroxyethyl methacrylate and urethane dimethacrylate (used in dental treatment) [27,28].

When vitamin C is present simultaneously with a genotoxic agent (rather than during a preincubation), potentiation of the damaging effect of the latter may be seen—even when the effect of preincubation is a protective one. Such a dual effect was reported by Wozniak and Blasiak [25] for $NiCl_2$. Vanadyl sulfate led to more DNA breaks in HeLa cells and lymphocytes when they were co-incubated with vitamin C for 1 h [29], perhaps as a result of a metal ion-vitamin C interaction. Both DNA breaks and oxidized purines were induced when HL-60 cells were incubated with vitamin C and copper (II) sulfate, but no such damage was caused by vitamin C alone [23]. Vitamin C was unable to protect human submandibular gland and oral epithelial cells against DNA damage induced by bracken fern, and in fact showed a synergistic effect on DNA breakage [30]. In contrast, co-incubation of HepG2 cells with both vitamin C and *N*-nitrosamines resulted in fewer DNA breaks/oxidized bases [20]—perhaps an effect of vitamin C mediated through xenobiotic metabolizing enzymes.

To summarize our results relating to DNA damage, in HeLa cells—which clearly are able to take up and accumulate vitamin C—we find no sign of either pro- or anti-oxidant effects.

There are some human intervention studies that suggest a possible regulatory role for vitamin C in the repair of oxidized DNA—a topic highlighted by Sram *et al.* in their recent review [8] as deserving further attention. Cooke *et al.* [31] measured 8-oxodGuo in lymphocyte DNA, serum and urine from 30 healthy volunteers involved in a 6 week placebo and 6 week vitamin C (500 mg/day) supplementation study (plus a washout period). They found a decrease in the levels of 8-oxodGuo in DNA and an increase in urine and serum. In addition to reservations about the less than ideal study design and the likely errors in the measurement of 8-oxodGuo, the interpretation of the results is questionable, since the presence of 8-oxodGuo in serum or urine does not directly reflect OGG activity; the base, not the nucleoside, is excised during BER. Tarng *et al.* [32] supplemented chronic hemodialysis patients with 300 mg of vitamin C, and found a significant upregulation of *hOGG1* mRNA at 24 h after vitamin C administration. Astley *et al.* [33] took lymphocytes from human volunteers after 3 weeks of supplementation with the modest dose of 60 mg vitamin C per 2 days. There was no significant effect on plasma vitamin C, and no change in repair capacity (detected as repair synthesis on an oxidatively damaged plasmid template).

Supplementation for 3 weeks with green kiwifruits led to a significant increase in plasma vitamin C, decreases in endogenous base oxidation and H_2O_2-induced damage *ex vivo*, and an enhancement of lymphocyte BER on a substrate containing 8-oxoGua [34]; however, golden kiwifruits modestly increased plasma vitamin C and showed protection against DNA oxidation but no effect on DNA repair [35]. Guarnieri *et al.* [36] supplemented volunteers with 0.5 g/day vitamin C in normal or slow release form (together with vitamin E); only the slow release form stimulated BER capacity in lymphocytes.

Reports in the literature on effects of vitamin C on DNA repair in cells in culture are sparse. Konopacka *et al.* [37] irradiated mouse lymphocytes with 2 Gy of γ-rays, and then incubated them with or without vitamin C, vitamin E and β-carotene; rejoining of strand breaks was faster in the presence of antioxidants.

We report here that vitamin C has no effect on cellular repair of SBs or oxidized bases in HeLa cells. The *in vitro* test for 8-oxoGua DNA glycosylase (OGG) activity could not be carried out, since it was evident that vitamin C itself can cause damage to nucleoid DNA (Figure 6), presumably acting as a pro-oxidant (as mentioned in the Introduction). This cleavage could be mediated via production of hydroxyl radicals in the presence of DNA-bound transition metal such as copper [14].

The reason for native nuclear DNA being resistant to attack by vitamin C, while nucleoid DNA is susceptible, is not clear, though it may be that this apparently pro-oxidant effect of vitamin C is prevented by the high concentrations of the thiol-rich antioxidant glutathione present in the intact nucleus. Bergstrom *et al.* [22,23] report the oxidation of dGuo *in vitro* by vitamin C. To summarize, we have found no evidence in HeLa cells for pro-oxidant effects of vitamin C at extracellular concentrations up to 200 μM, but also no evidence for antioxidant protection. Nor did we see any effect on the repair of SBs or oxidized bases. Vitamin C at low concentration is, however, capable of damaging nucleoid DNA. The same strategy was used in our laboratory to study the antioxidant/pro-oxidant effects of β-cryptoxanthin [13]. Our results showed that this carotenoid does not cause DNA damage but, in contrast to vitamin C, it protects HeLa cells from damage induced by H_2O_2 or photosensitizer plus light. In addition, it enhances DNA repair, as measured with the same assays as were used in the present report.

Acknowledgments

We thank F. Hoffmann-La Roche for the gift of Ro 19-8022, and the Research Council of Norway and the Throne Holstfond for financial support. AA thanks the Ministerio de Educación y Ciencia ("Juan de la Cierva" programme, 2009) of the Spanish Government for personal support. We confirm that there are no conflicts of interest. AA and ARC conceived the project and wrote the paper. AA also carried out experiments, with SC, YL and NEB; all authors contributed to analysis and interpretation of results.

References

1. Carr, A.; Frei, B. Does vitamin C act as a pro-oxidant under physiological conditions? *FASEB J.* **1999**, *13*, 1007–1024.
2. Green, M.H. L.; Lowe, J.E.; Waugh, A.P.W.; Aldridge, K.E. Effect of diet and vitamin C on DNA strand breakage in freshly-isolated human white blood cells. *Mutat. Res.* **1994**, *316*, 91–102.
3. Duarte, T.L.; Lunec, J. Review: Part of the series: From dietary antioxidants to regulators in cellular signalling and gene expression review: When is an antioxidant not an antioxidant? A review of novel actions and reactions of vitamin C. *Free Radic. Res.* **2005**, *39*, 671–686.
4. Moller, P.; Loft, S. Oxidative DNA damage in human white blood cells in dietary antioxidant intervention studies. *Am. J. Clin. Nutr.* **2002**, *76*, 303–310.
5. Møller, P.; Viscovich, M.; Lykkesfeldt, J.; Loft, S.; Jensen, A.; Poulsen, H.E. Vitamin C supplementation decreases oxidative DNA damage in mononuclear blood cells of smokers. *Eur. J. Nutr.* **2004**, *43*, 267–274.
6. Herbert, K.; Fletcher, S.; Chauhan, D.; Ladapo, A.; Nirwan, J.; Munson, S.; Mistry, P. Dietary supplementation with different vitamin C doses: No effect on oxidative DNA damage in healthy people. *Eur. J. Nutr.* **2006**, *45*, 97–104.
7. Podmore, I.D.; Griffiths, H.R.; Herbert, K.E.; Mistry, N.; Mistry, P.; Lunec, J. Vitamin C exhibits pro-oxidant properties. *Nature* **1998**, *392*, 559.
8. Sram, R.J.; Binkova, B.; Rossner, J. Vitamin C for DNA damage prevention. *Mutat. Res.* **2012**, *733*, 39–49.

9. Bjelakovic, G.; Nikolova, D.; Gluud, L.L.; Simonetti, R.G.; Gluud, C. Mortality in randomized trials of antioxidant supplements for primary and secondary prevention: Systematic review and meta-analysis. *JAMA* **2007**, *297*, 842–857.
10. McCall, M.; Frei, B. Can antioxidant vitamins materially reduce oxidative damage in humans? *Free Radic. Biol. Med.* **1999**, *26*, 1034–1053.
11. Azqueta, A.; Shaposhnikov, S.; Collins, A.R. DNA Repair Measured by the Comet Assay. In *DNA Repair*; Kruman, I., Ed.; InTech: Rijeka, Croatia, 2011.
12. Collins, A.R.; Azqueta, A.; Brunborg, G.; Gaivão, I.; Giovannelli, L.; Kruszewski, M.; Smith, C.C.; Stetina, R. The comet assay: Topical issues. *Mutagenesis* **2008**, *23*, 143–151.
13. Lorenzo, Y.; Azqueta, A.; Luna, L.; Bonilla, F.; Domínguez, G.; Collins, A.R. The carotenoid B-cryptoxanthin stimulates the repair of DNA oxidation damage in addition to acting as an antioxidant in human cells. *Carcinogenesis* **2009**, *30*, 308–314.
14. Halliwell, B. Vitamin C: Antioxidant or pro-oxidant *in vivo*? *Free Radic. Res.* **1996**, *25*, 439–454.
15. Rehman, A.; Collis, C.S.; Yang, M.; Kelly, M.; Diplock, A.T.; Halliwell, B.; Rice-Evans, C. The effects of iron and vitamin C co-supplementation on oxidative damage to DNA in healthy volunteers. *Biochem. Biophys. Res. Commun.* **1998**, *246*, 293–298.
16. ESCODD; Gedik, C.M.; Collins, A. Establishing the background level of base oxidation in human lymphocyte DNA: Results of an interlaboratory validation study. *FASEB J.* **2005**, *19*, 82–84.
17. Levine, M.; Conry-Cantilena, C.; Wang, Y.; Welch, R.W.; Washko, P.W.; Dhariwal, K.R.; Park, J.B.; Lazarev, A.; Graumlich, J.F.; King, J.; Cantilena, L.R. Vitamin C pharmacokinetics in healthy volunteers: Evidence for a recommended dietary allowance. *Proc. Natl. Acad. Sci. USA* **1996**, *93*, 3704–3709.
18. Duarte, T. Effects of Vitamin C on DNA Damage, Iron Homeostasis and Gene Expression Profiling in Human Fibroblasts. Ph.D. Dissertation, University of Leicester, Leicester, UK, 2006.
19. Welch, R.W.; Bergsten, P.; Butler, J.D.; Levine, M. Ascorbic acid accumulation and transport in human fibroblasts. *Biochem. J.* **1993**, *294*, 505–510.
20. Arranz, N.; Haza, A.I.; Garcia, A.; Rafter, J.; Morales, P. Protective effect of vitamin C towards *N*-nitrosamine-induced DNA damage in the single-cell gel electrophoresis (SCGE)/HepG2 assay. *Toxicol. In Vitro* **2007**, *21*, 1311–1317.
21. Duarte, T.L.; Jones, G.D. Vitamin C modulation of H_2O_2-induced damage and iron homeostasis in human cells. *Free Radic. Biol. Med.* **2007**, *43*, 1165–1175.
22. Bergström, T.; Bergman, J.; Möller, L. Vitamin A and C compounds permitted in supplements differ in their abilities to affect cell viability, DNA and the DNA nucleoside deoxyguanosine. *Mutagenesis* **2011**, *26*, 735–744.
23. Bergström, T.; Ersson, C.; Bergman, J.; Möller, L. Vitamins at physiological levels cause oxidation to the DNA nucleoside deoxyguanosine and to DNA—alone or in synergism with metals. *Mutagenesis* **2012**, *27*, 511–517.
24. Blasiak, J.; Sikora, A.; Wozniak, K.; Drzewoski, J. Genotoxicity of streptozotocin in normal and cancer cells and its modulation by free radical scavengers. *Cell Biol. Toxicol.* **2004**, *20*, 83–96.
25. Wozniak, K.; Blasiak, J. Free radicals-mediated induction of oxidized DNA bases and DNA-protein cross-links by nickel chloride. *Mutat. Res.* **2002**, *514*, 233–243.

26. Sharma, R.K.; Sharma, B. *In-vitro* carbofuran induced genotoxicity in human lymphocytes and its mitigation by vitamins C and E. *Dis. Markers* **2012**, *32*, 153–163.
27. Pawlowska, E.; Poplawski, T.; Ksiazek, D.; Szczepanska, J.; Blasiak, J. Genotoxicity and cytotoxicity of 2-hydroxyethyl methacrylate. *Mutat. Res. Genet. Toxicol. Environ. Mutagen.* **2010**, *696*, 122–129.
28. Poplawski, T.; Loba, K.; Pawlowska, E.; Szczepanska, J.; Blasiak, J. Genotoxicity of urethane dimethacrylate, a tooth restoration component. *Toxicol. In Vitro* **2010**, *24*, 854–862.
29. Wozniak, K.; Blasiak, J. Vanadyl sulfate can differentially damage DNA in human lymphocytes and HeLa cells. *Arch. Toxicol.* **2004**, *78*, 7–15.
30. Campos-da-Paz, M.; Pereira, L.O.; Bicalho, L.S.; Dórea, J.G.; Poças-Fonseca, M.J.; Santos Mde, F. Interaction of bracken-fern extract with vitamin C in human submandibular gland and oral epithelium cell lines. *Mutat. Res.* **2008**, *652*, 158–163.
31. Cooke, M.S.; Evans, M.D.; Podmore, I.D.; Herbert, K.E.; Mistry, N.; Mistry, P.; Hickenbotham, P.T.; Hussieni, A.; Griffiths, H.R.; Lunec, J. Novel repair action of vitamin C upon *in vivo* oxidative DNA damage. *FEBS Lett.* **1998**, *439*, 363–367.
32. Tarng, D.C.; Liu, T.Y.; Huang, T.P. Protective effect of vitamin C on 8-hydroxy-2(prime)-deoxyguanosine level in peripheral blood lymphocytes of chronic hemodialysis patients. *Kidney Int.* **2004**, *66*, 820–831.
33. Astley, S.; Elliott, R.M.; Archer, D.B.; Southon, S. Evidence that dietary supplementation with carotenoids and carotenoid-rich foods modulates the DNA damage:repair balance in human lymphocytes. *Br. J. Nutr.* **2004**, *91*, 63–72.
34. Collins, A.R.; Harrington, V.; Drew, J.; Melvin, R. Nutritional modulation of DNA repair in a human intervention study. *Carcinogenesis* **2003**, *24*, 511–515.
35. Brevik, A.; Gaivao, I.; Medin, T.; Jorgenesen, A.; Piasek, A.; Elilasson, J.; Karlsen, A.; Blomhoff, R.; Veggan, T.; Duttaroy, A.; Collins, A. Supplementation of a western diet with golden kiwifruits (*Actinidia chinensis* var.'Hort 16A':) effects on biomarkers of oxidation damage and antioxidant protection. *Nutr. J.* **2011**, *10*, 54.
36. Guarnieri, S.; Loft, S.; Riso, P.; Porrini, M.; Risom, L.; Poulsen, H.; Dragsted, L.O.; Møller, P. DNA repair phenotype and dietary antioxidant supplementation. *Br. J. Nutr.* **2008**, *99*, 1018–1024.
37. Konopacka, M.; Widel, M.; Rzeszowka-Wolny, J. Modifying effect of vitamins C, E and beta-carotene against gamma-ray-induced DNA damage in mouse cells. *Mutat. Res.* **1998**, *417*, 85–94.

10

The Effects of High Concentrations of Vitamin C on Cancer Cells

Seyeon Park

Department of Applied Chemistry, Dongduk Women's University, 23-1 Wolgok-dong, Sungbuk-ku, Seoul 136-714, Korea; E-Mail: sypark21@dongduk.ac.kr or seypark21@hotmail.com;

Abstract: The effect of high doses of vitamin C for the treatment of cancer has been controversial. Our previous studies, and studies by others, have reported that vitamin C at concentrations of 0.25–1.0 mM induced a dose- and time-dependent inhibition of proliferation in acute myeloid leukemia (AML) cell lines and in leukemic cells from peripheral blood specimens obtained from patients with AML. Treatment of cells with high doses of vitamin C resulted in an immediate increase in intracellular total glutathione content and glutathione-S transferase activity that was accompanied by the uptake of cysteine. These results suggest a new role for high concentrations of vitamin C in modulation of intracellular sulfur containing compounds, such as glutathione and cysteine. This review, discussing biochemical pharmacologic studies, including pharmacogenomic and pharmacoproteomic studies, presents the different pharmacological effects of vitamin C currently under investigation.

Keywords: high concentrations of vitamin C; pharmacogenomics; pharmacoproteomics

---

1. Introduction

There is increasing evidence that vitamin C (ascorbate) is selectively toxic to some types of tumor cells, functioning as a pro-oxidant [1–3]. Vitamin C at concentrations of 10 nM–1 mM induced apoptosis in neuroblastoma and melanoma cells [4] and was shown to be an important modulator for the growth of mouse myeloma cells in an *in vitro* colony assay [5]. Studies have established that the growth of leukemic progenitor cells from patients with acute myeloid leukemia (AML) and myelodysplastic syndromes (MDS) can be significantly modulated by vitamin C [6,7]. Intravenous (i.v.) administration of sodium 5,6-benzylidene-l-ascorbate (SBA) to inoperable cancer patients induced a significant reduction in tumor volume without any adverse side effects [8]. Furthermore, recent clinical studies have reported that manipulation of vitamin C levels *in vivo* can result in clinical benefit for patients with AML and solid tumors [9].

Recent pharmacokinetic studies reported that 10 g of ascorbate given by i.v. produced plasma concentrations of nearly 6 mM, which were 25-fold higher than concentrations resulting from the same oral dose [10–12]. Depending on the dose, as much as a 70-fold difference in plasma concentration was found between oral and i.v. administration [13]. Complementary and alternative medicine practitioners worldwide currently use ascorbate i.v. in patients, in part because there are no apparent harmful effects [14–16]. Physiological concentration of vitamin C is under 0.1 mM, while plasma vitamin C concentrations that cause toxicity to cancer cells *in vitro* (1 mM–10 mM, depending on cell lines) can be achieved clinically by intravenous administration, which means a high dose of vitamin C.

In this review, *in vitro* and *in vivo* studies are summarized, showing that ascorbate killed cancer cells (Table 1). In addition, the mechanisms and physiologic relevance under investigation are also described. The results suggest that doses of vitamin C induce oxidative stress in cancer cells. Our previous results indicated that treatment of malignant lymphocytic cell lines with vitamin C (0.25–1 mM) for 24 h led to a marked dose-dependent decrease of cell proliferation [17]. The responsive cell lines were human myeloid leukemia cell line HL-60, retinoic acid (RA)-sensitive acute promyelocytic leukemia (APL) cell line NB4 and RA-resistant APL cell line NB4-R1. Different types of leukemia cells, such as K562 (chronic myelogenous leukemia cell line) [17] and KG1 (myeloblast cell line) [18], were also responsive to vitamin C. A similar result was obtained with cells containing over 90% of blasts from patients with AML. In these cell lines, induction of apoptosis by vitamin C demonstrated a dose-dependent effect. In addition, vitamin C weakly induced apoptosis in ovarian cell lines, including SK-OV-3, OVCAR-3 and 2774 [17]. For many of the cancer cell lines, ascorbate concentrations caused a 50% decrease in cell survival. The half maximal concentration (IC_{50}) values were less than 5 mM, and all tested normal cells were insensitive to 20 mM ascorbate [13].

Table 1. Effects of vitamin C treatment on cell survival [13,17,18].

Cell Line	IC_{50} (mM)
HL-60	0.33 ± 0.18 *
NB4	0.76 ± 0.14 *
NB4-R1	0.45 ± 0.24 *
NB4-R2	0.75 ± 0.3 *
KG1	0.79 ± 0.22 *
K562	0.5 ± 0.11 *
U937	0.3 ± 0.16 *
Normal Bone Marrow	1 ± 0.3 *
Patient with AML	0.84 ± 0.16 *
OVCAR	>10 *
SK-OV3	>10 *
JLP119	<1

Table 1. *Cont.*

MCF7	2
MB231	7
Hs587T	20
KLN205	<1
RAG	<2
CT26	4
B16	7
LL/2	11
Hs587Bst	>20
CCD34SK	>20
Human normal lymphocyte	>20
Human normal monocyte	>20

The IC_{50} values are means ± standard deviations from triplicate experiments. HL-60, human myeloid leukemia; NB4, NB4-R1, NB4-R2, human acute promyelocytic leukemia (APL); KG1, human myeloblast; K562, human chronic myelogenous leukemia; U937, human histiocytic lymphoma; OVCAR, SK-OV3, ovarian cancer; JLP119, human lymphoma; MCF7, MB231, Hs587t, human breast cancer; KLN205, mouse lung cancer; RAG, mouse kidney cancer; CT26, mouse colon cancer; B16, mouse melanoma; LL/2, mouse lung cancer; Hs587Bst, human normal breast cells; CCD34SK, human normal fibroblast cells. * IC_{50} value was determined using H^3 incorporation proliferation assay for 24 h.

2. Molecular Mechanisms Induced by Vitamin C

In our previous study, vitamin C at concentrations of 0.25–2.0 mM significantly induced apoptosis in AML cell lines. Vitamin C induced oxidation of glutathione (GSH) to its oxidized form (GSSG). As a result, H_2O_2 accumulated in a concentration-dependent manner, in parallel with the induction of apoptosis. The direct role of H_2O_2 in the induction of apoptosis in AML cells was demonstrated by the finding that catalase could completely abrogate vitamin C-induced apoptosis [17].

A 30-min incubation of NB4 cells with 0–10 mM vitamin C resulted in its uptake in a concentration-dependent manner [17,19]. In accordance with its proposed pro-oxidant activity, vitamin C treatment reduced the GSH/GSSG ratio, which correlated with increased intracellular H_2O_2 in the NB4 cell line. Levine *et al.* suggested that the effect was due only to extracellular and not intracellular ascorbate, and that ascorbate-mediated cell death was probably due to protein-dependent extracellular H_2O_2 generation, via ascorbate radical formation from ascorbate as the electron donor [13].

Although H_2O_2 induced by ascorbate was first generated extracellularly, it is possible that it could diffuse across the plasma membrane into the intracellular space. Although studies in yeast and bacteria have shown that diffusion of H_2O_2 across membranes is limited, some reports have suggested that selected aquaporin homologues from plants and mammals can channel H_2O_2 across these membranes [20–25]. The susceptibility of cancer cells to ascorbate treatment might therefore be related to the permeability of hydrogen peroxide.

In our studies, vitamin C dramatically increased intracellular GSH oxidation and reactive oxygen species (ROS) levels within 3 h in a concentration-dependent manner. However, this GSH oxidation and the ROS accumulation did not last for a long period of time. After 3 h, the increase in GSH has been observed and hypothesized to be a defense mechanism [18]. No additional ROS accumulation resulted from the change in GSH. However, based upon our studies, the dramatic changes of intracellular oxidation state within 3 h seem to be enough to induce intracellular signaling. The studies showed that treatment with 1 mM vitamin C for only 30–60 min, followed by removal when replacing media, could induce apoptosis in both HL-60 and NB4 cells. This observation is consistent with initiation of apoptosis, resulting from generation of H_2O_2 after treatment with ascorbate. However, treatment with As_2O_3 resulted in less ROS accumulation than with vitamin C, and it was not in a concentration-dependent manner. However, ROS accumulation increased up to 24 h, with a long-lasting effect. Treatment with vitamin C combined with As_2O_3 increased ROS accumulation, as well as sustained the effect for up to 24 h. These results are consistent with cellular data showing that apoptosis induced by As_2O_3 is evident even at three days [26,27].

3. Proteomics Studies

Proteomics provides important qualitative information on post-translational modifications to proteins and quantitative data on protein expression in response to a particular stimulus. This information is particularly important when it provides data on early cellular events, such as the stimulus and signaling cascades triggered independently of protein neosynthesis. In accordance with its proposed pro-oxidant activity, vitamin C-mediated reduction in the GSH/GSSG ratio correlated with an intracellular H_2O_2 increase in the NB4 cell line [17,19]. This type of change in regional oxidation state could cause changes in the cellular milieu that could result in changes in protein structure. This is especially true of the oxidation state of cysteine sulfur, which is important for determining the tertiary structure of proteins. The immediate effects of cell stimuli are associated with protein post-translational modifications, such as phosphorylation, glutathionylation and cysteine oxidation. To study these early modifications, NB4 human leukemia cells were treated with 0.5 mM vitamin C and then analyzed by two-dimensional analysis. Approximately 240 different spots that were focused in a pH range of 4–7 were detected per sample.

After exposing cells to vitamin C, we observed one new spot, three intensified spots and five attenuated spots [19]. Each of these spots were excised, digested with trypsin and analyzed by matrix-assisted laser desorption/ionization-time of flight (MALDI-TOF). Peptide mass fingerprint analysis and non-redundant sequence database matching allowed the unambiguous identification of all of the analyzed species [19]. An important protein identified from the proteomic analysis was a thiol/disulfide exchange catalyst, protein disulfide isomerase (PDI), which was a marker of the effect of vitamin C on NB4 cells [19]. PDI belongs to the superfamily of thiol/disulfide exchange catalysts, which act as protein-thiol-oxidoreductase enzymes, sharing sequence homology with thioredoxin [28]. PDI is composed of four domains, which have similarities with thioredoxin folds (*i.e.*, a-b-b′-a′) [29]. In our study [19], the intensity of the spot corresponding to the PDI b subunit was decreased in vitamin C-treated cells as compared with control cells. These results demonstrated that thiol/disulfide exchange proteins are regulated in NB4 cells after vitamin C exposure. This is consistent with our study showing that intracellular GSH/GSSG exchange occurs shortly after vitamin C exposure [17].

When we measured cysteine uptake in leukemia cell lines exposed to vitamin C by using ^{35}S-labeled-L-Cys in the media, the time-dependent rate of cysteine uptake in the cell culture increased significantly. The rate of uptake, determined under conditions without vitamin C, was very low. The glutathione synthesis inhibitor, buthionine sulfoximine, potently inhibited this increase, suggesting that incorporation of cysteine that corresponded to the amount of increased glutathione was mediated by glutathione synthesis. Overall, our results indicated that vitamin C-induced glutathione synthesis was accompanied by intracellular cysteine uptake.

Glutathione-S transferases (GSTs) are enzymes that catalyze the conjugation of electrophilic substitution to GSH, which protects cells by removing reactive oxygen species and regenerating *S*-thiolated proteins [30]. Intracellular total GSH levels in AML cells incubated with vitamin C peaked around 3 h, then declined, while the increase in incorporated [^{35}S]-L-Cys peaked at 3 h and remained high. These results showed that [^{35}S]-L-Cys transported into cells through cysteine uptake was incorporated and transferred intracellularly, strongly suggesting that the sulfhydryl transfer system is affected by vitamin C [30].

We therefore hypothesize that the biochemical pathway leading to thiol/disulfide redox regulation could be activated by vitamin C. Interestingly, of the proteins whose expressions changed by vitamin C treatment, immunoglobulin heavy chain binding protein (BiP, identical to Hsp70 chaperone) [19], like PDI, is also a multi-domain chaperone. BiP associated with the α-subunit of prolyl 4-hydroxylase (P4-H) by a disulfide bond [31]. P4-H consists of two distinct polypeptides, the catalytically more important α-subunit and the β-subunit, which is identical to the multifunctional enzyme, PDI [31]. Thus, BiP associated with the α-subunit of P4-H, which is another partner of PDI. The interaction of PDI with its substrates was due to a change in disulfide bonds, indicating that intrachain disulfide bonds between domains and substrates had been reduced [19]. Taken together, these results suggested that vitamin C oxidizes intracellular-reduced glutathione and affects disulfide bond formation in proteins [30].

Tropomyosin was also identified as a marker of the oxidative effect of vitamin C in NB4 cells. The spot corresponding to tropomyosin was positioned at an isoelectric point (pI) of approximately 5.0 and was attenuated in vitamin C-treated cells. In addition, a new spot having almost the same molecular weight was detected, which was positioned at a pI of 4.9 [19]. This new spot was also identified as tropomyosin, suggesting that post-translational chemical modification had affected its pI value. This result is consistent with previous data showing that the extracellular signal-regulated kinase (ERK)-mediated phosphorylation of tropomyosin-1 promoted cytoskeleton remodeling in response to oxidative stress [32]. The acidic shift of the spot with pI 5.0 to the phosphorylated tropomyosin spot by treatment with vitamin C was found to be abrogated by co-treatment with PD98059 [19], demonstrating that phosphorylation of tropomyosin was responsible for the observed acidic shift.

The significance of this observation may be related to differences in the regulation of the actomyosin contractile system in non-muscle cells as compared with that present in muscle cells. In addition, proteins that specifically reacted with sera from chronic myeloid leukemia patients included structural proteins, such as β-tubulin and tropomyosin isoforms [33]. Although the function of these proteins in myeloid leukemia needs further investigation, tropomyosin may have value as a leukemia-associated antigen and as a molecular target in antigen-based immunotherapy. In this regard, it is important to note that vitamin C causes a tropomyosin isoform to be modified during the immediate early response.

4. *In Vivo* Studies

Levine *et al.* reported that reaction products obtained from ascorbate *in vitro* are also found *in vivo* [34]. They showed that after i.v. injection, ascorbate baseline concentrations of 50–100 μM in blood and extracellular fluids peaked to >8 mM. After intraperitoneal injection, peaks approached 3 mM in both fluids. They hypothesized that *in vivo*, ascorbate was a prodrug for selective delivery of ascorbate radical and H_2O_2 to the extracellular space. Moreover, a regimen of daily pharmacologic ascorbate treatment significantly decreased growth rates of ovarian ($p < 0.005$), pancreatic ($p < 0.05$) and glioblastoma ($p < 0.001$) tumors established in mice [35]. In addition to inducing oxidative stress, high concentrations of ascorbic acid inhibited cell migration and the gap filling capacity of endothelial progenitor cells (EPCs) [36], and it has been reported that ascorbic acid inhibited corneal neovascularization in a rat model [37].

High concentrations of ascorbic acid also inhibited tumor growth in BALB/C mice implanted with sarcoma 180 cancer cells [38]. The survival rate increased by 20% in the group that received high doses of ascorbic acid, compared to controls. Gene expression studies from biopsy and wound healing analysis *in vivo* and *in vitro* suggested that the carcinostatic effect induced by high doses of ascorbic acid were related to inhibition of angiogenesis [39]. In addition, intraperitoneal administration of high doses of ascorbic acid quantitatively upregulated Raf kinase inhibitory protein (RKIP) and annexin A5 expression in a group of BALB/C mice implanted with S-180 sarcoma cancer cells. The increase in RKIP protein levels suggested that these proteins are involved in the ascorbic acid-mediated suppression of tumor formation [39]. Moreover, high doses of ascorbic acid (~1 mM) enhanced the apoptosis of cancer cells during co-treatment with paclitaxel, and the combinational treatment of paclitaxel and ascorbic acid ameliorated the side effects caused by paclitaxel in BALB/c mice implanted with or without sarcoma 180 cancer cells [40].

5. Clinical Studies

Cases of apparent responses of malignancies to intravenous vitamin C therapy have been reported, although they were reported without sufficient detail [15,41–46]. A recent study showed that oral administration of the maximum tolerated dose of vitamin C (18 g/day) produced peak plasma concentrations of only 0.22 mM, whereas intravenous administration of the same dose produced plasma concentrations approximately 25-fold higher. Larger doses (50–100 g) given intravenously resulted in plasma concentrations of approximately 14 mM [41].

Some case reports stated that high dose i.v. vitamin C has been used by Complementary and Alternate Medicine (CAM) practitioners [47]. Phase I evaluation of intravenous vitamin C in combination with gemcitabine and erlotinib in patients with metastatic pancreatic cancer data did not reveal increased toxicity with the addition of ascorbic acid [48]. No side effects were reported for most patients, while 59 were reported to have lethargy or fatigue out of 11,233 patients that received intravenous vitamin C in 2006 and 8876 in 2008 [47]. Overall, it was reported that high dose intravenous vitamin C did not appear to cause serious side effects in patients.

Another clinical study reported the depletion of L-ascorbic acid alternating with its supplementation in the treatment of patients with acute myeloid leukemia or myelodysplastic syndromes [49]. During the supplementation phase, patients received daily i.v. administration of vitamin C. A pre-therapy *in vitro* assay was performed for vitamin C sensitivity of leukemic cells from individual patients. Of the nine patients with the *in vitro* assay indicating their leukemic cells were sensitive to vitamin C, seven exhibited a clinical response, compared with none of the six patients who were insensitive to vitamin C.

6. Conclusions

Previous studies have shown that vitamin C is involved in the mechanism of action of the intracellular microenvironment (oxidation) state changes that improve therapeutic potential, including apoptosis and necrosis. Although it is difficult to postulate precise vitamin C-specific mechanisms at this time, identification of genes or proteins that are specifically regulated by vitamin C in certain cellular phenotypes could improve the efficacy of therapies.

References

1. Bram, S.; Froussard, P.; Guichard, M.; Jasmin, C.; Auqery, Y.; Sinoussi-Barre, F.; Wray, W. Ascorbic acid preferential toxicity for malignant melanoma cells. *Nature* **1980**, *284*, 629–631.
2. Bruchelt, G.; Baader, L.; Reith, A.G.; Holger, N.L.; Gebhardt, S.; Niethammer, D. Rationale for the Use of Ascorbic Acid in Neuroblastoma Therapy. In *Human Neuroblastoma*; Schwab, M., Ed.; Harwood Academic Publishers: Newark, NJ, USA, 1993; pp. 34–40.
3. Fujinaga, S.; Sakagami, H.; Kuribayashi, N.; Takahashi, H.; Amano, Y.; Sakagami, T.; Takeda, M. Possible role of hydrogen peroxide in apoptosis induction by ascorbic acid in human myelogenous leukemic cell lines. *Showa Univ. Med. Sci.* **1994**, *6*, 135–144.
4. De Laurenzi, V.; Melino, G.; Savini, I.; Annicchiarico-Petruzzelli, M.; Finazzi-Agro, A.; Avigliano, L. Cell death by oxidative stress and ascorbic acid regeneration in human neuroectodermal cell lines. *Eur. J. Cancer* **1995**, *31*, 463–466.
5. Park, C.H.; Bergsagel, D.E.; McCulloch, E.A. Ascorbic acid: A culture requirement for colony formation by mouse plasmacytoma cells. *Science* **1971**, *174*, 720–722.
6. Park, C.H. The biological nature of the effect of ascorbic acids on the growth of human leukemic cells. *Cancer Res.* **1985**, *45*, 3969–3973.
7. Park, C.H.; Kimler, B.F.; Bodensteiner, D.; Lynch, S.R.; Hassanein, R.S. *In vitro* growth modulation by L-ascorbic acid of colony-forming cells from bone marrow of patients with myelodysplastic syndromes. *Cancer Res.* **1992**, *52*, 4458–4466.
8. Sakagami, H.; Asano, K.; Fukuchi, K.; Gomi, K.; Ota, H.; Kazama, K.; Tanuma, S.; Kochi, M. Induction of tumor degeneration by sodium benzylideneascorbate. *Anticancer Res.* **1991**, *11*, 1533–1538.
9. Park, C.H.; Kim, W.S.; Park, C.; Lee, M.H.; Boo, Y.C.; Yoon, S.S. Clinical disease suppression and reduction in acute myeloid leukemia and solid tumors by very high dose of L-ascorbic acid: A new concept and in search of molecular targets. *Clin. Cancer Res.* **1999**, *5*, 3784s.

10. Padayatty, S.J.; Sun, H.; Wang, Y.; Riordan, H.D.; Hewitt, S.M.; Katz, A.; Wesley, R.A.; Levine, M. Vitamin C Pharmacokinetics: Implications for Oral and Intravenous Use. *Ann. Intern. Med.* **2004**, *140*, 533–537.
11. Levine, M.; Conry-Cantilena, C.; Wang, Y.; Welch, R.W.; Washko, P.W.; Dhariwal, K.R.; Park, J.B.; Lazarev, A.; Graumlich, J.; King, J.; *et al.* Vitamin C Pharmacokinetics in healthy volunteers: Evidence for a recommended dietary allowance. *Proc. Natl. Acad. Sci. USA* **1996**, *93*, 3704–3709.
12. Levine, M.; Wang, Y.; Padayatty, S.J.; Morrow, J.D. A new recommended dietary allowance of vitamin C for healthy young women. *Proc. Natl. Acad. Sci. USA* **2001**, *98*, 9842–9846.
13. Chen, Q.; Espey, M.G.; Cherukuri, M.K.; Mitchell, J.B.; Corpe, C.P.; Buettner, G.R.; Shacter, E.; Levine, M. Ascorbic acid at Pharmacologic concentrations selectively kill cancer cells: Ascorbic acid as a pro-drug to deliver hydrogen peroxide to tissues. *Proc. Natl. Acad. Sci. USA* **2005**, *102*, 13604–13609.
14. Levine, M.; Rumsey, S.C.; Daruwala, R.C.; Park, J.B.; Wang, Y. Criteria and recommendation for vitamin C intake. *J. Am. Med.* **1999**, *281*, 1415–1423.
15. Riordan, N.H.; Riordan, H.D.; Casciari, J.J. Clinicla and experimental experiences with intravenous vitamin C. *J. Orthomol. Med.* **2000**, *15*, 201–203.
16. Riordan, H.D.; Hunninghake, R.E.; Riordan, N.H.; Jackson, J.J.; Meng, X.; Taylor, P.; Casciari, J.J.; Gonzalez, M.J.; Miranda-Massari, J.R.; Mora, E.M.; *et al.* Intravenous Ascorbic Acid: Protocol for its Application and Use. *P. R. Health Sci. J.* **2003**, *22*, 287–290.
17. Park, S.; Han, S.S.; Park, C.H.; Hahm, E.R.; Lee, S.J.; Park, H.K.; Lee, S.H.; Kim, W.S.; Jung, C.W.; Park, K.; *et al.* L-Ascorbic acid induces apoptosis in acute myeloid leukemia cells via hydrogen peroxide-mediated mechanisms. *Int. J. Biochem. Cell Biol.* **2004**, *36*, 2180–2195.
18. Park, S. Samsung Medical Center, Seoul, Korea. Unpublished work, 2004.
19. Park, S.; Lee, J.; Yeom, C.H. A proteomic approach to the identification of early molecular targets changed by L-ascorbic acid in NB4 human leukemia cells. *J. Cell. Biochem.* **2006**, *99*, 1628–1641.
20. Bienert, G.P.; Schjoerring, J.K.; Jahn, T.P. Membrane transport of hydrogen peroxide. *Biochim. Biophys. Acta* **2006**, *1758*, 994–1003.
21. Seaver, L.C.; Imlay, A.J. Hydrogen peroxide fluxes and compartmentalization inside growing *Escherichia coli. J. Bacteriol.* **2001**, *183*, 7182–7189.
22. Antunes, F.; Cadenas, E. Estimations of H_2O_2 gradients across biomembranes. *FEBS Lett.* **2000**, *475*, 121–126.
23. Makino, N.; Sasaki, K.; Hashida, K.; Sakakura, Y. A metabolic model describing the H_2O_2 elimination by mammalian cells including H_2O_2 permeation through cytoplasmatic and peroxisomal membranes: comparison with experimental data. *Biochim. Biophys. Acta* **2004**, *1673*, 149–159.
24. Sousa-Lopes, A.; Antunes, F.; Cyrne, L.; Marinho, H.S. Decreased cellular permeability to H_2O_2 protects Saccharomyces cerevisiaein stationary phase against oxidative stress. *FEBS Lett.* **2004**, *578*, 152–156.
25. Mathai, J.C.; Sitaramam, V. Strech sensitivity of transmembrane mobility of hydrogen peroxide through voids in the bilayer. *J. Biol. Chem.* **1994**, *269*, 17784–17793.

26. Zhu, X.H.; Shen, Y.L.; Jing, Y.K.; Cai, X.; Jia, P.M.; Huang, Y.; Tang, W.; Shi, G.Y.; Sun, Y.P.; Dai, J.; *et al.* Apoptosis and Growth Inhibition in Malignant Lymphocytes After Treatment With Arsenic Trioxide at Clinically Achievable Concentrations. *J. Natl. Cancer Inst.* **1999**, *91*, 772–778.
27. Dai, J.; Weinberg, R.S.; Waxman, S.; Jing, Y. Malignant cells can be sensitized to undergo growth inhibition and apoptosis by arsenic trioxide through modulation of the glutathione redox system. *Blood* **1999**, *93*, 268–277.
28. Noiva, R. Protein disulfide isomerase: The multifunctional redox chaperone of the endoplasmic reticulum. *Semin. Cell Dev. Biol.* **1999**, *10*, 481–493.
29. Kemmink, J.; Darby, N.J.; Dijkstra, K.; Nilges, M.; Creighton, T.E. The folding catalyst protein disulfide isomerase is constructed of active and inactive thioredoxin modules. *Curr. Biol.* **1997**, *7*, 239–245.
30. Park, S. Apoptosis of Leukemia Cells Induced by L-Ascorbic Acid and Arsenic Trioxide: The Effect of Oxidative Stress and Glutathione homeostasis.Albina. In *Cell Apoptosis and Cancer*; Taylor, A.W., Ed.; Nova Science Publishers, Inc.: New York, NY, USA, 2007; pp. 87–111.
31. John, D.C.; Bulleid, N.J. Intracellular dissociation and reassembly of prolyl 4-hydroxylase: The alpha-subunits associated with the immunoglobulin-heavy-chain binding protein (BiP) allowing reassembly with the β-subunit. *Biochem. J.* **1996**, *317*, 659–665.
32. Houle, F.; Rousseau, S.; Morrice, N.; Luc, M.; Mongrain, S.; Turner, C.E.; Tanaka, S.; Moreau, P.; Huot, J. Extracellular signal-regulated kinase mediates phosphorylation of tropomyosin-1 to promote cytoskeleton remodeling in response to oxidative stress: Impact on membrane blebbing. *Mol. Biol. Cell* **2003**, *14*, 1418–1432.
33. Zou, L.; Wu, Y.; Pei, L.; Zhong, D.; Gen, M.; Zhao, T.; Wu, J.; Ni, B.; Mou, Z.; Han, J.; *et al.* Identification of leukemia-associated antigens in chronic myeloid leukemia by proteomic analysis. *Leuk. Res.* **2005**, *29*, 1387–1391.
34. Chen, Q.; Espey, M.G.; Sun, A.Y.; Lee, J.H.; Krishna, M.C.; Shacter, E.; Choyke, P.L.; Pooput, C.; Kirk, K.L.; Buettner, G.R.; *et al.* Ascorbate in pharmacologic concentrations selectively generates ascorbate radical and hydrogen peroxide in extracellular fluid *in vivo*. *Proc. Natl. Acad. Sci. USA* **2007**, *104*, 8749–8754.
35. Chen, Q.; Espey, M.G.; Sun, A.Y.; Pooput, C.; Kirk, K.L.; Krishna, M.C.; Khosh, D.B.; Drisko, J.; Levin, M. Pharmacologic doses of ascorbate act as a prooxidant and decrease growth of aggressive tumor xenografts in mice. *Proc. Natl. Acad. Sci. USA* **2008**, *105*, 11105–11109.
36. Mikirova, N.A.; Ichim, T.E.; Riordan, N.H. Anti-angiogenic effect ofhigh doses of ascorbic acid. *J. Transl. Med.* **2008**, *6*, doi:10.1186/1479-5876-6-50.
37. Peyman, G.A.; Kivilcim, M.; Morales, A.M.; DellaCroce, J.T.; Conway, M.D. Inhibition of corneal angiogenesis by ascorbic acid in the ratmodel. *Graefe's Arch. Clin. Exp. Ophthalmol.* **2007**, *245*, 1461–1467.
38. Yeom, C.H.; Lee, G.; Park, J.; Yu, J.; Park, S.; Yi, S.Y.; Lee, H.; Hong, Y.; Yang, J.; Lee, S. High dose concentration administration of ascorbic acid inhibits tumor growth in BLAB/C mice implanted with sarcoma 180 cancer cells via the restriction of angiogenesis. *J. Transl. Med.* **2009**, *7*, doi:10.1186/1479-5876-7-70.

39. Park, S.; Ahn, E.S.; Lee, S.; Jung, M.; Park, J.H.; Yi, S.Y.; Yeom, C.H. Proteomicanalysis reveals upregulation of RKIP in S-180 implanted BALB/C mouse after treatment with ascorbic acid. *J. Cell. Biochem.* **2009**, *106*, 1136–1145.
40. Park, J.H.; Davis, K.R.; Lee, G.; Jung, M.; Jung, Y.; Park, J.; Yi, S.Y.; Lee, M.A.; Lee, S.; Yeom, C.H.; *et al.* Ascorbic acid alleviates toxicity of paclitaxel without interfering with the anticancer efficacy in mice. *Nutr. Res.* **2012**, *32*, 873–883.
41. Padayatty, S.J.; Riordan, H.D.; Hewitt, S.M.; Katz, A.; Hoffer, L.J.; Levine, M. Intravenously administered vitamin C as cancer therapy: Three cases. *CMAJ* **2006**, *174*, 937–942.
42. Riordan, H.D.; Jackson, J.A.; Riordan, N.H.; Schultz, M. High-dose intravenous vitamin C in the treatment of a patient with renal cell carcinoma of the kidney. *J. Orthomol. Med.* **1998**, *13*, 72–73.
43. Riordan, H.D.; Riordan, N.H.; Jackson, J.A.; Casciari, J.J.; Hunninghake, R.; Gonzalez, M.J.; Mora, E.M.; Miranda-Massari, J.R.; Rosario, N.; Rivera, A. Intravenous vitamin C as a chemotherapy agent: a report on clinical cases. *P. R. Health Sci. J.* **2004**, *23*, 115–118.
44. Riordan, H.D.; Jackson, J.A.; Schultz, M. Case study: High-dose intravenous vitamin C in the treatment of a patient with adenocarcinoma of the kidney. *J. Orthomol. Med.* **1990**, *5*, 5–7.
45. Jackson, J.A.; Riordan, H.D.; Hunninghake, R.E.; Riordan, N. High-dose intravenous vitamin C and long-time survival of a patient with cancer of the head of the pancreas. *J. Orthomol. Med.* **1995**, *10*, 87–88.
46. Riordan, N.H.; Jackson, J.A.; Riordan, H.D. Intravenous vitamin C in a terminal cancer patient. *J. Orthomol. Med.* **1996**, *11*, 80–82.
47. Padayatty, S.J.; Sun, A.Y.; Chen, Q.; Espey, M.G.; Drislo, J.; Levine, M. Vitamin C: Intravenous use by complementary and alternative medicine practitioners and adverse effects. *PLoS One* **2010**, *5*, e11411.
48. Monti, D.A.; Mitchell, E.; Bazzan, A.J.; Littman, S.; Zabrecky, G.; Yeo, C.J.; Pillai, M.V.; Newberg, A.B.; Deshmukh, S.; Levine, M. Phase I evaluation of intravenous ascorbic acid in combination with gemcitabine and erlotinib in patients with metastatic pancreatic cancer. *PLoS One* **2012**, *7*, e29794.
49. Park, C.H.; Kimler, B.F.; Yi, S.Y.; Park, S.H.; Kim, K.; Jung, C.W.; Kim, S.H.; Lee, E.R.; Rha, M.; Kim, S.; *et al.* Depletion of L-ascorbic acid alternating with its supplementation in the treatment of patients with acute myeloid leukemia or myelodysplastic syndromes. *Eur. J. Haematol.* **2009**, *83*, 108–118.

11

A Randomized Steady-State Bioavailability Study of Synthetic *versus* Natural (Kiwifruit-Derived) Vitamin C

Anitra C. Carr [1,*], Stephanie M. Bozonet [1], Juliet M. Pullar [1], Jeremy W. Simcock [2] and Margreet C. M. Vissers [1]

[1] Centre for Free Radical Research, Department of Pathology & Biomedical Science, University of Otago, Christchurch, PO Box 4345, Christchurch 8140, New Zealand; E-Mails: stephanie.bozonet@otago.ac.nz (S.M.B.); juliet.pullar@otago.ac.nz (J.M.P.); margreet.vissers@otag (M.C.M.V.)

[2] Department of Plastic and Reconstructive Surgery, University of Otago, Christchurch, PO Box 4345, Christchurch 8140, New Zealand; E-Mail: jeremy.simcock@cdhb.health.nz

* Author to whom correspondence should be addressed; E-Mail: anitra.carr@otago.ac.nz;

Abstract: Whether vitamin C from wholefoods has equivalent bioavailability to a purified supplement remains unclear. We have previously showed that kiwifruit provided significantly higher serum and tissue ascorbate levels than synthetic vitamin C in a genetically vitamin C-deficient mouse model, suggesting a synergistic activity of the whole fruit. To determine if these results are translatable to humans, we carried out a randomized human study comparing the bioavailability of vitamin C from kiwifruit with that of a vitamin C tablet of equivalent dosage. Thirty-six young non-smoking adult males were randomized to receive either half a gold kiwifruit (*Actinidia Chinensis* var. *Hort 16A*) per day or a comparable vitamin C dose (50 mg) in a chewable tablet for six weeks. Ascorbate was monitored weekly in fasting venous blood and in urine, semen, leukocytes, and skeletal muscle (*vastus lateralis*) pre- and post-intervention. Dietary intake of vitamin C was monitored using seven day food and beverage records. Participant ascorbate levels increased in plasma ($P < 0.001$), urine ($P < 0.05$), mononuclear cells ($P < 0.01$), neutrophils ($P < 0.01$) and muscle tissue ($P < 0.001$) post intervention. There were no significant differences in vitamin C bioavailability between the two intervention groups in any of the fluid, cell or tissue samples tested. Overall, our study showed comparable bioavailability of synthetic and kiwifruit-derived vitamin C.

Keywords: ascorbate; ascorbic acid; human; plasma; urine; semen; leukocytes; skeletal muscle

1. Introduction

Vitamin C (ascorbate) is an essential water-soluble micronutrient that is obtained through the diet primarily from fruits and vegetables [1]. The bioavailability of dietary vitamin C represents the proportion absorbed by the intestines and available for metabolic processes within the body. Vitamin C is actively transported into the body via two sodium-dependent vitamin C transporters, SVCT1 and SVCT2, which exhibit different tissue distributions and uptake kinetics [2,3]. SVCT1 is expressed in epithelial tissue and is primarily responsible for intestinal uptake and renal reabsorption of vitamin C, the latter maintaining whole body homeostasis [3]. SVCT2 is expressed in specialized and metabolically active tissues and is required for delivery of vitamin C to tissues with a high demand for the vitamin either for enzymatic reactions [4] and/or to help protect these tissues from oxidative stress [3].

Kiwifruit are rich in vitamin C [5] and we have previously used a genetically vitamin C-deficient mouse model (the *Gulo* mouse) to investigate the comparative bioavailability of synthetic *versus* kiwifruit-derived vitamin C [6]. Interestingly, we found that kiwifruit gel provided higher serum, leukocyte, heart, liver and kidney levels of ascorbate than equivalent amounts of purified vitamin C, suggesting a synergistic activity of the whole fruit in this model. Although synthetic and food-derived vitamin C are chemically identical, the bioavailability of vitamin C could potentially be affected by the numerous micronutrients and phytochemicals with antioxidant properties that are present in fruits and vegetables [7,8]. For example, kiwifruit contain reasonable amounts of vitamin E [9], which has been shown to spare vitamin C in an animal model [10]. Kiwifruit also contain numerous different flavonoids [9,11], some of which can inhibit the *in vitro* oxidation of vitamin C via direct scavenging of free radicals and/or chelation of redox-active metal ions [7,8].

To determine if the results of our animal study [6] are translatable to humans, we carried out a randomized human study comparing the bioavailability of vitamin C from gold kiwifruit (*Actinidia Chinensis* var. *Hort 16A*) with a tablet of equivalent dosage. We have previously shown that consumption of half a gold kiwifruit per day results in a significant increase in plasma ascorbate in individuals with low initial levels (<23 μmol/L) [12]. For this study, we chose a dose of half a kiwifruit per day and the equivalent 50 mg/day vitamin C since this dose lies on the steeply rising portion of the sigmoidal plasma bioavailability curve [13]. This enhances the likelihood of detecting a difference between the two interventions compared with doses >100 mg/day where plasma saturation is approached [13].

Several previous studies have tested the comparative bioavailability of synthetic *versus* food-derived vitamin C utilizing plasma and/or urine levels [14–18]. However, only one has investigated the comparative bioavailability of vitamin C in leukocytes [19]. Therefore, in addition to plasma and urine, we have monitored the bioavailability of vitamin C in peripheral blood mononuclear cells and neutrophils, seminal fluid and skeletal muscle tissue [20] before and after the six week intervention. We also monitored the participants' dietary intake of vitamin C using seven day food and beverage records.

2. Study Design and Methods

2.1. Participants

This study was conducted according to the guidelines laid down in the Declaration of Helsinki and all procedures involving human participants were approved by the Upper South Regional Ethics Committee (#URA/11/02/003). The study was registered with the Australian New Zealand Clinical Trials Registry (#ACTRN12611000162910).

Non-smoking males aged 18–35 years from local tertiary institutes were screened to ascertain their eligibility for the study. Exclusion criteria included recent smoker (within previous year), allergy/intolerance to kiwifruit, taking vitamin C-containing supplements (within past three months), taking prescription medication (within past three months), excessive alcohol consumption (>21 standard drinks/week), high fruit and vegetable consumption (>5 servings per day), diabetes mellitus, bleeding disorders, and fainting due to fear of needles. Anthropometric measurements were carried out to determine body mass index (BMI) and a fasting venous blood sample was drawn to determine plasma ascorbate levels as described below.

Sample size calculations indicated that at 80% power and alpha = 0.05, a sample size of 15 participants per intervention group would detect a minimum difference of 10 µmol/L ascorbate as determined using data derived from our previous vitamin C bioavailability study [12]. To allow for potential withdrawal during the study, 36 non-smoking participants (18 per group) with below average plasma ascorbate levels were enrolled for the study and provided written informed consent.

2.2. Study Design

The study employed a parallel arms design and the participants were randomized into a 50 mg vitamin C per day group or a half kiwifruit per day group using a random numbers chart. A parallel arms rather than cross-over study design was chosen to avoid potential confounding by kiwifruit-derived constituents, e.g., vitamin E, which may not wash out prior to the vitamin C supplement phase of a cross-over study. A lead-in phase of five weeks allowed the participants time to control their dietary vitamin C intake by eliminating juice and substituting high vitamin C foods, e.g., citrus and kiwifruit, with low vitamin C foods, e.g., apples and bananas (guidelines were provided as to the vitamin C content of common foods). This was followed by an intervention phase of six weeks and a washout phase of four weeks (Figure 1). Fasting venous blood samples were drawn weekly to monitor plasma ascorbate levels. Twenty four hour urine, semen, and leukocyte samples were collected at week five (baseline), week 11 (post-intervention) and week 15 (post-washout). Muscle biopsies were carried out at baseline and post-intervention. Participants also completed four seven-day food and beverage records (at the beginning of the study, pre- and post-intervention and post-washout).

Figure 1. Parallel groups study design. * Weekly plasma samples; ** urine, semen and leukocyte samples; *** urine, semen, leukocyte and skeletal muscle samples.

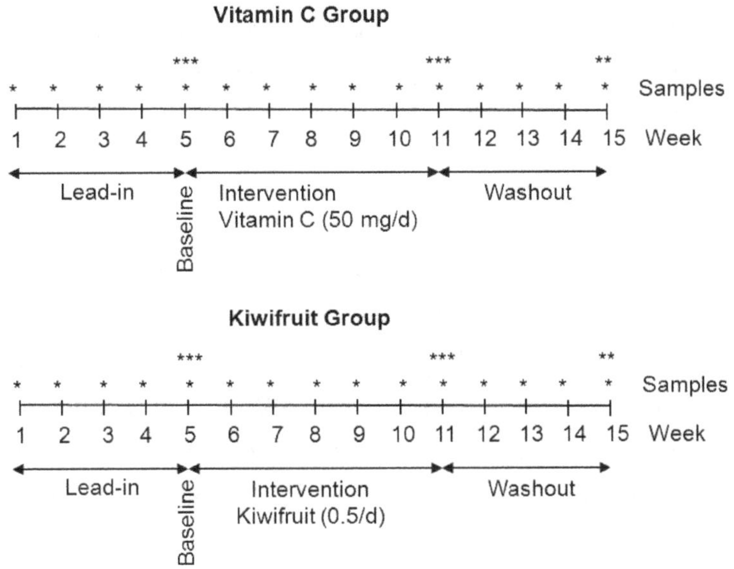

2.3. Interventions

Chewable orange-flavored vitamin C tablets were provided by Tishcon Corp., Westbury, NY, USA. Analysis of the tablets indicated that they contained 52 mg of vitamin C per tablet. Participants in the vitamin C tablet arm of the study were asked to consume one tablet per day.

Gold kiwifruit (*Actinidia chinensis* var. *Hort. 16A*) were provided by Zespri International Ltd., Mount Maunganui, New Zealand, and were stored at ≤4 °C. The vitamin C content of the kiwifruit was monitored by HPLC with electrochemical detection [12] and indicated that the kiwifruit flesh contained 116 ± 10 mg vitamin C per 100 g (mean ± SD, $n = 5$); this value did not change during cold storage of the fruit. Participants in the kiwifruit arm were asked to consume half a fresh kiwifruit daily, not including the skin. Therefore, the actual amount of vitamin C consumed was estimated to be ~53 mg per half a kiwifruit.

2.4. Sample Collection and Processing

2.4.1. Plasma, Urine and Semen

Peripheral blood was collected into 5 mL K_3-EDTA vacutainer tubes and plasma was isolated by centrifugation at 4 °C. Urine was collected over 24 h into pre-weighed collection bottles containing K_2-EDTA. Semen was collected into pre-weighed collection containers containing K_2-EDTA and kept cold until processed. The plasma, urine and semen samples were extracted with perchloric acid containing DTPA, as described previously [12], prior to storage at −80 °C until HPLC analysis.

2.4.2. Mononuclear Leukocytes and Neutrophils

White blood cells were purified from heparinized whole blood as described previously [20], the cell pellets counted and extracted with perchloric acid containing DTPA, and the supernatants stored at −80 °C until HPLC analysis.

2.4.3. Skeletal Muscle Tissue

A small piece of tissue (~14 mg) was removed from the *vastus lateralis* using a Quick-Core biopsy needle (14 gauge, 6 cm long with a 20 mm throw, from Cook Medical Inc., Bloomington, IN, USA), and processed as described previously [20], extracted with perchloric acid containing DTPA, and stored at −80 °C until HPLC analysis.

2.5. Analysis of Vitamin C by HPLC

The ascorbate content of the kiwifruit, plasma, urine, semen, leukocytes and muscle tissue was analyzed using reverse-phase HPLC with electrochemical detection as described previously [12]. Briefly, samples were separated on a Synergi 4 μ Hydro-RP 80A 150 × 4.6 mm column (Phenomenex NZ Ltd., Auckland, New Zealand) using a Waters 600 solvent delivery system with a Hitachi L-2200 refrigerated autosampler and an ESA Coulochem II electrochemical detector (+200 mV electrode potential and 20 μA sensitivity). The mobile phase comprised 80 mM sodium acetate buffer, pH 4.8, containing DTPA (0.54 mmol/L) and freshly added paired-ion reagent *n*-octylamine (1 μmol/L), delivered at a flow rate of 1.2 mL/min. A standard curve of sodium-L-ascorbate, standardized spectrophotometrically, was freshly prepared for each HPLC run in 77 mmol/L HPLC-grade perchloric acid containing DTPA (100 μmol/L).

2.6. Analysis of Food and Beverage Records

The vitamin C content of the food and beverage dietary records was estimated using *Diet Cruncher* software [21], and the New Zealand FOODfiles Food Composition Database (2006) as described previously [12].

2.7. Statistical Analysis

Data is represented as mean ± SD for group characteristics and mean ± SEM for comparison of group means. The differences between paired and unpaired data were determined by two-tailed Students's *t*-tests and *P* values ≤ 0.05 were considered significant. Analysis of variance with Fisher pairwise multiple comparison procedure was carried out using *SigmaStat* software [22].

3. Results

3.1. Participant Characteristics

One hundred and thirty four non-smoking individuals were screened and their fasting plasma ascorbate concentrations determined. The average ± SD plasma ascorbate concentration for these individuals was 48 ± 16 μmol/L (Table 1). Thirty six of the individuals with below average plasma ascorbate levels, who also satisfied the other inclusion criteria, were enrolled in the study and randomized into the vitamin C tablet group or the half kiwifruit per day group. The average ± SD fasting plasma ascorbate levels of the enrolled groups were 31 ± 11 μM and 34 ± 10 μM, with a range of 3 μM to 44 μM (Table 1). There were no significant differences between the two groups.

Table 1. Characteristics of individuals screened and enrolled in the study.

	Screened [a] (n = 134)	Vitamin C Group [a] (n = 18)	Kiwifruit Group [a] (n = 18)
Age (years)	21 ± 3	21 ± 3	22 ± 4
Weight (kg)	81 ± 16	84 ± 19	89 ± 23
Height (cm)	182 ± 7	181 ± 7	181 ± 7
BMI (kg/m^2)	24 ± 4	26 ± 5	27 ± 6 *
Ascorbate (μmol/L)	48 ± 16	31 ± 11 **	34 ± 10 **

[a] Data represent mean ± SD; * $P < 0.05$, ** $P < 0.001$ for unpaired t-test of intervention groups *versus* screened group. There were no significant differences between the intervention groups.

3.2. Dietary Intake of Vitamin C

Analysis of the food and beverage records indicated a vitamin C intake of ~30 mg/day at baseline (Table 2). Addition of the vitamin C tablet or half a kiwifruit per day to the daily diet of the two groups resulted in an increase in vitamin C intake, with both groups approaching ~75 mg (Table 2), and no difference between the two groups ($P = 0.512$). Following four weeks washout, the vitamin C intake had returned to baseline levels.

Table 2. Change in vitamin C intake and ascorbate concentration in body fluids, cells and tissue following supplementation with 50 mg vitamin C or half a kiwifruit per day for six weeks.

	Vitamin C group [a] (50 mg/day)			Kiwifruit group [a] (half/day)			Between group
	Baseline	Intervention	Washout	Baseline	Intervention	Washout	Intervention P value [b]
Intake (mg/day)	31.2 ± 3.1	76.7 ± 2.6 ***	29.1 ± 2.9	28.6 ± 3.1	73.4 ± 4.2 ***	31.4 ± 5.1	0.512
Plasma (μmol/L)	23.5 ± 2.5	51.3 ± 3.5 ***	34.3 ± 4.4 *	22.7 ± 2.5	45.5 ± 2.5 ***	30.5 ± 3.1	0.860
Urine (μmol/24 h)	42.8 ± 9.2	104.2 ± 27.6 *	59.5 ± 19.9	32.3 ± 8.1	70.5 ± 17.0 *	64.7 ± 29.8	0.503
Semen (μmol/L)	284.8 ±27.0	321.0 ± 33.3	264.4 ± 31.1 *	326.3 ± 47.5	378.8 ± 42.7	237.7 ± 19.6 *	0.676
Mononuclear cells (nmol/10^8 cells)	38.7 ± 6.2	84.5 ± 6.3 ***	78.5 ± 4.3 **	60.5 ± 6.1	90.9 ± 6.1 **	75.2 ± 5.2	0.227
Neutrophils (nmol/10^8 cells)	21.9 ± 3.1	39.6 ± 3.8 **	24.9 ± 2.1	13.7 ± 2.4	30.4 ± 2.5 ***	24.8 ± 1.7 ***	0.798
Skeletal muscle (nmol/g)	14.5 ± 2.0	61.3 ± 3.5 ***	nd	15.1 ± 2.5	52.8 ± 5.0 ***	nd	0.429

[a] Data represent mean ± SEM; [b] P values were determined by unpaired t-test of vitamin C group *versus* kiwifruit group post-intervention following subtraction of baseline values; * $P < 0.05$ and ** $P < 0.01$ and *** $P < 0.001$ for paired t-test of intervention *versus* baseline. nd = not determined.

3.3. Vitamin C Status of Plasma, Urine and Semen

Plasma ascorbate levels increased significantly during the six week intervention phase, from ~23 μmol/L to a maximum of ~50 μmol/L (Table 2). There were no significant differences between the two groups during this period or during the four week washout phase (Figure 2). Similarly, there were no significant differences between the two treatment groups for either urinary ascorbate excretion ($P = 0.503$) or seminal ascorbate levels ($P = 0.676$) (Table 2).

Figure 2. Plasma ascorbate concentrations in vitamin C group (50 mg/day, •) and kiwifruit group (0.5/day, ○). Data represent mean ± SEM. Two way analysis of variance with Fisher pairwise multiple comparison procedure indicated a significant increase in plasma ascorbate from one week post-intervention (week 6) onwards, but no significant difference between the two interventions.

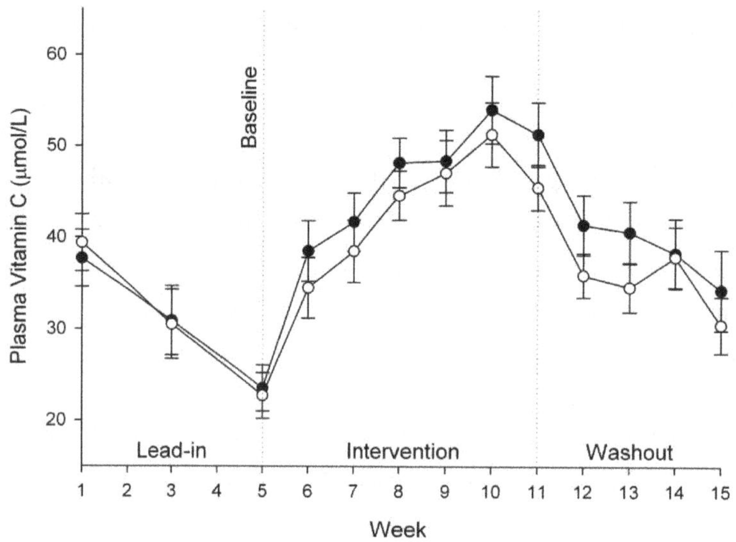

3.4. Vitamin C Status of Leukocytes and Skeletal Muscle Tissue

The ascorbate levels in mononuclear cells and neutrophils in both intervention groups increased following the six week intervention (Table 2), but there were no differences between the two interventions ($P = 0.798$). The baseline skeletal muscle tissue ascorbate levels were ~15 nmoL/g wet weight, and following intervention there were 3.5- to 4-fold increases in tissue ascorbate levels in both treatment groups (Table 2). Once again, there were no significant differences between the two intervention groups ($P = 0.429$).

4. Discussion

In direct contrast to our previous *Gulo* knockout mouse study, which showed clear differences in comparative vitamin C bioavailability [6], this investigation has shown no differences in the steady-state bioavailability of synthetic *versus* kiwifruit-derived vitamin C in plasma, semen, peripheral blood leukocytes and skeletal muscle of humans. Other comparative bioavailability studies in guinea pigs have shown similar results to our animal study [23–27]. Enhanced uptake of vitamin C into specific organs of guinea pigs (e.g., adrenals and spleen) was observed when administered with flavonoid-rich juices/extracts or purified plant flavonoids [23–27], although comparable vitamin C accumulation was observed in some organs (e.g., liver) in several studies [23–25,28], suggesting either tissue specific differences or effects of differences in study design.

In agreement with our current human study, others have shown little difference in steady-state plasma and/or urine bioavailability of synthetic vitamin C and that found in different fruits, fruit juices and vegetables [14–19]. Only one previous study has investigated the comparative bioavailability of synthetic *versus* natural vitamin C in leukocytes [19]. Although neutrophils express SVCT2 [29], when their respiratory burst is activated they primarily transport the oxidized form of ascorbate (dehydroascorbic acid) via the glucose transporters GLUT 1 and GLUT 3, followed by intracellular reduction [30]. In support of our observations with neutrophils and mononuclear cells, Pelletier *et al.* [19] found no difference in leukocyte ascorbate uptake between synthetic vitamin C (in the presence or absence of rutin) and that from orange juice. Interestingly, an *in vitro* study showed that the flavonoids myricetin and quercitin inhibited the uptake of both ascorbate and dehydroascorbic acid into monocytic (HL-60 and U937) and lymphocytic (Jurkat) cells [31]. Whether this occurs *in vivo* is, however, uncertain due to the low plasma bioavailability of flavonoids [32].

Although leukocyte ascorbate status is often used as an indicator of whole body status, whether this is an accurate model for other tissues and organs is uncertain. This premise is supported by our animal study which indicated that different organs exhibited maximal uptake at varying doses of vitamin C [6]. Therefore, we also investigated the previously unreported effects of synthetic *versus* natural vitamin C on skeletal muscle ascorbate status. Ascorbate is transported into muscle cells via SVCT2 [33,34]. In our study muscle tissue exhibited a greater relative uptake of ascorbate than leukocytes, however, there was again no difference in bioavailability between the synthetic and fruit-derived vitamin C.

We also investigated seminal fluid ascorbate status. Although the baseline seminal fluid ascorbate was lower than vitamin C replete and healthy non-smoking men [35–37], little change was observed with the low dose vitamin C tablet or half kiwifruit per day dose. Early studies have shown that vitamin C intakes of up to 250 mg/day are required to return depleted seminal ascorbate to normal levels [35,36,38], indicating that higher intakes of vitamin C, e.g., those that result in plasma saturation, are required to increase seminal fluid levels [39].

5. Conclusions

Numerous animal studies have shown differences between the tissue bioavailability of synthetic and natural or flavonoid-rich vitamin C. However, more evidence is accumulating to indicate that this is not the case in humans. Our current human study showed no difference in bioavailability to plasma, semen, peripheral blood leukocytes and skeletal muscle of kiwifruit-derived vitamin C compared with a chewable vitamin C tablet of equivalent dosage. Thus, other nutrients and phytochemicals present in kiwifruit appear to be neither enhancing nor inhibiting the uptake of vitamin C from the whole fruit. However, vitamin C is known to enhance the bioavailability of other nutrients, such as non-heme iron [40,41], and kiwifruit also contain numerous micronutrients and phytochemicals which will undoubtedly confer considerable health benefits in addition to the positive effects of the high levels of vitamin C also delivered by this fruit [42].

Acknowledgments

We are grateful to the young men who participated in this study, many of whom showed great dedication and perseverance. We acknowledge Maria Webb and Heather Webb for assistance with recruitment, Wathsala Kumarasinghe for the diet analysis, Jo Kepple for the use of Primorus Clinical Trials Unit, Lynley Drummond for consultation on study design, and John Pearson for consultation on statistical power. Role of each author: A.C.C. study design, recruitment, study co-ordination, sample processing, data analysis, writing manuscript; S.B. recruitment, sample processing and analysis, editing manuscript; J.P. editing manuscript; J.S. muscle biopsies, editing manuscript; M.C.M.V. study design, sample processing, editing manuscript. Sources of support included University of Otago, Dunedin, New Zealand and Zespri International Ltd., Mount Maunganui, New Zealand.

References

1. Carr, A.C.; Frei, B. Toward a new recommended dietary allowance for vitamin C based on antioxidant and health effects in humans. *Am. J. Clin. Nutr.* **1999**, *69*, 1086–1107.
2. Tsukaguchi, H.; Tokui, T.; Mackenzie, B.; Berger, U.V.; Chen, X.Z.; Wang, Y.; Brubaker, R.F.; Hediger, M.A. A family of mammalian Na^+-dependent L-ascorbic acid transporters. *Nature* **1999**, *399*, 70–75.
3. Savini, I.; Rossi, A.; Pierro, C.; Avigliano, L.; Catani, M.V. SVCT1 and SVCT2: Key proteins for vitamin C uptake. *Amino Acids* **2008**, *34*, 347–355.
4. Englard, S.; Seifter, S. The biochemical functions of ascorbic acid. *Annu. Rev. Nutr.* **1986**, *6*, 365–406.
5. Nishiyama, I.; Yamashita, Y.; Yamanaka, M.; Shimohashi, A.; Fukuda, T.; Oota, T. Varietal difference in vitamin C content in the fruit of kiwifruit and other *actinidia* species. *J. Agric. Food Chem.* **2004**, *52*, 5472–5475.
6. Vissers, M.C.M.; Bozonet, S.M.; Pearson, J.F.; Braithwaite, L.J. Dietary ascorbate affects steady state tissue levels in vitamin C-deficient mice: Tissue deficiency after sub-optimal intake and superior bioavailability from a food source (kiwifruit). *Am. J. Clin. Nutr.* **2011**, *93*, 292–301.
7. Beker, B.Y.; Sonmezoglu, I.; Imer, F.; Apak, R. Protection of ascorbic acid from copper(II)-catalyzed oxidative degradation in the presence of flavonoids: Quercetin, catechin and morin. *Int. J. Food Sci. Nutr.* **2011**, *62*, 504–512.
8. Clemetson, C.A.; Andersen, L. Plant polyphenols as antioxidants for ascorbic acid. *Ann. N. Y. Acad. Sci.* **1966**, *136*, 341–476.
9. Fiorentino, A.; D'Abrosca, B.; Pacifico, S.; Mastellone, C.; Scognamiglio, M.; Monaco, P. Identification and assessment of antioxidant capacity of phytochemicals from kiwi fruits. *J. Agric. Food Chem.* **2009**, *57*, 4148–4155.
10. Tanaka, K.; Hashimoto, T.; Tokumaru, S.; Iguchi, H.; Kojo, S. Interactions between vitamin C and vitamin E are observed in tissues of inherently scorbutic rats. *J. Nutr.* **1997**, *127*, 2060–2064.

11. Latocha, P.; Krupa, T.; Wolosiak, R.; Worobiej, E.; Wilczak, J. Antioxidant activity and chemical difference in fruit of different *Actinidia* sp. *Int. J. Food Sci. Nutr.* **2010**, *61*, 381–394.
12. Carr, A.C.; Pullar, J.M.; Moran, S.; Vissers, M.C.M. Bioavailability of vitamin C from kiwifruit in non-smoking males: Determination of "healthy" and "optimal" intakes. *J. Nutr. Sci.* **2012**, *1*, e14.
13. Levine, M.; Conry-Cantilena, C.; Wang, Y.; Welch, R.W.; Washko, P.W.; Dhariwal, K.R.; Park, J.B.; Lazarev, A.; Graumlich, J.F.; King, J.; *et al.* Vitamin C pharmacokinetics in healthy volunteers: Evidence for a recommended dietary allowance. *Proc. Natl. Acad. Sci. USA* **1996**, *93*, 3704–3709.
14. Mangels, A.R.; Block, G.; Frey, C.M.; Patterson, B.H.; Taylor, P.R.; Norkus, E.P.; Levander, O.A. The bioavailability to humans of ascorbic acid from oranges, orange juice and cooked broccoli is similar to that of synthetic ascorbic acid. *J. Nutr.* **1993**, *123*, 1054–1061.
15. Hartzler, E.R. The availability of ascorbic acid in papayas and guavas. *J. Nutr.* **1945**, *30*, 355–365.
16. Clayton, M.M.; Borden, R.A. The availability for human nutrition of the vitamin C in raw cabbage and home-canned tomato juice. *J. Nutr.* **1943**, *25*, 349–369.
17. Todhunter, E.N.; Fatzer, A.S. A comparison of the utilization by college women of equivalent amounts of ascorbic acid (vitamin C) in red raspberries and in crystalline form. *J. Nutr.* **1940**, *19*, 121–130.
18. Hawley, E.E.; Stephens, D.J.; Anderson, G. The excretion of vitamin C in normal individuals following a comparable quantitative administration in the form of orange juice, cevitamic acid by mouth and cevitamic acid intravenously. *J. Nutr.* **1936**, *11*, 135–145.
19. Pelletier, O.; Keith, M.O. Bioavailability of synthetic and natural ascorbic acid. *J. Am. Diet. Assoc.* **1974**, *64*, 271–275.
20. Carr, A.C.; Bozonet, S.M.; Pullar, J.M.; Simcock, J.W.; Vissers, M.C. Human skeletal muscle ascorbate is highly responsive to changes in vitamin C intake and plasma concentrations. *Am. J. Clin. Nutr.* **2013**, *97*, 800–807.
21. *Diet Cruncher*, version 1.6; Nutricomp: Dunedin, New Zealand, 2003.
22. *SigmaStat*, version 11; Systat Software Inc.: San Jose, CA, USA, 2009.
23. Wilson, H.K.; Price-Jones, C.; Hughes, R.E. The influence of an extract of orange peel on the growth and ascorbic acid metabolism of young guinea-pigs. *J. Sci. Food Agric.* **1976**, *27*, 661–666.
24. Douglass, C.D.; Kamp, G.H. The effect of orally administered rutin on the adrenal ascorbic acid level in guinea pigs. *J. Nutr.* **1959**, *67*, 531–536.
25. Papageorge, E.; Mitchell, G.L., Jr.; The effect of oral administration of rutin on blood, liver and adrenal ascorbic acid and on liver and adrenal cholesterol in guinea pigs. *J. Nutr.* **1949**, *37*, 531–540.
26. Cotereau, H.; Gabe, M.; Gero, E.; Parrot, J.L. Influence of vitamin P (vitamin C2) upon the amount of ascorbic acid in the organs of the guinea pig. *Nature* **1948**, *161*, 557–558.
27. Hughes, R.E.; Hurley, R.J.; Jones, P.R. The retention of ascorbic acid by guinea-pig tissues. *Br. J. Nutr.* **1971**, *26*, 433–438.
28. Todhunter, E.N.; Robbins, R.C.; Ivey, G.; Brewer, W. A comparison of the utilization by guinea

pigs of equivalent amounts of ascorbic acid (vitamin C) in lemon juice and in crystalline form. *J. Nutr.* **1940**, *19*, 113–120.

29. Corpe, C.P.; Lee, J.H.; Kwon, O.; Eck, P.; Narayanan, J.; Kirk, K.L.; Levine, M. 6-Bromo-6-deoxy-L-ascorbic acid: An ascorbate analog specific for Na^+-dependent vitamin C transporter but not glucose transporter pathways. *J. Biol. Chem.* **2005**, *280*, 5211–5220.
30. Washko, P.W.; Wang, Y.; Levine, M. Ascorbic acid recycling in human neutrophils. *J. Biol. Chem.* **1993**, *268*, 15531–15535.
31. Park, J.B.; Levine, M. Intracellular accumulation of ascorbic acid is inhibited by flavonoids via blocking of dehydroascorbic acid and ascorbic acid uptakes in HL-60, U937 and Jurkat cells. *J. Nutr.* **2000**, *130*, 1297–1302.
32. Lotito, S.B.; Frei, B. Consumption of flavonoid-rich foods and increased plasma antioxidant capacity in humans: Cause, consequence, or epiphenomenon? *Free Radic. Biol. Med.* **2006**, *41*, 1727–1746.
33. Savini, I.; Catani, M.V.; Duranti, G.; Ceci, R.; Sabatini, S.; Avigliano, L. Vitamin C homeostasis in skeletal muscle cells. *Free Radic. Biol. Med.* **2005**, *38*, 898–907.
34. Low, M.L.; Sandoval, D.; Aviles, E.; Perez, F.; Nualart, F.; Henriquez, J.P. The ascorbic acid transporter SVCT2 is expressed in slow-twitch skeletal muscle fibres. *Histochem. Cell. Biol.* **2009**, *131*, 565–574.
35. Jacob, R.A.; Pianalto, F.S.; Agee, R.E. Cellular ascorbate depletion in healthy men. *J. Nutr.* **1992**, *122*, 1111–1118.
36. Fraga, C.G.; Motchnik, P.A.; Shigenaga, M.K.; Helbock, H.J.; Jacob, R.A.; Ames, B.N. Ascorbic acid protects against endogenous oxidative DNA damage in human sperm. *Proc. Natl. Acad. Sci. USA* **1991**, *88*, 11003–11006.
37. Kandar, R.; Drabkova, P.; Hampl, R. The determination of ascorbic acid and uric acid in human seminal plasma using an HPLC with UV detection. *J. Chromatogr. B* **2011**, *879*, 2834–2839.
38. Jacob, R.A.; Kelley, D.S.; Pianalto, F.S.; Swendseid, M.E.; Henning, S.M.; Zhang, J.Z.; Ames, B.N.; Fraga, C.G.; Peters, J.H. Immunocompetence and oxidant defense during ascorbate depletion of healthy men. *Am. J. Clin. Nutr.* **1991**, *54*, 1302S–1309S.
39. Dawson, E.B.; Harris, W.A.; Rankin, W.E.; Charpentier, L.A.; McGanity, W.J. Effect of ascorbic acid on male fertility. *Ann. N. Y. Acad. Sci.* **1987**, *498*, 312–323.
40. Beck, K.; Conlon, C.A.; Kruger, R.; Coad, J.; Stonehouse, W. Gold kiwifruit consumed with an iron-fortified breakfast cereal meal improves iron status in women with low iron stores: A 16-week randomised controlled trial. *Br. J. Nutr.* **2011**, *105*, 101–109.
41. Hallberg, L.; Brune, M.; Rossander, L. Effect of ascorbic acid on iron absorption from different types of meals. Studies with ascorbic-acid-rich foods and synthetic ascorbic acid given in different amounts with different meals. *Hum. Nutr. Appl. Nutr.* **1986**, *40*, 97–113.
42. Stonehouse, W.; Gammon, C.S.; Beck, K.L.; Conlon, C.A.; von Hurst, P.R.; Kruger, R. Kiwifruit: Our daily prescription for health. *Can. J. Physiol. Pharmacol.* **2013**, *91*, 442–447.

Permissions

All chapters in this book were first published by MDPI; hereby published with permission under the Creative Commons Attribution License or equivalent. Every chapter published in this book has been scrutinized by our experts. Their significance has been extensively debated. The topics covered herein carry significant findings which will fuel the growth of the discipline. They may even be implemented as practical applications or may be referred to as a beginning point for another development.

The contributors of this book come from diverse backgrounds, making this book a truly international effort. This book will bring forth new frontiers with its revolutionizing research information and detailed analysis of the nascent developments around the world.

We would like to thank all the contributing authors for lending their expertise to make the book truly unique. They have played a crucial role in the development of this book. Without their invaluable contributions this book wouldn't have been possible. They have made vital efforts to compile up to date information on the varied aspects of this subject to make this book a valuable addition to the collection of many professionals and students.

This book was conceptualized with the vision of imparting up-to-date information and advanced data in this field. To ensure the same, a matchless editorial board was set up. Every individual on the board went through rigorous rounds of assessment to prove their worth. After which they invested a large part of their time researching and compiling the most relevant data for our readers.

The editorial board has been involved in producing this book since its inception. They have spent rigorous hours researching and exploring the diverse topics which have resulted in the successful publishing of this book. They have passed on their knowledge of decades through this book. To expedite this challenging task, the publisher supported the team at every step. A small team of assistant editors was also appointed to further simplify the editing procedure and attain best results for the readers.

Apart from the editorial board, the designing team has also invested a significant amount of their time in understanding the subject and creating the most relevant covers. They scrutinized every image to scout for the most suitable representation of the subject and create an appropriate cover for the book.

The publishing team has been an ardent support to the editorial, designing and production team. Their endless efforts to recruit the best for this project, has resulted in the accomplishment of this book. They are a veteran in the field of academics and their pool of knowledge is as vast as their experience in printing. Their expertise and guidance has proved useful at every step. Their uncompromising quality standards have made this book an exceptional effort. Their encouragement from time to time has been an inspiration for everyone.

The publisher and the editorial board hope that this book will prove to be a valuable piece of knowledge for researchers, students, practitioners and scholars across the globe.

List of Contributors

David Højland Ipsen, Pernille Tveden-Nyborg and Jens Lykkesfeldt
Department of Veterinary Disease Biology, Faculty of Health and Medical Sciences, University of Copenhagen, Ridebanevej 9, Frederiksberg C, 1870 Copenhagen, Denmark

Zhi-Hong Zhang, Xin-An Zeng, Zhong Han and Xia-Yu Xiong
College of Light Industry and Food Science, South China University of Technology, Guangzhou 510640, China

Charles S. Brennan
College of Light Industry and Food Science, South China University of Technology, Guangzhou 510640, China
Centre for Food Research and Innovation, Department of Wine, Food and Molecular Biosciences, Lincoln University, Lincoln 85084, New Zealand

Margaret Brennan
Centre for Food Research and Innovation, Department of Wine, Food and Molecular Biosciences, Lincoln University, Lincoln 85084, New Zealand

Daniel R. Gallie
Department of Biochemistry, University of California, Riverside, CA 92521-0129, USA

Anitra C. Carr, Stephanie M. Bozonet and Margreet C. M. Vissers
Centre for Free Radical Research, Department of Pathology & Biomedical Science, University of Otago, Christchurch, Christchurch 8140, New Zealand

Fiona E. Harrison
Division of Diabetes, Endocrinology and Metabolism, Department of Medicine, Vanderbilt University Medical Center, Nashville, TN 37232, USA

Gene L. Bowman
Brain Institute, Department of Neurology, NIA-Aging and Alzheimer's Disease Center Oregon Health and Science University, Portland, OR 97239, USA

Maria Cristina Polidori
Geriatrics Department, University of Cologne Medical Faculty, Cologne 50937, Germany

Alexander J. Michels and Balz Frei
Linus Pauling Institute, 307 Linus Pauling Science Center, Oregon State University, Corvallis, OR 97331, USA

Donald F. Brophy
Department of Pharmacotherapy and Outcomes Science, Virginia Commonwealth University, Richmond, VA 23298, USA

Bassem M. Mohammed
Department of Pharmacotherapy and Outcomes Science, Virginia Commonwealth University, Richmond, VA 23298, USA
Department of Clinical Pharmacy, Faculty of Pharmacy, Cairo University, Cairo 11562, Egypt

Bernard J. Fisher, Donatas Kraskauskas, Daniela Farkas, Alpha A. Fowler III and Ramesh Natarajan
Division of Pulmonary Disease and Critical Care Medicine, Virginia Commonwealth University, Richmond, VA 23298, USA

Amaya Azqueta
Department of Pharmacology and Toxicology, University of Navarra, C/Irunlarrea 1, 31009 Pamplona, Spain
Department of Nutrition, Institute of Basic Medical Sciences, University of Oslo, PB 1046 Blindern, 0316 Oslo, Norway

Yolanda Lorenzo, Nasser E. Bastani and Andrew R. Collins
Department of Nutrition, Institute of Basic Medical Sciences, University of Oslo, PB 1046 Blindern, 0316 Oslo, Norway

Solange Costa
Department of Nutrition, Institute of Basic Medical Sciences, University of Oslo, PB 1046 Blindern, 0316 Oslo, Norway
Environmental Health Department, National Institute of Health, Rua Alexandre Herculano 321, 4000-055 Porto, Portugal

Seyeon Park
Department of Applied Chemistry, Dongduk Women's University, 23-1 Wolgok-dong, Sungbuk-ku, Seoul 136-714, Korea

Juliet M. Pullar
Centre for Free Radical Research, Department of Pathology & Biomedical Science, University of Otago, Christchurch, Christchurch 8140, New Zealand

Jeremy W. Simcock
Department of Plastic and Reconstructive Surgery, University of Otago, Christchurch, Christchurch 8140, New Zealand

Index

N

O

P

R

S

T

www.ingramcontent.com/pod-product-compliance
Lightning Source LLC
LaVergne TN
LVHW060603210926
848485LV00005B/1360